Praise for *Go Dairy Free*

"This is the definitive bible for dairy-free living. Whether you have food allergies or are choosing to reduce or eliminate dairy for health or ideological reasons, Alisa walks you through every question, concern, and obstacle, and provides simple solutions in an informative yet easy-going and approachable way. With well-researched information, terrific tips, and righteous recipes, this brilliant book is a comprehensive road map to dairy-free divinity."

—**TESS MASTERS**, author of *The Blender Girl, The Blender Girl Smoothies,* and *The Perfect Blend*

"This book is the ultimate guide to going dairy free! Part guidebook and part cookbook, *Go Dairy Free* is the perfect resource for anyone wanting or choosing to reduce or eliminate the dairy in their diet. Alisa provides a wealth of well-researched information and helps you navigate the dairy-free world whether it be eating out at restaurants, going grocery shopping, or stocking your own kitchen. With over 250 delicious recipes, there are plenty of options to suit any taste. I can't wait to try out the Cinn-Full Overnight Cinnamon Rolls and the Crazy for Coconut Cream Pie!"

—**DR. SONALI RUDER**, The Foodie Physician

"This book is one of the most powerful resources available for anyone who is considering or is living dairy free. It is packed with insight, knowledge, wisdom, and practical solutions for 21st-century families. I am incredibly grateful for Alisa's steadfast leadership here!"

—**ROBYN O'BRIEN**, bestselling author, renowned activist, and founder of AllergyKids

"With her engaging and fully revised *Go Dairy Free*, Alisa Fleming has unveiled a remarkable road map to dairy-free living. Her array of 250 recipes is unbeatable—from plant-based 'mylks,' to creative mains, free-from ice creams, cakes, toddler foods, 'cheeze' wheels, and plenty more. She provides intelligent guidance on diet balance, calcium-rich foods, and setting up your pantry, while offering tips on dairy-free child-rearing and exploring research. Whether you have a child with a severe milk allergy, your own lactose intolerance, or a preference for life without dairy, look no farther: this is the book to for you."

—**GWEN SMITH**, chief editor of *Allergic Living* magazine

"For more than a decade, Alisa Fleming has led the dairy-free movement sharing recipes, product reviews, and lifestyle tips with millions of readers. Now, Alisa delivers the quintessential dairy-free resource with *Go Dairy Free*. This book will give you the confidence and necessary tools to go dairy free—for good!"

—**DREENA BURTON**, author of *Plant-Powered Families*, dreenaburton.com

"Ten years ago, I was relatively new to the dairy-free life and *Go Dairy Free* became my everyday reference. This 2nd edition fills in any blanks there may have been. This book is a must-have reference guide and a vital tool for everyone living a dairy-free life, as well as anyone considering making the leap. The depth of information is outstanding and the organization of such a wide breadth of knowledge makes *Go Dairy Free* an unparalleled essential on the topic. From the health conditions associated with dairy sensitivities and allergies, through to substitution recommendations and recipes to suit every diet, this book makes the what, why, and how of dairy-free living absolutely effortless."

—**MEGHAN TELPNER**, bestselling author of *The UnDiet Cookbook* and founder of the Academy of Culinary Nutrition

"I wish I had Alisa Fleming's book as a resource when I transitioned to a dairy-free lifestyle to help manage my chronic asthma almost a decade ago. Now, her community and books are a resource for my clients and audience. No one should be worried that removing dairy means deprivation or lack of joy in eating. *Go Dairy Free*'s tips and recipes show that you can still enjoy your favorite dishes and even expand your diet's variety and nutrient density."

—**KELLY JONES, MS, RD, CSSD, LDN**, sports nutrition consultant and intuitive eating expert

"*Go Dairy Free* is a comprehensive guide that teaches you how to navigate a dairy-free life fully without feeling deprived. Not only does Alisa teach you how to navigate grocery stores, food labels, and your own kitchen, but she also provides the evidence-based science behind why more and more individuals are forgoing dairy. As we continue to see the numbers of people going dairy free increase for a variety of reasons, this book will prove to be a valuable tool for so many individuals."

—**AMY GOOD, RD, LD**

"When I realized it was truly time to kick the dairy if I wanted to feel better, I needed two things: information that would fully convince me it was a good idea and a guide to make it seem less intimidating. I found both of those in *Go Dairy Free* and it made the journey so much easier."

—**AMANDA BROOKS**, owner of RunToTheFinish.com

"Whether you're new to going dairy-free or just need some fresh recipe inspiration, Alisa has got you covered with this comprehensive collection of easy and delicious recipes. Her real world tips are sure to help make the transition to this lifestyle easier, without missing out on any of the essential nutrients your body needs."

—**MEGAN GILMORE**, author of *Everyday Detox* and *No Excuses Detox*

GO
DAIRY
FREE

GO DAIRY FREE

*The Ultimate Guide and Cookbook for Milk Allergies,
Lactose Intolerance, and Casein-Free Living*

ALISA FLEMING

BenBella Books, Inc.
Dallas, TX

BenBella

BenBella Books, Inc.
10440 N. Central Expressway, Suite 800
Dallas, TX 75231
www.benbellabooks.com
Send feedback to feedback@benbellabooks.com

Printed in the United States of America
10 9 8 7 6 5 4 3 2 1

Library of Congress Cataloging-in-Publication Data
Names: Fleming, Alisa Marie, author.
Title: Go dairy free : the ultimate guide and cookbook for milk allergies,
     lactose intolerance, and casein-free living / Alisa Marie Fleming.
Description: Dallas, TX : BenBella Books, Inc., [2018] | Includes
     bibliographical references and index.
Identifiers: LCCN 2017056216 (print) | LCCN 2018005911 (ebook) | ISBN
     9781946885241 (ebook) | ISBN 9781944648916 (trade paper : alk. paper)
Subjects: LCSH: Milk-free diet. | Milk-free diet--Recipes. | Cooking. |
     LCGFT: Cookbooks.
Classification: LCC RM234.5 (ebook) | LCC RM234.5 .F55 2018 (print) | DDC
     641.5/63971--dc23
LC record available at https://lccn.loc.gov/2017056216

Editing by Karen Levy
Copyediting by Karen Wise
Proofreading by Sarah Vostok and Lisa Story
Indexing by WordCo Indexing Services, Inc.
Text design and composition by Silver Feather Design
Front cover design by Oceana Garceau
Full cover design by Sarah Avinger
Printed by Versa Press

Distributed to the trade by Two Rivers Distribution, an Ingram Brand
www.tworiversdistribution.com

Special discounts for bulk sales (minimum of 25 copies) are available.
Please contact Aida Herrera at aida@benbellabooks.com.

This book is dedicated to my incredibly supportive husband and colleague, Anthony.

Go Dairy Free was created as a positive and helpful resource for those who need to, or might choose to, reduce or eliminate the dairy in their diet for any reason. Nonetheless, it was written for educational purposes only. The information supplied is not intended to diagnose, treat, cure, or prevent any disease; nor is it intended to replace the advice of a physician. Always consult a physician regarding any health problem and before altering your diet, starting an exercise program, making changes in prescribed medications, or taking supplements of any kind.

CONTENTS

SECTION 5:
THE RECIPES

THE GO DAIRY FREE JOURNEY

Two roads diverged in a wood, and I—
I took the one less traveled by,
And that has made all the difference.
—Robert Frost

By my late twenties, I had held a great career as a financial analyst in Silicon Valley, married the man of my dreams, and run a successful business with him. We went on a traveling sabbatical in South America and, upon returning, took some time to evaluate our next steps.

There were many logical ideas discussed—safe paths for our long-term goals. But when dairy-free living was thrust into my life, a new direction emerged. Unlike the wide-open trail of tech, this route was off the beaten track. It had twists and turns that kept me from seeing where I might be going, and many obstacles to climb. But despite the obvious challenges that lay ahead, I knew it was a trek worth taking.

My initial research on dairy-free living yielded very meager results. In the early 2000s, there were a few trailblazing vegan websites with bites of information and recipes. But most of my searches resulted in people with dairy-free questions, followed by no real answers. Beyond vegans, there were countless individuals dealing with lactose intolerance, milk allergies, or honest concerns about long-term health.

It became my mission to find those answers for myself, and for them. I started a website at **GoDairyFree.org**, where every morsel of my dairy-free knowledge was posted. And readers devoured it. Emails with more questions kept pouring in, and I continued to research, cook, and write about whatever they were seeking.

It was then that I found myself at a crossroads. Whichever path I started down, I knew I wasn't likely to come back. A new tech business venture would be all-consuming, and wouldn't allow enough spare time to continue supporting the dairy-free community. But if I took much more time off from my stable career path, my knowledge would most likely become dated.

Yet as that inquisitive group banded together, I knew that my destiny lay ahead in the dairy-free unknown. Though reluctant at first, my husband eventually followed, and neither of us has ever looked back.

Truth be told, when I released the first edition of *Go Dairy Free* a decade ago, I wasn't sure how many people it would help. Sure, there were statistics emerging on health conditions related to dairy, but how many of those affected were committing to their well-being, and did they know that dairy-free living was feasible?

To my pleasant surprise, tens of thousands quickly purchased my book, and millions more began flooding my website. I had spoken up for dairy-free needs, and the conversation was taking hold.

But a lot has happened on the dairy-free trail since the first edition of *Go Dairy Free* was released. Grass is no longer growing underfoot, and we've made it to many blissful vistas. A large number of new studies have been presented, thousands of dairy-free products have emerged, and the very topic of dairy-free food has been enriched with innovation.

I still don't know exactly how many of you live dairy free or even dairy low. But the dairy alternative market is expected to reach *$16 billion* in sales this year, so it's definitely a mighty crowd.

Our society has taken notice of dairy-free living, and now I've got even more to say.

WHAT'S NEW IN THE SECOND EDITION

The first edition of *Go Dairy Free* was released back in 2008. As I type this, a decade later, I'm proud of the wonderful new facts and features I've been able to add for you.

MORE OF EVERYTHING: The first edition was scrunched and squeezed to fit into a standard-size book. But now I'm able to fit in every helpful tidbit and have expanded this to be the largest and most extensive dairy-free living book available.

OVER 250 RECIPES: This isn't just a guide, it's also a rather sizable cookbook. This edition includes over 100 *new and improved* recipes, plus many of your favorites. I've added fresh homemade alternatives and several sweets and savories to make the transition even tastier. If you're hungry for more, I've also added a cookbook, *Eat Dairy Free*, to my collection this year, which offers over 100 more brand-new recipes from my kitchen.

MILK BEVERAGE MANIA: Since so many of you loved the dairy alternative section in the original *Go Dairy Free*, I've expanded it and added a whole new chapter on plant-based "milks." It includes homemade tips, tasting notes, nutritional highlights, and much more.

PAMPERING PARENTS: With the help of some experienced milk allergy moms, I was able to add more ideas for infants and toddlers. Plus, I've included quite a few kid-friendly options for snacking and meals.

UPDATED RESEARCH: Related studies on the market and health just keep popping up, and I wanted to make sure you know about them. Each informational section has been updated with the latest and greatest findings.

VEGAN-FRIENDLY: Every single recipe in this book now includes a tested, fully vegan option. It is still a general dairy-free cookbook for all, but I wanted to make sure all of my plant-based friends could enjoy each nibble, too.

MORE GLUTEN-FREE & FOOD ALLERGY OPTIONS: Starting on page 167, you will find an easy to cross-reference special diet chart for every recipe in this book. It covers gluten-free, egg-free, nut-free, peanut-free, and soy-free options. And I've added even more gluten-free and allergy-friendly options to this edition. Plus, you will find ample information in the first portion of this book for almost every dietary need.

ONLINE RESOURCES: I've added several pages on **GoDairyFree.org** specifically for this book, and also several for *Eat Dairy Free*. You will see those URLs referenced in this book for your use. They include printables, product recommendations, and more.

This book has every tool needed to *go* dairy free, but is also an indispensable guide and cookbook to help you *be* dairy free every day. I still reference it regularly myself!

WHY DAIRY FREE?
IT'S PERSONAL

At the age of 33, as I was in the midst of working on the first edition of this guidebook, my father handed me a baby book, which he found while cleaning out some boxes. It was mine, but I had never seen it before. It fell open in my hands to a page with just five words on it: "4 months—Allergic to Milk." I am not sure whether I was more amazed that it flipped right to that note or that it took me decades to discover this fact for myself, the one that was so casually and plainly written in those memoirs.

My parents knew that I had a milk allergy as an infant, but the doctors assured them that such a thing is always quickly outgrown—not lasting beyond the first year—so no testing was required. In my childhood, it was never spoken of.

You might be wondering how someone could live so long with a milk allergy and not know it. But there were actually *many* signs and symptoms. My near-constant ear infections (including surgery), eczema, frequent and often violent illness, gastrointestinal symptoms, sudden bouts of weakness, narcolepsy, a weakened immune system, and sporadic breathing difficulties were all written off as an unlucky childhood.

All the way through to my teens, I missed more days of school than my classmates. In fact, during the final quarter of my senior year in high school, the vice principal called me in to offer a kind word of warning that I was just one sick day away from not graduating, even though I liked school, was active in sports, and maintained good grades.

Yet I still wasn't prepared for what lay ahead, in my twenties.

Instinctively, I hated almost all dairy. My body knew what no one else could deduce. So when I went away to university and had full control over my diet, I gradually stopped eating it. My symptoms diminished, but I didn't make the connection. I was too busy enjoying the freedom of young adulthood and assumed that my body just liked sunny California better than dreary Oregon.

After several years of active warm-weather living, I decided to take up running. But the mild knee pain that had plagued me since my early teens turned up a notch. An orthopedic doctor took a full bone scan, which showed I had healthy bones for my age— above average in my hips, in fact! Everything was strong. The issue was simply my natural alignment fighting the pavement-pounding repetition. But because I come from a very petite family, the doctor was appalled that I wasn't drowning myself in dairy. He insisted that I must increase my dairy intake "for the sake of my bones."

Back then, I implicitly trusted physicians, and dairy was a highly revered food group. So I reluctantly obliged, adding tolerable things, like frozen yogurt and chocolate milk, to my daily regimen. And with the help of my husband, Tony, who loved to cook, I started to integrate small servings of cheese into meals.

The next five years brought a continuous downward spiral in my health. During everyday activities, I would suddenly become severely ill, followed by weakness and debilitating pain. And if I tried to stand, I would often lose consciousness and awake in a hospital bed. On a few unfortunate occasions, I even had convulsions.

My trips to the emergency room were becoming more frequent, until not a week passed without a visit. Yet the doctors had no answers. There were blood tests, MRIs, EKGs, and heart monitors, but I was deemed "healthy." I was scared, and Tony could no longer hide his own fear. So far, I was able to gradually recover from each episode, but what if the next time, I didn't wake up?

It was only by luck that I stumbled across a doctor who believed in alternative medicine and diet as treatment. In my first visit, he sat with me and Tony for a full 90 minutes, asking all types of questions, from medical to psychological. At the end of the time, he said, "Have you tried cutting out milk?"

I thought he was insane. That's it? I am having what feel like near-death experiences, and that's all you've got?! I was seconds away from walking out when Tony said, "Why not? We should give it a try." Yes, that wonderful man went completely dairy free with me.

Within three days, all of my symptoms ceased, and to this day, they have not returned. It felt like nothing short of a miracle. Of course, since I still wanted "real proof" (stubborn as I am), the doctor ordered a food allergy test. Sure enough, I was in fact allergic to milk, specifically casein (milk protein). Those test results could have brought on disappointment and stress, but I was elated. I had an answer, and both Tony and I felt better than we had in years.

So you see, *Go Dairy Free* isn't just a book. It's a piece of my daily dedication. Every hour of work, every meal consumed, every trip I take, and every connection I make is now a part of my mission to support the dairy-free community. My life depended on becoming strictly dairy free, but it also showed me the way to helping millions of people improve their quality of life.

If ONE simple change could resolve most of your symptoms and prevent various illnesses, why not try it? I'll show you how.

SECTION 1

UNDERSTANDING DAIRY & DAIRY FREE FROM A HEALTH PERSPECTIVE

CHAPTER 1
WHAT IS DAIRY?

Whether you're new to the world of dairy free or already culturing your own coconut yogurt, it's important to ensure that we are all on the same page. To get there, let's open with a baseline definition:

Dairy products are foods or beverages produced from the milk of mammals.

With respect to the American diet, dairy most often refers to cow's milk and its derivatives. Typical dairy foods produced from cow's milk include cheese, butter, yogurt, and ice cream, but milk has many purposes in our food supply well beyond these obvious applications. The proteins, fats, and sugars within cow's milk are commonly extracted for use in processed foods (even "natural" ones) to add flavor, structure, or other enhancements. Other types of mammal milk, which I will address later in this chapter, may also fall under the dairy header.

Individuals who follow a general nondairy diet may opt to restrict only whole dairy foods, such as milk, cheese, and cream. Those who follow a strict dairy-free diet would also cut out foods that are made with any milk-derived ingredients. If severe milk allergies or intolerances come into play, it may be essential to scrutinize products down to the manufacturing processes. Even trace amounts of milk (parts per million) from cross-contamination during production may elicit a reaction in the highly sensitive.

To the best of my knowledge, any ingredient used within this book is made without any derivatives of milk. However, you should always check the label prior to consumption and, if necessary, contact the company to address their manufacturing procedures and any cross-contamination concerns. Always remember that ingredients and processes are subject to change by the manufacturer at any time!

UNSCRAMBLING EGGS AND DAIRY

Though frequently found in or near the dairy case, eggs are *not* a dairy food. In fact, most milk-producing mammals do not lay eggs (there are a few extreme species in and around Australia that multitask). Aside from those who follow a vegan diet or who have an egg allergy or intolerance, eggs are suitable for dairy-free dieters.

Nevertheless, since egg allergies coexist with milk allergies at a higher rate than other top allergens, I have written this guide to accommodate egg-free and vegan needs, too. Select recipes do contain or suggest eggs for a superior product, but in those cases a fully tested, egg-free option is provided. I've also provided egg substitute suggestions online at GoDairyFree.org/egg-subs.

WHAT MAKES MILK SO SPECIAL?

Raw, completely unprocessed cow's milk has many nutrients. After all, its natural purpose is for the rapid growth of calves, just as human breast milk is intended for the development of babies.

Interestingly, humans are the only mammals that routinely consume milk past infancy, let alone milk from another species. Nonetheless, since milk has become such a staple in the American diet, it is important to understand which nutrients we have come to rely on it for, and how to ensure that a milk-free diet provides adequate nutrition.

Cow's milk can be broken down into the following seven major components.

Water

Cow's milk is approximately 88 percent water. Obvious as it may seem, if you have been consuming one or more glasses of cow's milk in a day, be sure to replace it with another hydrating liquid. Of course, plain old water will do the trick.

Did you know that it takes up to 2,000 gallons of water (for the day-to-day functions of a dairy cow) to produce just one gallon of milk? That's enough water to quench your thirst (8 cups per day) for 11 years!

Protein

Cow's milk contains roughly 3 to 4 percent protein, of which about 80 percent is casein and 20 percent is whey. Unfortunately, both casein and whey are top allergen sources. Meat, seafood, and eggs are milk-free complete protein sources. For vegans, beans, nuts, seeds, and even select grains (quinoa is a personal favorite) can serve as excellent sources of protein. To offer more specific ideas, I address protein-rich foods and protein powders beginning on page 76.

Fat

The natural fat content of cow's milk can range from 3 to 6 percent. In the United States, whole milk must contain at least 3.25 percent milk fat, while caps of 2 percent, 1 percent, and 0.5 percent milk fat are regulated for reduced-fat, low-fat, and skim varieties, respectively. This may sound quite low, but these percentages are by weight (diluted by all of the water in milk), not by calories. Whole milk derives 50 percent of its calories from fat, 2 percent milk gets 35 percent of its calories from fat, 1 percent milk weighs in with 23 percent of its calories from fat, and skim milk is the lone lightweight with 5 percent of its calories from fat. Also, approximately 70 percent of the fat in milk is saturated.

While many Americans are attempting to shed fat from their diets, I receive numerous emails from people attempting to pack on pounds. During growth and even times of illness, adequate intake of fat can be a crucial concern. Since North Americans and Europeans tend to rely heavily on dairy products for dietary fat, I've included a deeper discussion on good sources of dairy-free fat (starting on page 74), plus information on the various types of oils and butter alternatives (page 143).

Carbohydrates

When it comes to fiber and complex carbohydrates, milk is not a top contender. Approximately 5 percent of milk is sugar—lactose, to be specific. In fact, 1 cup of milk contains more than half the sugar found in an equivalent serving of soda pop!

Lactose is also a significant source of suffering for up to 70 percent of the world's population. More on this topic later, but for now, let's assume that consuming enough sugar probably isn't high on your list of worries.

Water-Soluble Vitamins

Natural, raw milk contains a fair amount of B and C vitamins. However, during pasteurization, most of the vitamin C is weakened or destroyed, and about 38 percent of the B vitamins suffer a similar fate. Better sources of these vitamins can be found in a diet full of fresh fruits, vegetables, and grains, with the exception of vitamin B12. Vitamin B12 is primarily found in animal-based foods, such as meat, fish, and dairy, but there are a few alternative sources. Nutritional yeast (see page 153) is usually enriched with a generous supply of B vitamins, including B12, and many breakfast cereals and milk substitutes are fortified with B12. Nonetheless, vegans or those who seldom consume animal products may need to consider supplementation of vitamin B12.

Fat-Soluble Vitamins

Cow's milk contains vitamins A, D, E, and a very small amount of K. However, these vitamins are mostly removed with the fat in the production of reduced-fat, low-fat, and skim milks.

To counteract one of these deficiencies, dairy farmers typically fortify low-fat and skim milk with 2,000 to 3,000 IU of vitamin A per quart. Retinol, one of the "preformed" animal types of vitamin A, is most commonly used for fortification rather than beta-carotene, which is a precursor that our bodies use to create vitamin A. Unfortunately, a moderate to high intake of retinol has now been linked to a potential increase in hip fracture risk. Scientists speculate that the vitamin A used to fortify most milk may actually interfere with the activity of vitamin D, a crucial bone-building nutrient. For this reason, many physicians now caution against retinol supplementation and encourage patients to naturally consume beta-carotene, which is incredibly abundant in greens (such as spinach and kale), carrots, red bell peppers, and sweet potatoes.

As for vitamin D, dairy farmers may choose to fortify with 400 to 600 IU of the "sunshine vitamin" per quart. Most dairy-free milk alternative manufacturers also fortify their products with vitamin D, but for many people, just 15 minutes of outdoor time per day (or even just a few times per week) can result in adequate levels of this essential compound. If you live in a gloomy place, your doctor may recommend that you take a vitamin D supplement. If you are a vegan living in a gloomy place, a multivitamin might be prescribed.

Minerals

The primary minerals in milk are phosphorus and calcium. The body needs to maintain a perfect balance of phosphorus and calcium; when too much of one is present, it depletes the other. High blood phosphate levels are a top concern in Westernized diets, which are rich in dietary phosphorus in the form of carbonated beverages and processed foods. Too much phosphorus can reduce the body's ability to utilize vitamin D (convert it into its active form), reduce blood calcium levels, and eventually lead to poor bone mineral content. As you might expect, this could have a negative effect on the growth and development of little ones, and could promote osteoporosis later in life.

Since Westernized diets tend to rely on milk for the bulk of calcium intake, the calcium-phosphorus balance can be further upset when dairy-free consumers replace milk with carbonated beverages, which happens all too often. Carbonated beverages are typically high in phosphoric acid, yet void of calcium.

Luckily, some wise food and beverage choices can ensure that your mineral intake is adequate for healthy bones while maintaining a milk-free diet. For starters, skip the soda. Enjoy some good old H_2O as a beverage substitute for milk, and consume a balanced diet that includes healthy, dairy-free sources of calcium. An entire chapter is dedicated to the discussion of calcium later in this book (beginning on page 46), which includes a chart of milk-free foods that can help you reach your calcium quota.

So what does make milk so special? It certainly isn't the protein, saturated fat, sugar, phosphorus, or vitamin A. Dairy milk is touted almost exclusively for its calcium, B vitamins, fortified vitamin D, and water. Most dairy-free milk beverages on the market are fortified with some level of calcium, vitamin D, and B vitamins, but proper hydration, a well-balanced diet, and some occasional sunshine can alternately supply the dairy-free individual with each of these essential nutrients. If in doubt, consult your physician about taking a multivitamin—even milk drinkers do!

WHEN TO CONSIDER ORGANIC

Organic milk is still dairy milk. It contains all of the same proteins, fats, sugars, and cholesterol that may be problematic for milk allergies, intolerances, special diets, or general health concerns. However, for those who can and do consume even small amounts of dairy, organic milk products may be worth the extra expense.

Dairy products repeatedly make the top lists of foods you should buy organic, and for good reason. Beyond dangerous pesticides, organic milk in the United States is also produced without the use of antibiotics and synthetic hormones. Are these drugs a true concern in the dairy supply, or has the issue been exaggerated by organic farmers and anti-milk campaigners? I was curious to know, so I pooled some unbiased facts as evidenced by regulations and scientific studies.

Why Dairy Farmers Use Synthetic Hormones

- Bovine growth hormone (BGH) is a naturally occurring hormone in cows that stimulates the production of another hormone, IGF-1 (insulin-like growth factor-1). IGF-1 in turn initiates the production of milk.

- The U.S. Food and Drug Administration (FDA) approved the use of rBGH (also known as rBST), a genetically engineered version of BGH, in 1993. The injection of rBGH into cows has become standard practice on many dairy farms, as it has the ability to increase a cow's output of milk by up to 20 percent (according to the rBGH manufacturer, Monsanto). Higher production per cow means a better bottom line for the dairy farmer.

The Effects of Synthetic Hormone Use on Humans

- Cows treated with rBGH produce greater levels of IGF-1. In fact, numerous studies have confirmed that cows treated with rBGH produce milk with two to ten times the levels of IGF-1 found in untreated cow's milk.

- The IGF-1 found in cows is a bio-identical hormone to the IGF-1 produced by humans.

- Dairy supporters argue that the IGF-1 in milk is not absorbed into the body; however, the consumption of cow's milk has been scientifically shown to increase the serum level of IGF-1 in humans by 10 percent. In contradiction to their prior claims, the National Dairy Council has even utilized a study confirming this increase in IGF-1 as a supporting document for bone health.

- Higher levels of IGF-1 in humans have been linked to a statistically significant increase in the risk of prostate, colon, lung, and breast cancers.

Other Consequences of Hormone Use

- Cows treated with rBGH were found to have a nearly 25 percent increased risk of acquiring an udder infection (mastitis). Other major side effects (as noted by the manufacturer of rBGH) include infertility, lameness, cystic ovaries, uterine disorders, digestive disorders, lacerations, and calluses of the knee.

Cue the Antibiotics

- An increase in infections results in greater antibiotic use, both legal and illegal.

- Antibiotic residues in milk may cause allergic reactions in sensitive individuals, and may be an important factor in the growth of antibiotic-resistant bacteria.

- Testing for antibiotics is limited in its effectiveness. Mandatory screenings by milk processors are for only a few select antibiotics (while dozens of types are in use). Additional testing is randomized and on more of an "audit" level.

- Even for those batches that pass inspection, low levels of antibiotic residues are typically permitted. The effects of these low levels, in addition to the potential antibiotic levels of untested milk, are largely unknown.

- In 2001, 6.7 million pounds of milk were dumped in Minnesota alone due to the detection of antibiotic residue—and this was only from the 10 percent of loads randomly inspected on a quarterly review. You might be shocked by the idea of how much "tainted" milk may have gone untested and continued on into our milk supply, or by the incredible amount of waste. In an odd twist of fate, the waste may have potentially negated the "increased production" from the use of rBGH. And so the cycle continues.

Though hotly contested by the United States, the European Union has maintained a ban on the use of rBGH since 1985. They have deemed rBGH as unsafe for public health and from a veterinary perspective. In 1999, the Codex Alimentarius Commission (established by the Food and Agriculture Organization of the United Nations and the World Health Organization) ruled in favor of the European moratorium on hormone-treated milk products. Australia, New Zealand, Japan, and Canada have upheld a similar ban on the use of hormones in the dairy industry. So why on earth did the FDA approve rBGH, and why are dairy farmers in the United States, Mexico, and South Africa still routinely administering it? Consumers are still waiting for that answer.

In recent years, many conventional U.S. dairy producers have opted to shun the use of this synthetic hormone and have won the right to proclaim "rBST free" on their packaging. On the surface, milk labeled as rBST free might seem like a good compromise, but keep in mind that it is still "conventional" milk and may have the same antibiotic and heavy pesticide concerns.

And even with organic milk, it remains unclear how the growth hormones that naturally occur in the milk of all cows can affect humans in the long run. Should we be consuming a food with enough hormones to help a calf gain 1 to 2 pounds per day? Some may opt to follow a dairy-free diet for this reason alone.

THE RAW DEBATE

All FDA-approved dairy products, whether organic or conventional, must be pasteurized, and the majority of milk is also homogenized. These standard processing methods essentially turn raw milk into a "packaged food," which has stirred up concern among staunch health advocates.

What Is Pasteurization?

According to the U.S. Centers for Disease Control (CDC), pasteurization is "the process of heating milk or other liquids to destroy microorganisms that can cause disease or spoilage." During pasteurization, raw milk is heated to 145°F for 30 minutes, 163°F for 15 seconds (flash pasteurization), or 285°F for a second or two (UHT, or ultra-high temperature pasteurization).

Pasteurization is a handy way to increase the shelf life of refrigerated milk and to destroy most unwanted microorganisms. On the typical dairy farm, unpasteurized milk can be a source of tuberculosis, diphtheria, salmonellas, typhoid fever, undulant fever,

Q fever, and listeria. It is estimated that pasteurization kills 95 to 99 percent of pathogenic bacteria in milk, which is why the FDA requires that all packaged or bottled milk shipped interstate be pasteurized.

What Could Be Wrong with Pasteurization?

This is a controversial question. A few of the typical responses are:

- It encourages relaxed regulations on the sanitary practices of dairy farms.
- It allows otherwise "unfit" milk to be released to the general public.
- It strips away some essential vitamins.
- It destroys "beneficial" bacteria, yet isn't fully effective against all known hazardous strains (note the 1 to 4 percent of pathogens remaining after pasteurization).
- Its introduction can be directly correlated with a sudden increase in the incidence of heart disease.
- It alters the nutrients in milk, resulting in more allergies.

To date, the link between pasteurization and conditions such as heart disease and food allergies remains weak in the scientific literature. Nonetheless, milk producers do know that the high-heat processing doesn't discriminate, destroying and potentially altering some beneficial nutrients along with the bad guys.

What Is Homogenization?

Homogenization is really just "pretty packaging." Natural milk separates, leaving skim milk on the bottom and a thick layer of cream on top. This cream can be easily skimmed off, similar to the layer of coconut cream that forms atop an unshaken can of coconut milk. However, the Westernized palate looked down on this type of presentation, causing the milk industry to respond with a consistent, creamy look achieved via the process of homogenization.

Homogenized milk has been forced through ultrafine mesh at high pressure to break up the milk fat globules and disperse them evenly throughout the milk, thereby creating a uniform product. While homogenized milk does in fact look better, it doesn't take a heart surgeon to point out (although a good one will) that whole foods are a much better choice than processed foods. Processing can destroy naturally occurring vitamins and minerals and, in the case of homogenization, may actually alter the state of some nutrients, including milk proteins, in a way that is not fully understood.

Since homogenization showed up on the scene around the same time as pasteurization, and it directly involves altering the fat globules, some physicians believe it may also be linked to the sudden rise in high cholesterol and heart disease rates. Homogenized milk has also been accused of increasing the allergenicity of milk and contributing to the substantial surge in milk allergies over the past few decades. However, further research would be needed to substantiate these claims.

Is Raw Milk a Good Alternative?

Raw milk isn't homogenized or pasteurized, and is therefore banned at the federal level. This prevents raw milk from crossing state lines, but approximately thirty U.S. states have some type of legalized raw milk sales within their boundaries. Raw milk sales remain illegal in the populous parts of Canada, but are legal in most European nations.

Proponents of raw milk often tout it as a healthy solution for the prevention of milk allergies and heart disease. Since raw milk is in fact cow's milk, many more studies would need to be conducted before these bold claims could be validated. Raw milk still harbors a good amount of lactose and allergenic proteins, and it may not be suitable for those who forgo milk for environmental, political, religious, or other health reasons. Plus, raw milk can be very difficult to find and expensive to purchase. And the jury is still out on whether it is truly "fit" for human consumption.

The U.S. Department of Health and Human Services expresses strong concern that contaminated raw milk may be a source of harmful bacteria and illness. Though raw, un-pasteurized dairy products account for just 1 to 3.5 percent of all dairy products consumed in the United States, the CDC reported that 60 percent of the outbreaks from the consumption of dairy products during a thirteen-year study period were attributed to unpasteurized milk products. In addition, the unpasteurized outbreaks had a higher rate of hospitalization.

UNMASKING MODIFIED MILKS

In their quest to capture every last consumer, dairy producers have created some mighty spins on ordinary milk. In this section, I'll address the potential heroes, and which are simply allergy and intolerance villains hiding behind health claims.

Acidophilus Milk

When I wrote the first edition of this book, acidophilus milk was a top inquiry among my readers. It has since slipped from its prominent position, but is still available and worth addressing. Acidophilus milk has the same nutritional makeup as the milk from which it is made, most often cow's milk. It differs in that the bacterium *Lactobacillus acidophilus*, a common probiotic, has been added to theoretically aid in digestion.

Traditionally, the bacterium was added to the milk, which was then fermented to create acidophilus-cultured milk. This process did lower the lactose level in the milk with increased lactase activity (the enzyme that binds to lactose), but it also increased the acidity of the milk, consequently resulting in a sour flavor that was unappealing to most taste buds.

To combat the flavor issues, a new process was developed to grow the bacterial culture first and then add it to the milk, skipping the acid-forming fermentation altogether. This resulted in the product we see most commonly on store shelves today, sweet acidophilus milk (SAM).

SAM proponents argue that the acidophilus aids in digestion regardless of the production process. However, a study reported in the *American Journal of Nutrition* showed that

SAM does not have enough lactase activity to enhance lactose digestion—in fact, it has far less than yogurt. However, SAM made with sonicated or "disrupted" cells, also known as SAM-S, did aid in lactose digestion for several of the study subjects.

If you are lactose intolerant and very interested in finding a cow's milk option, then it may be worth your while to seek out traditionally fermented acidophilus milk or SAM-S, but ordinary SAM will likely yield no benefits. None of these options will be suitable for those who are milk allergic or who are cutting milk for other health, social, or religious reasons.

Kefir

In the past decade, kefir has picked up where traditional acidophilus milk left off. It is a cultured milk product with the consistency, taste, and probiotic power of a tart drinkable yogurt, and studies have shown that it typically produces minimal to no digestive symptoms when ingested by many lactose-intolerant individuals. Kefir has not been qualified as a "cure" for lactose intolerance, nor is it lactose free, but rather a tolerant food with temporary benefits for some who crave mammal milk. Use caution, though, as neither yogurt nor kefir is a symptom-free haven for every lactose-intolerant person.

Originally, kefir was produced from camel's milk. Today, you are more likely to find commercially available kefir that is made from the milk of sheep, goats, or cows, though dairy-free soy, coconut, and even water versions of kefir have emerged. The dairy-free versions are often labeled as "drinkable yogurt" or "probiotic beverages" and should specifically state that they are dairy-free or vegan.

Both kefir and regular yogurt can provide a helpful dose of probiotics, but kefir reportedly contains a wider array of these digestion-boosting bacteria.

Store-bought kefir, aside from the dairy-free versions, is not believed to be a good choice for those who are seeking a milk alternative for reasons other than lactose intolerance. While you can make homemade kefir using liquids such as coconut water, almond milk, and even lemonade, it is very difficult to find truly dairy-free kefir starter powder or granules. For performance reasons, kefir starter is usually grown on a dairy medium (even some that are labeled as dairy free) and stored in milk for reuse. I have been told that any traces of dairy from the starter are eliminated during the fermentation process, but it is up to the individual to decide whether this is a worthwhile and safe option.

Lactose-Free Milk

There are no special secrets to lactose-free milk; it's simply plain old dairy milk minus the symptom-producing lactose. So how do they do it? First, dairy processors turn up the heat to ultra-pasteurize the milk. They then add lactase, a natural enzyme that converts lactose into glucose and galactose. Since lactose-intolerant individuals are short on their own internal lactase supplies, this step essentially predigests the lactose for them.

Lactose-free milk is another product that should be considered only by the lactose intolerant. It won't be suitable for those with milk protein allergies or those who forgo dairy for religious, social, or other health reasons.

A2 Milk

There are three types of casein proteins in milk: alpha, kappa, and the very abundant beta-casein. A1 and A2 are the most common types of beta-casein, but the amount of each can vary among mammal types and even by region. It has been found that cattle in Asia and Africa typically produce only A2 beta-casein, while A1 is far more common in dairy cows in the Western world. However, milk designated as A2 milk by the a2 Milk Company has been specifically tested to ensure that it contains only the A2 type of beta-casein rather than A1.

Why is this important? Rumors have circulated that A2 milk might be less allergenic than A1 milk for those who have an allergy to the casein proteins in cow's milk. Unfortunately, this theory has not been formally tested or proven, and even the a2 Milk Company has stated that these claims are unwarranted. On their website, they recommend against feeding A2 milk to someone with a milk protein allergy.

Furthermore, in contrast to the aforementioned milk products, A2 milk has shown no benefits for those with lactose intolerance. It differs only in its protein makeup, and still contains comparable levels of lactose to standard cow's milk. The a2 Milk Company has funded studies to support the digestive benefits of A2 milk over A1 milk, but they report that their findings are specifically for individuals who have an "A1 intolerance." At the time of writing, A2 milk was available in Australia and New Zealand, with increasing distribution in the United States.

UDDER OPTIONS

With the sharp rise in cow's milk allergy diagnoses, many claims emerged about the hypoallergenic nature of other mammal milks. Although these "better than cow's milk" statements may sound like a stretch, research has shown that a few might actually hold a grain (or should I say drop?) of truth.

In theory, all proteins have the potential to become allergenic, but a study out of the Institute of Food Research (now the Quadram Institute Bioscience) in Norwich, England, and the Medical University of Vienna found that the ability of a particular animal food protein to trigger a food allergy might correlate with its "evolutionary distance" from a human equivalent.

The researchers sought to define how closely an animal protein must resemble its human protein counterpart to lose its allergenic potential. In general, proteins that were more than 62 percent identical to a human equivalent were rarely allergenic, while those that fell below the 54 percent marker had a much higher ability to become allergenic. The more distant proteins may hinder the ability of the human immune system to discriminate between foreign and self-proteins, resulting in immune responses that are otherwise known as allergy symptoms.

This study does shed light on why cow's and goat's milks, which both fall under the 54 percent identical mark, are fairly prevalent food allergens, while mare's (horse's) milk is up to 66 percent identical to human milk proteins and can often be tolerated by the milk allergic.

Though horse's milk may sound unappealing to many, quite a few "odd" mammal milks are consumed by humans in different parts of the world, and research coupled with demand is bringing many of the following nearer to our grocery stores.

Goat's Milk

Goat's milk is slightly closer in composition to human milk than cow's milk is, with proteins that may be easier to digest, but it isn't typically recommended for those with a cow's milk allergy. Though one study showed that an estimated 25 percent of cow's milk–allergic individuals do not react to goat's milk, another investigation of 26 children with cow's milk allergy yielded no tolerance for goat's milk. Nonetheless, because goat's milk products have become more readily available worldwide, many allergists do include it on their test panel.

For those who can tolerate goat's milk, there are some potential benefits worth noting. Unlike cow's milk, goat's milk does not contain agglutinin, a substance that clusters fat globules together and makes them more difficult to digest. Goat's milk is also higher in calcium, vitamin B6, potassium, and niacin than cow's milk. However, it is significantly lower in vitamin B12 and folic acid.

The lactose levels in goat's milk versus cow's milk are very similar (4.1 percent and 4.7 percent, respectively), so lactose-intolerant individuals might experience little to no relief from making the switch.

Sheep's Milk

Sheep's milk is considered by many to be highly nutritious, and it is richer in certain vitamins (A, B, and E) and minerals (calcium, phosphorus, potassium, and magnesium) than cow's milk. It has also been noted that the fat globules in sheep's milk are smaller than the fat globules in cow's milk, potentially promoting easier digestion. Nonetheless, sheep's milk is much higher in both fat and protein than either goat's or cow's milk, and it has yet to receive the go-ahead in milk allergy research. For this reason, it would rarely be a good option for the milk allergic or other dairy-free dieters.

The commercial sheep dairy industry is concentrated in Europe and in countries surrounding the Mediterranean Sea. Sheep's milk is slowly hitting the mainstream in North America, most often in the form of cheese.

Camel's Milk

Camel's milk has slowly migrated to the United States from the Middle East, where it has long been a staple of the Bedouins. The gradual acceptance of, and emerging demand for, camel's milk in the Western world is due in part to recent studies on its potential "curative" properties.

In a study of 8 children with severe food allergies (including milk), all reacted well to a camel's milk diet and even recovered fully from their allergy symptoms. Further research with 35 cow's milk–allergic children confirmed that while it isn't the solution for all, 80 percent tolerated camel's milk.

The success of camel's milk may lie in its compositional differences from cow's milk. Camel's milk is free of the specific beta-casein protein and beta-lacto-globulin protein (whey) that are known instigators of milk allergies. In addition, the immunoglobulins in camel's milk are similar to those in human breast milk, and immunoglobulins reduce children's allergic reactions and strengthen their future response to foods.

Raw camel's milk (pasteurization may destroy some of its immune-boosting benefits) is now available in North America, but it doesn't come easy or cheap. Camels are much harder to milk than cows, and camel farms are still sparse in the United States. Even so, it might not be long before we see camel's milk ice cream and "camelbert" cheese in the dairy case.

Mare's Milk

As previously mentioned, the affinity of mare's milk to human milk has sparked some curiosity in the scientific and milk allergy communities. In one study of 25 children with severe cow's milk allergy, over 90 percent were able to safely consume mare's milk.

While this type of mammal milk may sound like a very new concept in English-speaking countries, it is old school throughout other parts of the world. It just happens to be enjoying a revival in continental Europe, including Belgium, France, the Netherlands, and Norway. Mare's milk is also fairly common in central Asia, but it is typically served in a fermented form, similar to kefir, called koumiss or airag.

In addition to its possibilities for milk allergies, some believe that mare's milk holds curative properties for digestive problems. This theory is still quite anecdotal. In fact, in my search to discover the lactose levels of mare's milk, I read that it is both much higher in lactose than cow's milk and much lower in lactose than cow's milk—within the same article!

As you can imagine, milking a horse could pose many more challenges than a cow, so mare's milk is still quite scarce and expensive. However, if the food allergy studies continue to prove fruitful for mare's milk, then we might eventually see its availability on a grander scale to consumers.

Donkey's Milk

Yes, donkey's milk. At present, you will run across it only when traveling, perhaps in France, Belgium, Italy, or Ecuador. However, speculators say that it may be on its way to North America, so I will briefly address it.

Researchers in Italy have given donkey's milk considerable attention in recent years due to its very close chemical composition to human milk, including the types and levels of proteins. It was proposed as a suitable substitute for cow's milk in allergic children, and a 2012 food allergy study confirmed its tolerance in approximately 90 percent of the participants.

Due to the very low milking output of donkeys, donkey's milk doesn't hold as much potential for broad distribution as other mammal milks do, but it is reportedly gaining traction as a specialized pediatric beverage in Italy.

Even More Mammal Milks

Beyond those noted above, buffalo, yak, water buffalo, reindeer, zebra, wallaby, and even moose have been known to provide milk used by humans for dairy products. While each may vary in composition, they are all mammal milks containing water, fat, lactose, whey, and casein in higher amounts than are found in human milk. Like cow's milk, these various milks may elicit allergic reactions, may upset lactose intolerance, and may not be suitable for those who forgo dairy for social, political, religious, or other health reasons. Research on each would be required before any opposing claims could be made.

Back to Human Milk

Isn't it strange how so many people recoil with an "Ew!" when someone asks why breast milk isn't readily sold in retail? Societal influence has made it seem normal to consume milk from a lactating cow, but not a human, past infancy. Nonetheless, human breast milk is a hot topic on many bodybuilding forums, and I periodically receive questions on this matter from health-oriented and allergic readers.

It certainly makes more sense, from an allergy perspective, to consume milk designed for humans. But drinking it past weaning and, furthermore, once we are fully grown, is still an issue of debate. All mammal milk naturally contains hormones designed to aid in rapid growth. These hormones have been linked to hormonal cancers in adults (we're done growing, but perhaps the hormones still need something to do!), and it remains to be seen if human breast milk wouldn't have the same connection.

Keep in mind that all mammal milks still possess the lactose, proteins, fat, and hormones that do, in fact, make them milk. To date, the only mammal milk that seems to be inarguably healthy for human consumption during infancy in most cases (see galactosemia on page 33 and lactose intolerance on page 27) is human breast milk. If you are interested in exploring other mammal milks, consult a physician first.

CHAPTER 2
WHY WE LIVE DAIRY FREE

Just twenty years ago, the concept of living without milk was viewed as radical and even impossible by some. But by 2006, the Vegetarian Resource Group estimated that over 22.8 million Americans were already following a nondairy lifestyle. And the upward trend for this once-ignored diet has continued to grow at near exponential rates. In 2015, the dairy alternative sector topped $2 billion in annual sales and was labeled "one of the largest markets in the North American food and beverage industry" by research analysts at MarketsandMarkets. This year, as mentioned previously, the industry is expected to reach $16 billion in annual sales.

It's impossible to point to a single movement behind this dietary shift, as the reasons for living dairy free are as diverse as the people themselves. But to put it in perspective, this chapter focuses on the most common motives for living sans dairy.

MILK ALLERGIES

Dairy milk contains over twenty-five different molecules that have the potential to elicit an allergic reaction, helping to make it one of the top allergenic foods worldwide. In fact, many doctors, scientists, and health specialists now recommend going dairy free as an initial test if a food allergy is suspected.

When the first edition of this book was released, most physicians still had a black-and-white understanding of food allergies—either you tested positive to a food allergen via an IgE skin prick test or you didn't have a "true" food allergy. But researchers were already arguing that many shades of gray were being missed. Most of their scientific findings were initially written off as insignificant at best, but it is now medically understood that there are at least two categories of food allergies, IgE-mediated and the much broader non-IgE-mediated. Both fall under the definition of food allergy:

a damaging immune response by the body to a substance to which it has become hypersensitive

The phrase *immune response* is a crucial key that connects these two rooms of science, but it excludes food intolerance or, as it relates to milk, lactose intolerance. I will explain lactose intolerance beginning on page 27, but first, let's dive into the details behind the types of milk allergies, related symptoms, and where the medical community is at with regard to treatments.

IgE-Mediated Milk Allergies

Antibodies are blood proteins used by our immune systems to help identify and neutralize pathogens, such as bacteria and viruses. But one type of antibody, immunoglobulin E (IgE), has its sights set on allergens. Though it's present in very minute amounts in our bodies, IgE binds to allergens and triggers the release of substances that can cause a cascade of allergic reactions.

Resultant symptoms from an IgE-mediated allergic reaction can be as mild as watery eyes from airborne pollen or as severe as life-threatening anaphylaxis from a peanut. Ironically, by trying to protect us from "invaders," our immune system can in turn cause internal harm. And contrary to common beliefs, milk is a top offender for IgE allergies and can trigger anaphylaxis in the severely allergic. In fact, some of the most highly publicized losses from allergic reactions were due to milk allergies.

The two leading allergy offenders within milk are the protein types known commonly as casein and whey. Casein is the curd that forms when milk is left to sour. Whey is the watery part that is left after the curd is removed. In IgE-mediated milk allergies, the body responds to one or more of these proteins immediately or typically within two hours following ingestion. But a reaction "aftershock" can occur up to twenty-four hours after the initial reaction.

Non-IgE-Mediated Milk Allergies

When a milk allergy is suspected but there is no immediate reaction and the patient tests negative for IgE activity, it is often classified as a non-IgE-mediated allergy (also referred to as a cell-mediated allergy).

Like IgE allergies, non-IgE food allergies also trigger a potentially damaging immune response to an allergen, which is typically casein and/or whey protein in the case of milk. But rather than busy antibodies, non-IgE-mediated allergies are believed to be primarily cell-mediated. White blood cells, known as T cells, take their time in launching an attack on allergens, resulting in a delayed onset of symptoms, which typically occur anywhere from 1 hour to 1 day after ingestion. Some reports state that symptoms may take up to 3 days to become fully apparent.

Though non-IgE food allergies can also result in anaphylaxis, such severe reactions are believed to be rare. Nonetheless, cell-mediated reactions share many common symptoms with IgE-mediated food allergies, with a greater focus on the digestive tract, and can result in long-term health problems, such as failure to thrive (in children) and anemia.

Note that some literature may refer to cell-mediated food allergies as "intolerances," but this is an understatement of the condition. "Intolerance" refers to an inability to properly metabolize or absorb a substance, resulting in symptoms; it does not imply any type of immune response coming into play.

The label confusion may stem from our still-limited knowledge of cell-mediated food allergies. Extensive research has been conducted to define nearly every aspect of IgE-mediated food allergies, but non-IgE is a broader category that has gained notable attention only in recent years. Yet current research has already identified several conditions with strong affiliation to cell-mediated food allergies:

Atopic Dermatitis (AD)

Also referred to as atopic eczema, AD is a fairly common chronic inflammatory disease of the skin that is more frequently diagnosed in children, but can occur at any age. Research has shown a strong link between AD and food allergies, particularly cell-mediated food allergies. In a Korean study of over 2,400 patients with AD, more than 50 percent tested positive for at least one food allergy. And, among those, nearly 95 percent had a cell-mediated food allergy, with another 3 percent presenting with "mixed allergies." Milk was one of the top offending foods, affecting approximately 21 percent of the allergic participants.

Food Protein–Induced Enterocolitis Syndrome (FPIES)

FPIES specifically affects the gastrointestinal tract, with symptoms that can range from mild reflux or runny stools to severe vomiting and diarrhea. The worst-case scenarios can result in dehydration and potentially life-threatening shock. In chronic cases, failure to thrive is observed, as this is a condition that is primarily seen in infants. Cow's milk and soy are the top two allergens associated with FPIES, which typically arises in formula-fed babies. According to some international studies, FPIES typically resolves by the age of 3, but in the United States, and particularly with cow's milk allergies, FPIES tends to persist longer and can leave a legacy. Approximately 25 percent of children with FPIES develop food-specific IgE antibodies, which can transition into IgE food allergies. Furthermore, approximately 30 percent of infants with FPIES develop atopic diseases, such as AD, asthma, or hay fever.

Eosinophilic Esophagitis (EE or EoE)

EE is a relatively "new kid on the block" in terms of scientific discovery, but it seems to be making up for lost time with an increasing rate of diagnosis. EE is an immune condition that causes inflammation of the esophagus, and studies have shown that it can be triggered by both IgE- and non-IgE-mediated food allergies, with a high incidence of cow's milk allergy. The symptoms of EE are often similar to those of gastroesophageal reflux disease (GERD), but do not respond to anti-reflux medication. They often include difficulty swallowing, abdominal pain, food impactions, vomiting, weight loss, anemia, and failure to thrive in children. Though EE can arise at any age, the mean age of diagnosis is 33.

There are additional eosinophilic gastrointestinal disorders (EGIDs) that can affect different parts of the digestive tract, such as eosinophilic gastroenteritis, eosinophilic gastritis, and eosinophilic colitis. These conditions also have a strong trigger correlation to food allergies, but they have not garnered the same medical attention in recent years as EE has.

Food-Induced Pulmonary Hemosiderosis (Heiner Syndrome)

Heiner syndrome is a rare disorder that primarily presents with respiratory symptoms, but may play out with recurrent infections and GI-related concerns, such as anemia and failure to thrive. It typically affects children aged 6 months to 2 years, and evidence suggests a strong link to milk allergy.

What about Milk Soy Protein Intolerance (MSPI)?

MSPI was a blanket term used for gastrointestinal symptoms caused by milk protein rather than lactose. As we are learning, the term *intolerance* is being phased out in cases where the reaction is believed to be caused by an immune or allergic response, as in FPIES, EE, and other EGID conditions.

How Many People Have Milk Allergies?

Most of the reports on milk allergy prevalence are based on personal accounts, rather than actual tests, resulting in very broad ranges and requiring big margins for error. However, in 2010 the World Allergy Organization gathered five European studies in which infants were tested for cow's milk allergy. The results showed an incidence of approximately 2 to 5 percent. These numbers most likely include both IgE- and non-IgE-mediated milk allergies, as oral food challenges were used for allergy confirmation in all of these studies.

For infants who present with IgE-mediated milk allergies specifically, the Johns Hopkins Children's Center conducted prolonged research to establish the age at which most children outgrow these milk allergies, and discovered that it was much later than estimates originally stated. According to their findings, the rates of milk allergy resolution were found to be 19 percent by the age of 4, 42 percent by the age of 8, 64 percent by the age of 12, and 79 percent by the age of 16.

Nonetheless, it is possible for older kids or adults to develop a milk allergy (IgE- or non-IgE-mediated) with or without a childhood history of allergies. And the majority of allergy researchers seem to agree that while patient reports of milk allergy may be high, cell-mediated milk allergies in kids and adults are probably underdiagnosed by the medical community.

Milk Allergy Symptoms

Reactions to milk can vary based on many factors, including the type of allergy (IgE, non-IgE, or both), the form and quantity of the allergen consumed, and the patient's own biology. I've provided some generalized symptom information in the preceding sections, but the following is a summary list of potential symptoms relating to milk allergy (per medical documentation):

SKIN: itchy, red rash; atopic dermatitis/eczema; acute urticaria/hives; pruritus/generalized itching

DIGESTIVE: abdominal pain/cramps; reflux; colic (in babies); bloating and gas; nausea; vomiting; diarrhea; loose or bloody stools; constipation; difficulty swallowing; fat malabsorption

RESPIRATORY: tingling or swelling of the lips, tongue, mouth, or throat; coughing or wheezing; shortness of breath or chest tightness; sinusitis

OTHER: irritability; night waking; anxiety; failure to thrive; unexplained weight loss; anemia; dizziness; watery eyes; recurrent ear infections/otitis media; migraine headaches

I've read several observational reports of other symptoms relating to milk allergy, such as dark under-eye circles, lethargy, congestion, muscle or joint pain, and runny nose, but found little research to either back up or refute these claims.

For individuals with severe IgE-mediated milk allergies, anaphylaxis is a potential reality. Anaphylaxis is a sudden systemic allergic reaction that may involve multiple areas of the body, including the skin, cardiovascular system, respiratory tract, and gastrointestinal tract. Anaphylactic reactions can be mild, but some cases are potentially fatal, and therefore require epinephrine and urgent medical attention. If you are concerned that you or a loved one may be at risk for anaphylactic reactions, consult a doctor immediately.

Milk Allergy Testing

When it comes to our health, we want definitive answers. We expect to walk into a doctor's office with a list of symptoms and leave with a 100 percent accurate diagnosis. Wouldn't that be nice? Unfortunately, as with most medical conditions, food allergy testing still has many limitations. Allergists do have a few good evaluation tools to choose from, but I think many of you will be surprised that the medical "gold standard" for allergy testing isn't very scientific at all.

Elimination Test and Oral Challenge

Your doctor might start with other types of testing, but at some point, this "gold standard" elimination test is often employed. Doctors know that symptom relief has the potential to tell a much bigger story than specific scientific tests can.

With an elimination test, suspicious foods are temporarily removed from the patient's regular diet to see if symptoms resolve. Depending on the doctor used, the recommended period of elimination may be anywhere from one week to one month, or possibly longer. Then, under the direct supervision of a physician, the suspect foods are slowly reintroduced one at a time to see whether symptoms are reproduced. The reintroduction phase is known as an oral challenge. Allergists also use an oral challenge to help confirm if a known allergic patient has outgrown a particular allergy.

It is important to note that reactions may be heightened following a period of elimination. If a significant change in symptoms is seen during the period of elimination, then your doctor may opt to skip the challenge phase altogether, and recommend a continued elimination of the suspect food(s). A detailed journal of diet and symptoms should be kept for one to two weeks prior to the elimination diet, during the period of elimination, and throughout the reintroduction/challenge phase.

A free, downloadable journal is offered at **GoDairyFree.org/journal** to help you log your diet and track symptoms. This journal offers 14 days of detail that you can access to download and/or print at any time.

Elimination tests and oral challenges do take longer than a blood test, and I've received numerous emails from people who are hesitant to rely on such a simple, free, unscientific assessment. But a food elimination challenge is still considered the "gold standard" of food allergy testing for both IgE-mediated and cell-mediated allergies among most of the medical community. In fact, it is typically used in research as the control by which other tests are evaluated.

Skin Prick Test

This old-school testing method has been used by allergists for decades as a fairly reliable tool for diagnosing IgE-mediated allergies to food, plants, mold, and even pets. It involves placing a very tiny drop of a suspect allergen on a person's arm or back and pricking the skin, thereby allowing a minute amount to penetrate the skin's surface. If a red spot, or wheal, flares up, then an allergic reaction is indicated. The results are almost immediate, as reactions should occur within about 15 minutes.

Allergists like skin prick tests for assessing several allergens at once because they rarely produce false negatives. However, there can be false positives due to the larger undigested nature of the food proteins, cross-reactivity with an allergen in the same "family," or medications. Anti-allergy medications, such as over-the-counter antihistamines, may need to be discontinued 2 to 3 days before the skin prick test, as they can interfere with the results. Cold medications, some antidepressants, beta-blockers, and other medications may also promote inaccuracy.

Though they may sound simple, skin prick tests cannot be easily mimicked at home and should always be administered by a physician. Even in a medical setting, this type of testing is sometimes ill advised for those who may have a life-threatening reaction to milk or other food allergens being tested. In those cases, blood tests are usually the preferred method.

Atopy Patch Test

This method is very similar to skin prick testing, but the potential allergens are applied via a large patch that is left on the skin for 48 hours to help identify delayed allergic reactions. Though results from atopy patch tests can overlap with skin prick tests and blood tests, recent studies have shown them to be more helpful in accurately identifying cell-mediated food allergies in patients with atopic dermatitis. Atopy patch testing has also shown usefulness in diagnosing certain cell-mediated food allergies in patients who present with gastrointestinal symptoms in cases of EE and FPIES, but it has produced some inadequate results with respect to identifying non-IgE-mediated milk allergy.

As with skin prick tests, atopy patch testing must be administered under physician supervision, and carries the same precautions and limitations.

Blood Tests

The RAST (radioallergosorbent test), otherwise known as the CAP-RAST, or ImmunoCAP test, is a key food allergy blood test that involves sending a small blood sample to a medical laboratory to be analyzed for reactivity to a set of food allergens. The results of the RAST are usually received within one week. Similar to skin prick tests, the RAST measures only IgE antibodies to detect allergies to specific foods.

Though the RAST test is not perfect (it is also known to produce false positives with some regularity), many doctors prefer the test for its relatively high level of accuracy for ruling out allergens and for ruling them in when IgE levels are high. The RAST is often useful for determining if an oral challenge (discussion coming up!) will be safe when testing to see if a child has outgrown a severe food allergy. The RAST is also helpful for patients who have eczema or other skin problems that may complicate reading the results of a skin prick test. Plus, this blood test is not affected by the presence of medications.

The RAST is not a useful test for non-IgE-mediated food allergy diagnosis and, unfortunately, the science behind cell-mediated blood tests is still somewhat lacking.

The ELISA (enzyme-linked immunosorbent assay) is often touted as a more complete food allergy blood test because it measures both IgE and immunoglobulin G (IgG) antibodies in response to suspect allergens. IgG antibodies are found in the most abundance in our bodies, and they are powerful soldiers in the fight against bacterial and viral infections. Proponents of the ELISA test suggest that they also play an indicative role in delayed food allergies.

Though scientists have not fully ruled out IgG antibody evaluation in food allergy research, their general diagnostic value for patients has not yet been proven. In fact, the first large-scale study of IgG antibody testing for food allergies showed that food-specific IgG levels were variable in both healthy and symptomatic adults, with limited correlation to dietary elimination results. In fact, the researchers were not able to conclusively state whether food-specific IgG antibodies necessarily play an allergenic role or if their presence actually indicates tolerance in certain subgroups.

A third, and even more controversial, food allergy blood test is the ALCAT test (sometimes referred to as a leucocytotoxic or NuTron test). Rather than looking for elevated antibodies, the ALCAT measures the reactivity of leukocytes, white blood cells in the immune system that are responsible for defending the body against foreign materials. The ALCAT is relatively popular among alternative health practitioners, but it is not as readily accepted by allergists. Due to the potential inaccuracies of both ALCAT and IgG testing, and the fact that they can suggest a substantial number of food allergens in a single patient, many physicians also worry that these tests may lead to overzealous elimination diets.

Gastrointestinal Tests

When a gastrointestinal disorder, such as EE or FPIES, is suspected, the patient may be referred to a gastroenterologist for evaluation. To aid in diagnosis, the gastroenterologist might order an endoscopy, pH monitoring, general blood tests, stool analysis, and/or imaging. If an EGID, Heiner syndrome, or FPIES is confirmed, the patient is often referred back to an allergist to help pinpoint any potential allergen triggers of symptoms.

Other Allergy Tests

You may come across a few other types of food allergy tests if you're venturing into naturopathy. These could include the Vega test, kinesiology, or hair analysis, among others. From my research, I found little, if any, concrete evidence to back up these types of assessments. Be sure to consult a physician before undergoing any type of allergy testing.

Can Milk Allergies Be Treated?

As with most allergies, avoiding the offending substance is the top recommended form of treatment. And in the case of food allergies, it's currently the only concrete way to prevent a reaction.

To date, there isn't an FDA-approved "cure" for milk allergies, but studies have ramped up in recent years to work toward treatment and even prevention of IgE-mediated food allergies. By the time you read this, there could be even more in the pipeline, but thus far, these are the most promising bodies of research underway:

Probiotic Formula

As I write, news is circulating about a new dietary intervention study out of the University of Chicago targeting milk allergy. For one year, 12 infants with cow's milk allergy were fed an extensively hydrolyzed casein formula supplemented with the probiotic *Lactobacillus rhamnosus* GG. By the end of the treatment, 5 (42 percent) had developed tolerance to cow's milk proteins, compared to none of the 7 milk-allergic controls who did not receive the formula.

The small-scale study focused on patients diagnosed exclusively with non-severe IgE-mediated cow's milk allergy; those with known non-IgE-mediated allergic conditions or a prior history of anaphylaxis were excluded. So the depth of the findings is limited, but still promising in the grand scheme of food allergy research.

Immunotherapy

For many years, a procedure known commonly as "desensitization" has been used as a treatment for environmental allergies. It involves subjecting the patient (under strict medical supervision) to minute amounts of their known allergen in gradually increasing quantities over time, with a goal to increase their tolerance to the allergen. Though not always successful, desensitization does work for many individuals, resolving or lessening the severity of their symptoms, at least temporarily.

Environmental allergy desensitization, or immunotherapy, is most typically performed via injections. But for food allergies, the administration methods being tested are oral immunotherapy (OIT) and sublingual immunotherapy (SLIT). In OIT, a food allergen (in a powdered mix) is administered slowly, in small but steadily increasing doses over time, and under physician supervision to monitor for a reaction. SLIT is similar, but the food allergen is dissolved in a solution that is placed under the tongue. OIT has been shown to be more effective in studies than SLIT, but it is also more likely to cause serious allergic reactions.

One of the first notable studies to demonstrate the potential of food allergy immunotherapy was released in 2008. A desensitization program was administered to 30 children with severe IgE-mediated allergies to cow's milk proteins. After one year, 11 (36 percent) of the children had become completely tolerant, 16 (54 percent) could tolerate limited amounts of milk (5 to 150 mL/0.1 to 5.0 oz.), and 3 (10 percent) were not able to complete the program due to persistent respiratory or abdominal complaints.

Further research has shown that OIT and SLIT might hold promise for IgE-mediated food allergy treatment, but the results have remained mixed on safety and efficacy. Beyond reactions that can occur during immunotherapy, in many patients, the success appears to be temporary. Several test subjects who appeared to gain tolerance to their food allergen had allergy symptoms return (in some cases severe, as in anaphylaxis) within the study period following their immunotherapy. Drug therapies are being researched in combination with immunotherapy in the hopes of achieving greater long-term success.

Chinese Herbs

At Mount Sinai Hospital in New York, Dr. Xiu-Min Li has spearheaded research on a revolutionary East-meets-West herbal therapy, which she believes could act as a cure for IgE-mediated food allergies. Named the food allergy herbal formula-2 (FAHF-2), Dr. Li's protocol is already showing promise for ease, safety, and efficacy and has garnered a great deal of support from the medical community. At last check, she was in phase 2 of clinical trials.

For non-IgE-mediated, or cell-mediated, food allergies, I was unable to find any solid research on potential treatments beyond allergen avoidance. With some conditions related to cell-mediated food allergies (like AD and EE), drugs such as antihistamines and steroids may be prescribed to aid in symptom relief, but for the most part, these have shown minimal effectiveness.

LACTOSE INTOLERANCE

As mentioned in the previous section, a food *allergy* is identified as an abnormal and heightened response of the immune system to certain components (most notably proteins) within the offending food. In contrast, a food *intolerance* is indicated when symptoms develop after eating a food that your body simply can't cope with effectively, but it does not involve an immune response. In the case of milk, lactose is typically the intolerance culprit.

Otherwise known as "milk sugar," lactose is the primary carbohydrate in milk products. During the digestion process, lactose is broken down into glucose and galactose for proper absorption. This step occurs in the small intestine with the assistance of an enzyme known as lactase. Many people have or develop a shortage of lactase, and therefore are unable to properly digest some or all of the lactose they consume. The unabsorbed lactose passes into the colon, where havoc ensues. This lactase deficiency and any resulting gastrointestinal symptoms are what we typically refer to as lactose intolerance.

If you are not lactose intolerant yourself, odds are you know someone who is. A 1994 report from the National Institute of Diabetes and Digestive and Kidney Diseases (NIDDK) estimated that 30 to 50 million people in the United States alone are lactose intolerant. Look around. That is about 1 in every 8 people you see.

Could It Just Be Maldigestion?

The true prevalence of lactose intolerance has been put into question by the dairy industry. The National Dairy Council suggests that most people are not actually lactose intolerant, but rather they are suffering from lactose "maldigestion."

If you want to get technical about it, they may be correct. According to the very sparse literature I was able to uncover on the term *lactose maldigestion* or *malabsorption* (pretty much the National Dairy Council website and one study in Sicily), "Lactose maldigestion occurs when digestion of lactose is reduced as a result of low activity of the enzyme lactase." In other words, maldigestion is a reduction in the ability to digest lactose, while intolerance is the complete inability to digest lactose.

As confirmed by their very definitions, both maldigestion and intolerance "can cause uncomfortable gastrointestinal symptoms and overall poor health." Since you may experience some very strange looks if you told people you were a lactose maldigester, and since both intolerance and maldigestion can cause discomfort following milk consumption, I think this may be a case of splitting hairs with terminology. To keep things simple, I will use the most commonly understood expression, lactose intolerance, to refer to lactose maldigesters of all magnitudes.

Who Is Most Likely to Be Lactose Intolerant?

As you may have noted, the NIDDK report is a little dated. Though it is a fairly common issue, studies on lactose intolerance have been quite limited in the past thirty-plus years. Nonetheless, the National Institutes of Health (NIH) released an Executive Summary in 2011 evaluating the research on lactose intolerance. Their report, along with cited studies, uncovered the following statistics on the subject of prevalence:

- Among adults in the United States with reported GI symptoms, lactose malabsorption (as determined by hydrogen breath tests) occurred in approximately 6 to 24 percent of Caucasians, 50 percent of Mexican Americans, and 70 percent of African Americans. The rate may be even higher (some say 90 percent) among Asian Americans.

- Northern Europeans tend to have the lowest overall rates of lactose intolerance, while Africa, Asia, and Latin America have prevalence rates ranging from 15 to 100 percent, depending on the specific population studied.

- The occurrence of lactose malabsorption tends to be relatively low in young children, particularly under six years of age. But in populations with high adult rates of lactose malabsorption (such as African Americans and Mexican Americans), rates peaked between ten and sixteen years of age.

Internationally, it has been estimated that a whopping 65 percent of the world's population has a reduced ability to digest lactose past infancy, which can progress with age. Rates of lactose intolerance seem to be equivalent among men and women, although some women may temporarily regain the ability to digest lactose during pregnancy.

Lactose Intolerance Symptoms

Lactose intolerance symptoms may vary from person to person, and can range from mildly uncomfortable to quite severe, but are specific to the gastrointestinal tract. The most notable by-products of lactose intolerance are abdominal pain, abdominal cramps, intestinal bloating, gas/flatulence, diarrhea, and nausea. One or more of these symptoms may emerge about 30 minutes to 2 hours after ingesting lactose-laden foods.

How Does Lactose Intolerance Develop?

For most, lactose intolerance is developed through the progression into adulthood; for some, it is acquired as a result of an acute illness; and for a very few, lactose/lactase issues may be present from birth.

Primary lactose intolerance stems from a natural and gradual decrease in lactase activity after weaning. This is the most common cause of lactose intolerance. Due to the progression, symptoms may develop as early as five years old, and often worsen with age. Some may have a complete loss of lactase activity, but many will retain 10 to 30 percent of their initial level of the enzyme activity (those maldigesters again). This may allow for digestion of very low levels of lactose.

Secondary lactose intolerance may occur during episodes of acute illness. This can happen at any age, and following full recovery it is possible for the damage to be reversed. A few potential causes of secondary lactose intolerance are irritable bowel syndrome, acute gastroenteritis, celiac disease, cancer, and chemotherapy. The lactose intolerance may subside once the underlying condition has resolved, though for many it persists.

Congenital lactose intolerance is a very rare metabolic disorder in which a baby is born with lactose intolerance. Congenital lactose intolerance must be passed through the generations via autosomal recessive inheritance. In other words, both the mother and the father must possess and pass on the defective form of the gene in order for their child to be affected. Infants with congenital lactose intolerance are actually intolerant of the lactose in their mother's breast milk, too, and will typically present with symptoms (diarrhea, vomiting, dehydration, and failure to thrive) within a few days following birth. This condition seems to be most common in Finland.

Is Lactose Intolerance Normal?

Contrary to popular belief, primary lactose intolerance is not a disease, but rather a natural process in human development. Unlike milk proteins, which can vary in composition among different mammals, lactose is lactose—a basic blend of two simple sugars that is essentially the same, whether the milk is from a cow, camel, or human.

After weaning, lactase production typically decreases as the need for an infant to digest mother's milk is no longer present. But thousands of years ago, when groups of Northern Europeans made the shift from hunting and gathering to livestock and farming, the small number in the domesticated bunch that had "lactase persistence" were able to thrive. The genetics passed on, resulting in a high rate of lactose tolerance among Northern European populations specifically. It's believed that cross-cultural migrations are the primary reason that this genetic mutation for digesting milk has reached other ethnic populations to some degree.

Lactose Intolerance Testing

Lactose intolerance can be diagnosed through one of the following commonly utilized tests, performed on an outpatient basis at a hospital, clinic, or doctor's office:

The Lactose Tolerance Test

This test begins with a 24-hour fasting period. At the end of this fast, the patient's blood is drawn, and the glucose level is tested. The patient then receives a lactose-rich beverage, and for the next 2 to 3 hours blood samples are taken to check their glucose level. Normally, when lactose reaches the digestive system, the lactase enzyme breaks it down into glucose and galactose. The liver then changes the galactose into more glucose, which in turn enters the bloodstream and raises the patient's blood glucose level. If lactose is incompletely broken down, then the blood glucose level does not rise as it should, and a diagnosis of lactose intolerance may be confirmed.

The lactose tolerance test is not given to infants and very young children who are suspected of having lactose intolerance. The large lactose load administered may be dangerous for very young individuals, since they are more prone to the dehydration that can result from lactose-induced diarrhea.

The Hydrogen Breath Test

Very little hydrogen is detectable in the breath of someone who has a normal healthy gut. However, in lactose-intolerant individuals, bacteria ferments undigested lactose in the colon and hydrogen is produced.

In the hydrogen breath test, the patient drinks a lactose-rich beverage, and their breath is analyzed at regular intervals. Increased levels of hydrogen in the breath indicate improper digestion of lactose and may confirm a diagnosis of lactose intolerance. Prior to the hydrogen breath test, certain foods, medications, and cigarettes should be avoided, as they may interfere with the accuracy of the results.

Like the lactose tolerance test, the hydrogen breath test is considered too dangerous to administer to infants and very young children.

The Stool Acidity Test

Undigested lactose fermented by bacteria in the colon also creates lactic acid, which can be detected in a stool sample. This third test is suitable for infants and young children and may be an easy option to help identify the presence of lactose intolerance.

Some pediatricians may simply recommend that a baby or young child be switched to a lactose-free diet as a trial to see if the symptoms subside. Likewise, many doctors feel that this short-term "elimination" diet may be a good testing option for adults who believe they are suffering with lactose intolerance. A doctor should be consulted regarding whether any of the above tests, including an elimination diet, would be appropriate.

Lactose Intolerance Treatment Options

Unfortunately, scientists have not yet discovered a way to boost the body's ability to produce lactase, so the best treatment is dietary avoidance of lactose-laden foods. As mentioned, many people are not completely intolerant and are thus able to digest limited quantities of lactose. However, there are a few things to keep in mind.

Naturally low-lactose dairy foods can include butter, hard cheeses, and yogurt. Yet most doctors would be hesitant to recommend cheese and butter for daily consumption or as major sources of calcium. They are rich in animal-based saturated fats, proven instigators of heart disease. Plain yogurt, specifically with live yogurt cultures (aka probiotics), may be well tolerated. However, the yogurt we Americans love is typically loaded with fruit, flavors, and sweeteners (sometimes in the form of milk solids/lactose), combating the power of these digestion-boosting bacteria.

Unlike milk allergies, primary lactose intolerance (the most common type) isn't typically outgrown. In fact, lactase production usually decreases with age. It is not uncommon for individuals to experience a worsening of lactose-intolerant symptoms or, for those with a previous record of good digestion, to suddenly begin experiencing symptoms of lactose intolerance. In other words, that hunk of cheese may be okay today, but it might spell disaster tomorrow. It really is a system of trial and sometimes-unpleasant error for lactose-intolerant individuals who choose to consume dairy.

For those who must have that ice cream sundae, lactase enzymes are available over the counter. However, these are not 100 percent effective, and dosage can be a tricky balancing act. Lactase enzymes function well only in very acidic environments (such as the human gut), but too much acid can denature them. For this reason, it is best not to take them on an empty stomach. However, the enzymes will not be effective if they don't reach the small intestine before the problematic food arrives. So they must be taken prior to, or at the time of, each bout of dairy intake. There is also the risk that the enzymes will not provide enough lactase to digest the lactose being consumed, allowing the symptoms to ensue regardless.

Some people have such severe lactose intolerance that a strict dairy-free diet is the only way to go, but I have received numerous stories from *moderately* lactose-intolerant people who have simply chosen to go dairy free. In general, they found that complete avoidance broke their cheesy cravings, the experimentation was more of a hassle than it was worth, and while they were able to "tolerate" some milk products, they actually felt better when they didn't bother to consume any. Nonetheless, if you have lactose intolerance and prefer to eat some dairy foods, it helps to know which options have the most and the least lactose.

Lactose Levels in Specific Dairy Foods

Like milk protein, lactose is a water-soluble molecule that is not found in the fat portion of milk. Therefore, curdling processes and fat percentages can have a big impact on the prevalence of lactose. Unlike many weight-loss dieters, lactose-intolerant individuals may find that low-fat and nonfat products are their nemesis. Furthermore, lower-fat dairy foods often have milk solids or other dairy derivatives added back in to enhance sweetness, which may consequently increase the lactose content.

Surprisingly, determining consistent lactose percentages in dairy foods is no easy feat. Because processes can vary among dairies and manufacturers, and with so many new types of dairy products continually coming on the market, reported lactose levels can vary. For the most extensive data, I turned to the *American Journal of Clinical Nutrition* and the lactose intolerance guru, Steve Carper. Steve left a legacy of well-researched information online and literally wrote the book on the subject of lactose intolerance, *Milk Is Not for Every Body*.

The following is intended as a general guide to lactose levels in dairy products; it should not be taken as absolute. Also, lactose levels below 2 percent are typically considered low lactose, and may be well tolerated by many lactose-intolerant people when consumed in reasonable quantities.

WHEY (52.0 to 80.0 percent): Dry whey is very high in lactose, whether it is sweet, sour, or reduced lactose. The only exceptions are whey protein concentrate (ranging from 10 to 55 percent), whey protein isolate (around 0.5 percent), and liquid whey (4.5 to 5.0 percent).

DRY MILK POWDERS (36.0 to 55.0 percent): This concentrated form of milk is very high in lactose and best avoided by lactose-intolerant individuals. Dry milk powders include nonfat and buttermilk versions (which are on the high end of the scale) and whole milk powder.

CONCENTRATED MILK (9.7 to 16.3 percent): Sweetened condensed milk and evaporated milk (whole and skim) contain more lactose than regular cow's milk, with sweetened condensed milk being the highest offender.

HUMAN BREAST MILK (9.0 percent): While milk protein–allergic infants are able to thrive on Mom's breast milk, lactose-intolerant infants simply cannot digest lactose, regardless of the source. Human milk contains nearly double the lactose of many other mammal milks.

COW'S MILK (3.7 to 5.7 percent): This range applies to whole, low-fat, and nonfat/skim milk and buttermilk, but in general lowering the fat results in a slight bump up in lactose levels. It should also be noted that the lactose levels for the milk of other mammals, including goat, sheep, buffalo, and yak, are similar to cow's milk, varying only by fractions of a percentage.

ICE CREAM (3.1 to 8.4 percent): This includes ice cream and ice milks, but sherbet often weighs in with less than 2 percent lactose. Low-lactose or lactose-free ice cream is also available.

CREAM (2.8 to 4.3 percent): As in milk, the fat in cream matters when it comes to lactose. Whipping cream falls at around the 3.0 percent mark, while light cream is closer to 4.0 percent, and half-and-half weighs in at over 4.0 percent. Sour cream also fits comfortably into this range, with roughly 3.0 to 4.0 percent lactose.

"CULTURED" PRODUCTS (1.9 to 6.0 percent): This range is wide due to the variability among commercial yogurts. Sweet acidophilus milk (SAM) and part-skim kefir have lactose levels of around 4.0 percent.

CHEESE (0.0 to 5.1 percent): Cheese is tricky, as the lactose percentages don't just vary by the type of cheese, but also by how the cheese is manufactured. Hard and soft ripened cheeses that are produced via traditional methods are often better tolerated than milk, as the fermentation processes and higher fat content contribute to lower lactose levels. Moreover, the traditional aging of some cheeses (over 2 years) reduces the lactose content to near zero. However, modern processes used in the production of most cheeses today rarely assist in lactose reduction, and typically involve minimal aging. Swiss cheese, for example, could easily range from zero lactose to as much as 3.4 percent lactose, depending on how it was manufactured. Cheeses that are usually moderately high in lactose are lower-fat soft cheeses, such as ricotta, feta, and cottage cheese. Highly processed cheeses (such as processed American and Velveeta) also tend to be very high in lactose and are best avoided by the lactose intolerant.

LACTOSE-REDUCED MILK (0.0 to 1.6 percent): Not all lactose-reduced milk is completely lactose free, but it can usually be considered a low-lactose beverage.

BUTTER AND MARGARINE (0.0 to 1.0 percent): In a perfect world, butter would be completely lactose-free, but this rarely happens. However, both butter and margarine are considered low-lactose foods. And ghee will bring you even closer to that zero lactose mark.

DAIRY INTOLERANCE

The term *dairy intolerance* is used by many individuals who suffer dairy woes. But until recently, it lacked scientific backing. In an ongoing 2017 study out of the University of Auckland, researchers found that some participants who didn't have lactose intolerance (as confirmed by hydrogen breath tests) still experienced acute stomach pain, flatulence, bloating, and distension when they consumed milk. This suggested digestive reactions to something else in milk rather than lactose. The researchers concluded that dairy intolerance is a real phenomenon and "not in people's heads." They hope to further identify which specific component(s) in milk might be causing the observed dairy intolerance.

I do think it's important to note that the study did not state if the participants were evaluated for cell-mediated milk allergies (page 20). Based on the report released, it seems plausible that they were observing non-IgE milk allergy symptoms rather than dairy "intolerance." Either way, their findings are a big step forward for acknowledging that dairy digestive issues do extend beyond lactose intolerance.

GALACTOSEMIA

Galactosemia is a very rare metabolic disorder that affects how the body processes galactose, one of the simple sugars created when lactose is broken down in the digestive system. Not to be confused with lactose intolerance, galactosemia is a much more serious medical disorder. While those with galactosemia may have no problem digesting lactose, they have a shortage or absence of the liver enzyme GALT, which is needed to break down galactose. As a result, galactose accumulates in the body, where it may damage the liver, kidneys, eyes, central nervous system, and other body systems.

The classic form of galactosemia presents itself quite soon after birth, with symptoms of vomiting, diarrhea, jaundice, and failure to thrive. Diagnosis is usually made during the first week of life with a heel prick blood test as part of standard newborn screening. Since galactose is a lactose by-product, babies with the more severe forms of galactosemia are not able to consume any lactose-containing foods, including their own mother's breast milk.

Treatment requires the strict lifetime exclusion of lactose/galactose from the diet. This includes milk products, but it can also include processed foods, some fruits and vegetables, meats, and some children's medicines. Even with prompt diagnosis and treatment, galactosemic children are known to have long-term complications.

As mentioned, galactosemia is very rare, with the classic form affecting only 1 in 30,000 to 60,000 newborns. For more information on galactosemia, visit the Galactosemia Foundation website at **Galactosemia.org**.

THE VEGAN DIET

While vegetarians typically shun meat and fish, strict vegans consume a diet that is free of all animal products. This includes (or should I say excludes) meat, seafood, eggs, dairy products, and often honey.

The vegan diet was once associated almost exclusively with socially aware individuals who were concerned about animal rights, but in recent years, millions of people have trialed a plant-based diet (rich in vegetables, fruits, grains, nuts, and seeds) for health reasons. This shift has helped the number of vegans in the United States rise from 1.4 percent of the population in 2006 to 2.5 percent by 2011, according to Harris Interactive polls (reported by the Vegetarian Resource Group). And many now consider vegan to be "the new vegetarian."

The vegan diet has received considerable scientific backing for its potential strength in battling heart disease and diabetes. In a 2006 study, the vegan diet even beat out the American Diabetes Association (ADA) diet in the treatment of diabetes. Not only was the vegan diet much more effective in shedding pounds and reversing type 2 diabetes symptoms, but the researchers also noted that it seemed easier to follow. Unlike the ADA diet, the vegan diet was simple and straightforward, with no calories to count, portion sizes to measure, or carbohydrates to limit.

A 2009 study confirmed the weight loss and potential glycemic and cholesterol-lowering benefits over the ADA diet. This was followed by a 2015 study showing weight loss and lowered cholesterol as well as a potential decline in diabetic nerve pain with a plant-based diet.

Vegan websites and cookbooks are fantastic tools for all dairy-free dieters, omnivorous or not, since a primary difference between vegan and vegetarian diets is the dairy. For those who do consume meat and/or fish, it is easy to use vegan recipes as the base for meals, adding in your protein of choice.

As a dairy-free consumer, I owe a great deal of thanks to the vegan community for bringing so many wonderful recipes and foods to the mainstream.

AUTISM

Public awareness of autism has expanded exponentially since the U.S. Centers for Disease Control (CDC) released its first reports announcing the increased prevalence of autism. In 2003 and 2004, two national health organizations interviewed the parents of approximately 98,000 school-aged children, combined. The results estimated that nearly 1 in every 175 children is living with autism. In a follow-up study in 2007, the CDC revised these numbers upward, to close to 1 in 150 children. In 2014, another revision was released: the CDC reported that 1 in 68 children were now identified with autism spectrum disorder. This equates to roughly 1.47 percent of all school-aged children, or around 1 million kids.

According to the medical community, autism refers to a neurodevelopmental disorder that typically makes its presence known in early childhood. It affects several crucial areas of development, including social interaction, communication, behavior, creativity, and imagination. Autism was formally identified around the mid-1900s, but it still isn't fully understood.

For decades, the parents of autistic children have experimented with various medical and alternative treatments to address problematic symptoms. Their network of trial and error has yielded some surprising and positive results.

In 2005, the Autism Research Institute published their findings from an ongoing study, focused on the usefulness of different interventions. Overall, they questioned nearly 23,700 parents of autistic children. The parents were asked to rate the therapies they had trialed according to effectiveness. The options fell into three major categories: drugs; biomedical non-drug therapies, such as vitamin supplements; and special diets.

Much to the dismay of major drug companies, the results swung largely in favor of alternative therapies and diet.

Approximately fifty different drugs were reported as tested. On average, 30 percent of the cases showed an improvement of symptoms; however, 31 percent actually got worse while on one or more of the drugs. Biomedical non-drug therapies fared far better; 45 percent of the cases reported a decline in symptoms, with only 5 percent exhibiting an increase. Yet amazingly, special diets rated as the most successful treatment category overall. Among the autistic children who were put on a special diet, 50 percent of the cases exhibited signs of improvement, while only 2 percent experienced a rise in problematic symptoms.

The simple removal of dairy products was the special diet option tried most, with over 5,500 parental reports. In this group, 49 percent found it improved their child's symptoms, with a worsening of symptoms in only 2 percent of the cases. Of those who were willing to take it a step further to a gluten-free/casein-free (GFCF) diet, a resounding 65 percent saw an improvement in symptoms. Gluten is a protein found in wheat and other flours.

Another study in the same year, out of the New Jersey Medical School Department of Pediatrics, also reported positive results with dietary intervention. They found that a casein-free diet (in some cases coupled with additional food avoidance based on test results) led to the resolution of GI symptoms and improvement in behavioral symptoms in 97 percent of the autistic children who presented with digestive symptoms at the beginning of the study.

Gradually, the gluten-free/casein-free diet is inching into the mainstream as a recommendation for autistic children and adults. Other alternative therapies are beginning to receive similar recognition, particularly in the areas of reducing chemical exposure (in food, water, and the environment) and detoxification. However, no modification is one size fits all, so experts recommend consulting a gastroenterologist before embarking on a new dietary plan.

ADHD

Attention deficit hyperactivity disorder (ADHD) is frequently coupled in studies with autism, as these two developmental disorders seem to share many similarities in terms of symptoms. In fact, a study conducted in Norway found that, as with autism, a casein-free diet might improve mental health in children with ADHD. This ten-year study, led by Dr. Karl Ludvig Reichelt, placed 23 Norwegian children diagnosed with hyperactive disorders on milk-free and/or gluten-free diets. Twenty-two of the children who were taken off milk products and other casein-containing foods exhibited almost immediate improvement in their mental health and overall behavior, with longer attention spans and increased learning capabilities. However, the symptoms returned as soon as the milk-based foods were reintroduced into their diets. Most of the children involved in this study had also been taking behavioral medications, such as Ritalin, prior to changing their diets. However, after following a casein-free diet, they were soon taken off the medications.

Long-term follow-up with these children has found their disorders to be manageable, with the virtual disappearance of past behavioral challenges.

Reichelt believes that people with ADHD lack an enzyme that breaks down proteins like casein. As a consequence, the inability to efficiently digest these proteins may inhibit optimal brain function. By reducing the intake of these aggravators, he feels that hyperactivity can be brought under control—and based on his research findings this may very well be true.

THE PALEO DIET

In the late 1980s, Dr. Loren Cordain's dietary research evolved into the paleo diet, a way of eating based on what our Paleolithic ancestors consumed. His findings didn't immediately gather a huge following, but in recent years, the paleo diet has caught on like wildfire.

The basic necessities of the paleo diet focus on the following whole foods: grass-fed meats, seafood, eggs, fruits, vegetables, nuts, seeds, and healthful oils (such as olive, walnut, flaxseed, macadamia, avocado, and coconut). Banished foods include dairy, grains, legumes (including peanuts), refined sugar, potatoes, refined oils, and salt. I had the opportunity to speak with Robb Wolf, a student of Dr. Cordain and *New York Times* best-selling author of *The Paleo Solution*, and he said that in his opinion, dairy free, gluten free, and legume free are the three most important keys to the paleo diet.

Please note that the primal diet, created more recently by Mark Sisson, is different from the paleo diet, and is rather vague on dairy. When Sisson first launched his paleo spin-off, dairy was forbidden, but in recent years he has put ghee and fatty, grass-fed dairy on the "occasional" list. When asked if dairy is good nutrition, Sisson simply replied, "I don't know."

WEIGHT LOSS

In 2007, the dairy industry lost some serious promotional footing when the Physicians Committee for Responsible Medicine (PCRM) petitioned the Federal Trade Commission (FTC) to shut down their infamous milk/weight-loss campaigns. According to Dan Kinburn, PCRM's general counsel, "Milk and cheese are more likely to pack on pounds than help people slim down." It seems the FTC believed that Mr. Kinburn might be right, because the campaigns were halted. And from my personal experience, I agree with Mr. Kinburn wholeheartedly.

When my husband opted to go dairy free, he dropped over 10 pounds in two months (all from his waist) without changing any other aspect of his diet or lifestyle. It was then that I began to think about the true purpose of milk. Calves weigh roughly 50 to 100 pounds at birth, but they grow within a year to around 500 pounds (continuing on to their full weight of around 1,500 pounds, give or take a few hundred), primarily with the assistance of their mother's milk . . . the stuff that we consume by the gallon. Cow's milk is used as a shortcut for growth in our own species, but what happens when we are done growing and are still consuming milk with all of its natural (and sometimes synthetic) hormones, fats, and proteins?

I frequently receive emails and comments from Go Dairy Free readers who proclaim how good they feel and how much weight they have lost since they cut out dairy. For most, it wasn't their original intent. They changed their diet for a milk allergy, intolerance, veganism, or other health or social reason. But to their great surprise a side benefit emerged—unwanted pounds melted away. This real-world evidence speaks volumes, but there are also studies to both directly and indirectly back up the dairy and weight correlation.

How to Lose 36 Pounds Per Year

On the surface, it appears that Americans have taken on healthier eating habits in recent decades. Coffee jitters have been traded in for antioxidant-rich tea, red meat has taken a back seat to lean proteins such as fish and poultry, superfood sales are soaring, and cartons of nonfat milk crowd out whole milk on grocery store shelves. So what gives with the rapidly rising obesity rates? Underneath the nutritious facade, our society's fat, sugar, and overall calorie consumption has increased dramatically.

Some may point to alcohol and butter consumption, which are both on the rise. Yet they are mere slugs compared to the growing popularity of the number one fat offender: cheese. According to the United States Department of Agriculture (USDA) Economic Research Service, the average American's appetite for cheese grew from 7.7 pounds per year in the 1950s to 36 pounds per year in 2014. That is a 468 percent increase! Imagine the damage that 36 pounds of cheese (approximately 60,300 calories and 4,900 grams of fat) could do to your waistline.

How does one person eat this much cheese? Are consumers literally sitting around eating big wedges? Maybe some, but in this day and age approximately two-thirds of cheese consumption is in the form of commercially manufactured and prepared foods, such as frozen pizzas, sauces, instant pasta meals, bagel spreads, and packaged snack foods. Consequently, many who choose a nondairy lifestyle not only cut out the fat and calories of cheese, but may also decrease their intake of refined sugars and hydrogenated oils from highly processed foods.

Is Low-Fat Dairy Better?

There may be a bit more to the weight-dairy connection than merely fat. Some studies, including the following, have linked milk consumption (whether low-fat, skim, or whole) specifically to weight gain and obesity-related diseases such as diabetes and heart disease.

Dairy Effects on Diabetes, Obesity, and Heart Disease in Women

The British Women's Heart and Health Study examined 4,286 British women ranging in age from 60 to 79 for links to metabolic syndrome. Metabolic syndrome was defined as women who had type 2 diabetes or pre-diabetes (insulin resistance or high fasting glucose) and at least two of the following: obesity, hypertension, and lipid disorders (such as high triglycerides or low levels of healthy HDL cholesterol). The women who avoided milk were about half as likely to have metabolic syndrome when compared to milk drinkers. The non-milk drinkers benefited from lower insulin resistance levels, lower triglyceride levels, lower body mass index (BMI), and higher HDL levels.

Children & Milk Consumption: Are They Growing Up or Out?

A large study led by Catherine S. Berkey of Harvard Medical School and Brigham & Women's Hospital in Boston followed the diets and weight of 12,829 U.S. children. The children were diversified across all 50 states, and ranged in age from 9 to 14 years when the study began in 1996. Data was collected from the children through 1999, and the results were a bit of a surprise. Children consuming more than three servings of milk per day were approximately 35 percent more likely to become overweight than children who drank just one or two glasses of milk per day, even though most of the children were drinking low-fat milk.

GENERAL HEALTH & DISEASE PREVENTION

A growing number of nutrition-oriented doctors are recommending dairy-free diets to encourage better overall health and disease prevention. From their perspective, every calorie we consume takes on an internal function. Unfortunately, for many individuals, the proteins, sugar, and fat found in milk products can act in a very counterproductive role. The consumption of dairy may cause, aggravate, or inflame a serious medical condition. This section covers a few of the more common health concerns that may prompt recommendations of a dairy-free or dairy-low diet.

Ovarian Cancer

It is no secret that some rather large studies have identified dairy consumption as one of the strongest links to ovarian cancer. But the real kicker is that a significant increase in ovarian cancer risk was shown in women who consumed higher levels of low-fat and nonfat milk. Prior research had already suggested that a high consumption of whole milk, yogurt, and cheese may increase the risk of ovarian cancer, but now the fat-free varieties might be implicated, too.

One U.S. study of over 80,000 women showed that those who consumed just one or more servings of skim or low-fat milk daily had a 32 percent higher risk of developing any ovarian cancer and a 69 percent higher risk of serous ovarian cancer when compared to women who consumed three or fewer servings per month. Another study from Sweden of over 60,000 women confirmed these results. Their researchers found that women who consumed more than four servings per day of dairy products had twice the risk of serous ovarian cancer compared to women who consumed fewer than two servings of dairy products per day. To further the case against milk in particular, it was found that women who drank as little as two or more glasses of cow's milk per day were twice as likely to develop ovarian cancer as women who consumed little to no milk.

For once, added fat and hormones may not be to blame. The main theory circulating indicates galactose as the true culprit. As mentioned previously, galactose is one of the two main components produced when lactose is broken down in our digestive systems. Many researchers believe that high levels of galactose overstimulate, overload, or damage the ovaries, thus contributing to the development of ovarian cancer.

Prostate Cancer

Though controversy abounds on this topic, numerous studies have shown a solid connection between dairy consumption and the risk of prostate cancer. Prior theories circled around the increase in IGF-1 (insulin-like growth factor 1) hormone levels seen in milk drinkers. High levels of IGF-1 have been directly linked to various hormonal cancers. Although this theory may still hold some validity, research has uncovered a potential cause that has further heated the debate on dairy and prostate cancer: calcium.

A study led by the Harvard School of Public Health in 2001 observed over 20,000 men and concluded that men who consumed more than 600 milligrams of daily calcium from dairy products had a 32 percent higher risk of prostate cancer than men who consumed less than 150 milligrams of daily calcium from dairy products. The results of this study came as quite a shock for a couple of reasons. First, the researchers noted that the men who consumed the most dairy per day tended to be, by definition, healthier. On average, they smoked less, exercised more frequently, and were more likely to pop a multivitamin than their nondairy counterparts. Second, it presented a conflict in the medical world, since the USDA has recommended a minimum of 1,200 milligrams of daily calcium for men over 50, and 1,000 milligrams for men aged 19 to 50.

A cohort study published in mid-2005 by the *American Journal of Clinical Nutrition* showed that men with the highest dietary intake of dairy foods were 2.2 times more likely to develop prostate cancer than men with the lowest dietary intake of dairy foods. This dramatic increase in prostate cancer risk held true for men with the highest dietary calcium intake over those with the lowest.

A report in April 2008 detailed the work of researchers at the National Cancer Center in Tokyo, who followed over 43,000 Japanese men aged 45 to 74 for an average of 7.5 years. They found that the prostate cancer risk increased by more than 50 percent in those whose intake of dairy products was in the highest quartile, compared to those in the lowest quartile.

The Tokyo study was quickly followed by a June 2008 report in the *British Journal of Cancer*. The investigators utilized the European Prospective Investigation into Cancer and Nutrition database of 145,250 participants to study the relationship between diet, lifestyle, environmental factors, and cancer. In this group, 2,722 men had been diagnosed with prostate cancer at the time of follow-up. While there was no association between meat, fish, or eggs and the risk of prostate cancer, there was a strong correlation with dairy protein and dairy calcium intake. Dairy products and yogurt showed an increased risk of prostate cancer, as did calcium intake from dairy foods (but not calcium intake from nondairy foods).

And for those who have been diagnosed with prostate cancer, dairy products appear to continue presenting risks. A 2015 study followed 926 male physicians who had been diagnosed with non-metastatic prostate cancer. The patients who consumed three or more servings of dairy products per day had a 141 percent higher risk for death from prostate cancer and a 76 percent increased risk for earlier mortality when compared with men who ate less than one serving of dairy per day.

Luckily, the news on prostate cancer isn't all bad. Several other nutrients, vitamins, and minerals have been given a gold star for their potential to reduce the risk of prostate cancer. They include fructose (found in fruit), selenium (high in seafood, mushrooms, grains), vitamin D (produced from sunshine), vitamin E (high in nuts, seeds, and greens), lycopene (high in tomatoes), and soy. Wait, did I just mention soy in a discussion of men's health? Yes, it seems that a prospective study in the United States indicated a 70 percent reduction in the risk of prostate cancer among men who consumed more than one serving of soymilk per day.

Acne

While the acne-milk link is frequently dismissed as an old wives' tale, several medical studies have demonstrated the validity of this association. The most notable was a portion of the landmark Nurses' Health Study involving 47,355 women in 1998. The good news is that this enormous body of research did not find a link between chocolate and acne. However, it did find one with high milk consumption.

The researchers hypothesized that the hormones in milk, not the fat, were the true acne instigators. It has been estimated that 75 to 90 percent of milk and milk products on our shelves comes from pregnant cows. This milk contains progesterone and other hormones that are known precursors to DHT, the primary acne-producing hormone in humans.

In addition to the hormones mentioned above, there are about sixty growth hormones and growth factors present in dairy products. One of these, IGF-1, may be at least partially responsible for acne during the teen years. Back in the 1960s, Dr. Jerome K. Fisher conducted a clinical study on the cause-and-effect relationship between milk and acne for a presentation to the American Dermatological Association. His research looked at more than 1,000 teenage acne patients over a ten-year period. He concluded that the severity of their acne was directly correlated to their milk consumption. Dr. Fisher hypothesized that along with the hormones in milk, milk sugar (lactose) and butterfat might be acne triggers.

To further Dr. Fisher's findings, two more recent studies, in 2006 and 2008, evaluated the possible link between dietary milk and acne in kids. A team of medical researchers gathered data from thousands of adolescent girls and boys and did identify a solid correlation between reported acne and milk consumption.

These days, most dermatologists recognize the crucial role that diet plays in skin conditions, and many do cite milk products as the top food culprit in acne. I've also received numerous personal accounts from both teens and adults who've seen their acne clear with a dairy-free diet. But if your physician does recommend trying a dairy-free diet to help heal your skin, please note that it should be tested with patience. A dietary change may prevent new outbreaks, but it could take a few months for the already established acne to "cool."

Headaches and Migraines

The majority of research does suggest that food intolerances, allergies, and other hypersensitivities are frequent triggers of headaches and migraines. Although each migraine sufferer may react to a different food or group of foods, a few seem to pop up as frequent offenders: dairy (including milk, cheese, and yogurt), wheat, eggs, soy, corn, citrus, chocolate, coffee, beef, yeast, red wine, and processed foods with additives and preservatives.

In order to identify the culprit(s) from among these top instigators, scientists and physicians often put their patients on an oligoantigenic diet. This is a hypoallergenic "elimination" diet, consisting of a selection of foods that are presumably well tolerated. During the studies, patients are told to eat only the "safe" foods outlined on their version of the oligoantigenic diet in an effort to eliminate any symptoms. Once the symptoms have gone into remission, the "high risk" foods are reintroduced into the diet one at a time to assess their potential trigger effect on symptoms. This type of diet should be undertaken with the assistance of a physician, in order to ensure adequate nutritional intake. In each of the three case studies that follow, some form of an oligoantigenic diet was used.

In one study, 60 migraine patients followed an elimination diet after a five-day withdrawal from their normal diet. Upon reintroduction, specific foods elicited migraine reactions in a significant percentage of patients: wheat (78 percent), oranges (65 percent), eggs (45 percent), tea and coffee (40 percent each), chocolate and milk (37 percent each), beef (35 percent), and corn, cane sugar, and yeast (33 percent each). When an average of ten common trigger foods were avoided, there was a dramatic decline in the number of headaches per month, and 85 percent of patients actually became headache free! Another benefit was welcomed by the 25 percent of these patients who also had hypertension: their blood pressure returned to normal levels.

In a clinical trial, 93 percent of 88 children who suffered frequent and severe migraines recovered on oligoantigenic diets. Most of the patients responded to several foods, which suggested the probability of an allergic rather than a metabolic cause. An added bonus was that abdominal pain, behavior disorder, fits, asthma, and eczema also improved in several of these patients.

A research study tested an oligoantigenic diet on 63 children with epilepsy, 45 of whom also suffered from migraines, hyperkinetic behavior, or both. The 18 children who had epilepsy alone saw no improvement on the oligoantigenic diet. However, of the 45 children with additional symptoms, 25 ceased to have seizures and 11 had fewer seizures while on this diet. Migraines, abdominal pain, and hyperkinetic behavior halted in the 25 children who stopped having seizures, and also in some of those who did not stop having seizures. Reintroduction of foods one by one confirmed that the seizures, migraines, hyperkinetic activity, and abdominal pain these children were experiencing were related to 42 different "trigger" foods.

Why do so many people suffer from migraines and other headaches when they consume these foods? The medical community is getting closer to an answer. Researchers in Germany have discovered a genetic mutation believed to be responsible for the "faulty wiring" and the subsequent pain. Although clinical scientists have known for a while that migraines are often hereditary, the exact "defect" being passed on was previously unknown.

Irritable Bowel Syndrome

Irritable bowel syndrome (IBS) is a group of digestive symptoms that occur without evidence of damage from a disease. In other words, it's a vague diagnosis of recurrent pain or discomfort in the abdomen usually accompanied by constipation, diarrhea, or both.

These symptoms tend to be chronic, but may come and go over a period of several months or years. Research estimates that 10 to 20 percent of adults within the United States suffer from IBS, placing it at the top of the list for the most common functional gastrointestinal disorders.

Dairy is a potential offender for many IBS sufferers; however, it is rarely due to the milk protein. Though food allergies can certainly play a part in digestive upset, it's the sugar and fat in milk that are most often pinpointed as IBS triggers.

Lactose Intolerance

Lactose intolerance has the ability to mimic or aggravate IBS symptoms. The International Foundation for Functional Gastrointestinal Disorders references two studies on lactose intolerance/malabsorption in which patients diagnosed with IBS were given a hydrogen breath test to clinically identify lactose intolerance. The first study estimated that almost 25 percent of IBS patients had evidence of lactose malabsorption. The second study was performed on IBS patients who had no noticeable symptoms related directly to the ingestion of milk. Lactose malabsorption was identified in 68 percent of these patients. Symptoms improved on a lactose-limited diet.

These findings tie in to a relatively new and quite successful treatment for IBS, the low-FODMAP diet. FODMAPs are certain types of carbohydrates (including lactose) found in foods that may not be digested or absorbed well by some people. When eaten in excess, the undigested portions can be fermented by bacteria in the gut, resulting in some unpleasant symptoms.

High Fat Content

Eating foods that are too high in fat is a frequently cited instigator of IBS symptoms for many people. The majority of dairy foods consumed have a relatively high fat content, including cheese, ice cream, and other whole milk products.

Inflammatory Bowel Disease

Not to be mistaken for IBS, inflammatory bowel disease (IBD) is the name given to a group of more serious disorders that cause the intestines to become inflamed. Although less common than IBS, the prevalence of IBD is quickly growing, with recent estimates of around 3 million in North America, and an even higher rate of occurrence in Europe. General symptoms tend to "flare up" periodically, and may include abdominal cramping, abdominal pain, diarrhea, weight loss, and bleeding from the intestines. The two best-known types of IBD are Crohn's disease and ulcerative colitis, both of which must be diagnosed by a physician.

Though IBD is an immune response, it is not believed to be related to food allergies. In fact, the cause of IBD is still a mystery. However, many individuals find some symptom relief through dietary modifications under the supervision of their physician. In terms of dairy, research has shown a significant increase in the prevalence of lactose malabsorption among patients with Crohn's disease. For this reason, some doctors recommend a lactose-limited diet to individuals with Crohn's disease.

High Cholesterol

Studies in relation to dairy consumption and cholesterol have been sparse over the years. Nonetheless, the purpose of this guide is to help people, and if just one person discovers the cure for their own high cholesterol based on my family's personal experiences, then I feel it is a story worth sharing.

In my early twenties, I had my first cholesterol test. Though I was slight of build and athletic, my total cholesterol was high—bordering on very high—at 240. This included 200 LDL ("bad cholesterol") and 40 HDL ("good cholesterol"). If you are not familiar with cholesterol numbers, let's just say this is not a good ratio for anyone, let alone someone so young. Yet it wasn't too much of a shock, since high cholesterol runs in my family.

My doctor made dietary recommendations (more oats, low fat, etc.) and sent me on my way with a warning that I would need to start medication soon. Of course, my diet was already in line with a "good cholesterol diet," so I was stumped. For the next five years every test came back with the exact same numbers, but I refused to start on the medication. I just knew there had to be a natural answer . . . but I never would have guessed that it would be a strict dairy-free diet.

My annual cholesterol test came up just three months after I leapt into the dairy-free diet with both feet. To everyone's shock, my cholesterol dumped 100 points! I had not changed anything else in my diet, exercise habits, or lifestyle, but I was down to 100 LDL and 40 HDL. Since that time, my total cholesterol has not only continued at this "healthy" level, but the ratio has also improved. The "good cholesterol" numbers have risen to over 60 while the "bad cholesterol" numbers have fallen to just over 80.

I had my father try the dairy-free diet before one of his annual cholesterol checks. He also saw a surprise plummet in his numbers, and gradually went off his medication. Over the years, I have received two other personal stories from readers who gave up all dairy, only to discover a side benefit in their cholesterol.

But it wasn't until a 2014 study, partially funded by the Dairy Farmers of Canada, that a possible reason emerged. The researchers found that dairy intake was associated with an increase in plasma levels of total cholesterol and LDL cholesterol in individuals who were carriers of a specific cholesterol transport gene.

Parkinson's Disease

In 2016, the Mayo Clinic released a study that showed a significant increase in the incidence of Parkinson's disease, particularly in men, from 1976 to 2005. This thirty-year rise has prompted more research into possible causes and, surprisingly, dairy keeps popping up.

Most recently, a 2017 study of nearly 130,000 male and female participants found that people who consume at least three servings of low-fat dairy a day had a 34 percent increased risk of developing Parkinson's when compared to people who didn't consume any dairy. The results were similar for both men and women.

Those researchers then combined their study with four previously published studies on total milk intake or total dairy intake and Parkinson's risk. The pooled data showed a 56 percent increased risk with total milk intake and a 27 percent increased risk with all types of dairy.

OTHER UNEXPLAINED CONDITIONS

With the ever-changing landscape of medical conditions, sometimes even doctors admit that trial and error is the best hope for treatment. For many of my readers, it has led them to a dairy-free diet.

Scientific studies on dietary intervention are actually not that common, especially when compared to drug and other medical therapies. So in some cases, it can be valuable to hear successful anecdotal stories like the ones that follow.

Restless Leg Syndrome

As a child, I suffered with that horrible twitching and vibration known as restless leg syndrome (RLS). It brings new meaning to "not able to sit still." Fortunately, I outgrew it, but many don't. RLS can even pop up for the first time in adulthood, and it can come and go sporadically. I found very little research on RLS treatments, but have had numerous people come to Go Dairy Free with stories of RLS relief when they cut out dairy.

Narcolepsy

This condition hits home for me. From the age of twelve until the day I strictly cut dairy from my diet, I suffered with narcolepsy, a condition characterized by an extreme tendency to fall asleep whenever in relaxed or mundane surroundings.

Despite sleeping well and seeming quite alert, I would spontaneously nod off in class, during lectures, while reading, in the midst of working on tedious spreadsheets, and unfortunately, even while driving. Luckily, the only accident it caused was a non-injury one, and no other people were involved. But I learned to limit my driving to no more than twenty minutes at a time from that day forward. That is, until the condition magically vanished after the day I went dairy free.

Now, I can drive an entire day solo without the slightest bit of fatigue. To verify the culprit, I did have a dairy challenge under supervision and the narcolepsy quickly returned.

I've since heard several stories of people with severe narcolepsy reportedly triggered by dairy. Even one of my physicians, who commuted several hours to a rural hospital ER each week, said he couldn't consume any dairy before he hit the road.

Chronic Fatigue Syndrome

Rather than sudden sleepiness, chronic fatigue syndrome (CFS) is a constant feeling of exhaustion, which can vary from mild to extreme. CFS was once viewed as imaginary—"Oh, you're just tired," friends and physicians would say. But it's now known to be a true debilitating disorder, and the Internet abounds with personal success stories from dietary intervention, often including dairy elimination.

As a delicious side note, a couple of studies in the United Kingdom found dairy-free dark chocolate to be beneficial in treating CFS. The researchers did not find the same benefits with dairy milk chocolate.

Fibromyalgia

Like CFS, fibromyalgia was once believed to be a "mental disorder," but it has since been medically recognized as a true physical condition. Still, little is known about this mysterious widespread pain. Many people have reported success in resolving symptoms of fibromyalgia with dietary intervention and I've had several readers write that they have found relief with dairy-free living. In fact, a reader's personal story on Go Dairy Free called "Dairy Free = Pain Free (for me)" continually receives positive outpourings from others.

Arthritic Pain

This inflammation of the joints can be due to gradual wearing, as in osteoarthritis (OA), or an autoimmune "attack," as in rheumatoid arthritis (RA). In terms of food allergies, researchers have given the most attention to RA, but the results have been mixed. For every study pointing to milk as a potential pain trigger, another rebuts it. Even so, I've received, heard, and read many stories of RA patients who eliminate dairy to keep their symptoms at bay.

FEELING GOOD

It seems that we always need a medical explanation or a profound external influence to fend off the "embarrassment" of following a special diet. Buy why?

When I was in a funk, an alternative doctor recommended that I cut out sweeteners for a little while. I wasn't diagnosed with any type of insulin or sugar issue, but I thought, "Why not give it a try?" Within a week, my energy perked up dramatically. I simply felt better.

When asthma, allergies, or general malaise have someone down, medical and holistic practitioners often recommend a trial of avoiding dairy products. If they begin feeling better, it doesn't necessarily mean that they have a milk allergy or lactose intolerance. Perhaps dairy just doesn't work well for them, as is true for so many people.

It's hard to argue with a diet that optimizes your general well-being and improves your quality of life. From my point of view, that's reason enough. But of course, it's still something you should discuss with your physician.

CHAPTER 3
STRONG BONES, CALCIUM & BEYOND

What if I told you that citrus may be better for your bone health than milk? What if I even suggested that milk might not be a good option for fighting osteoporosis? Would you think I was insane? If so, I wouldn't blame you. Fifteen years ago, I too would have balked at the very notion that any food could be more powerful at battling brittle bones than the almighty glass of milk.

More often than not, the media has led us to believe that dairy is the superior, and perhaps the only suitable, choice for building and maintaining strong bones. Yet in recent years this notion has been put to the test, and shown by many studies to be alarmingly false. According to the enormous twelve-year Harvard study of 77,761 female nurses:

> *Women consuming greater amounts of calcium from dairy foods had significantly increased risks of hip fractures, while no increase in fracture risk was observed for the same levels of calcium from nondairy sources.*

Yes, you read that correctly: dairy products could actually be a *cause* of hip fractures from osteoporosis. This landmark study has raised more than a few eyebrows in the medical community, and although it was a giant study in its own right, it certainly does not stand alone.

In a review of thirty-four published studies in sixteen different countries, researchers at Yale University discovered that the countries with the highest rates of osteoporosis—including the United States, England, Sweden, and Finland—were also the highest consumers of dairy products. As further proof, countries with historically low rates of osteoporosis and hip fracture, such as China, are seeing a proportionate increase in the incidence of osteoporosis with the adoption of Westernized dietary habits, such as milk consumption.

To further these findings, a 2014 Swedish study of over 61,433 women and 45,339 men found that not only did higher milk intake correlate with an increased fracture incidence in women, but it was also associated with higher mortality in both men and women.

How is this possible? According to the USDA, isn't milk one of our major food groups? The answer is not completely clear, but there are a couple of sound theories circulating in the scientific community.

For starters, high dairy intake provides a good dose of animal protein, which in turn is rich in sulfur-containing amino acids. The body buffers the effects of these amino acids by releasing calcium from the bones and excreting it from the body. In addition, animal-based foods, particularly milk, contain very high levels of phosphorus, which may interfere with calcium absorption. Some researchers also believe that calcium consumption may be receiving too much of the focus rather than the right balance of vitamins and minerals to increase effectiveness.

The tides are turning on the osteoporosis front. Many renowned researchers are changing their healthy bone vote from milk to plant-based foods, such as vegetables, fruits, and nuts. Consequently, I have abundant information to share on this topic for dairy-free consumers.

SURPRISING SECRETS FOR STRONG BONES

Don't get me wrong: calcium is very important. After all, when combined with phosphorus, it composes approximately 80 to 90 percent of the mineral content of our bones. Yet, over the years, study after study has revealed that maintaining strong bones isn't as much about our intake of calcium as it is about how well we absorb it, and at what level we are able to keep it in our bones. The following suggestions include baseline tips for building and maintaining strong bones, followed by some potential bone "superfoods" that I hope you will find as interesting as I did.

Exercise

Exercise is recognized throughout the medical community as essential for keeping calcium in its place. "Use it or lose it" really is the name of the game; active people tend to absorb and keep calcium in their bones, while sedentary people lose it. Our bones may be thought of as hard and inflexible, but in reality they are constantly being remodeled with new bone cells replacing old ones. The impact of weight-bearing exercise assists in the bone-building cycle. This may include the obvious strength training, but for those of you who loathe the weight room, baseball, basketball, soccer, tennis, aerobics, dancing, running, jumping, and walking are all considered weight-bearing activities. However, "easy on the joints" sports, such as swimming and cycling, are not.

Keep a Balanced Diet

Magnesium, potassium, iron, zinc, copper, sodium, vitamin D, vitamin K, and antioxidant vitamins (such as C and E) each play a vital role in calcium absorption and/or retention. Enjoying a healthy, varied diet rich in these essential nutrients is definitely an insurance policy worth taking out. Eat a wide selection of fruits, vegetables (including loads of leafy greens and cruciferous types), beans, nuts, seeds, and whole grains.

Keep in mind that it is better to obtain vitamins and minerals via your diet rather than supplements, whenever possible. When consumed as food, there is far less risk for toxicity of a particular vitamin or mineral. Also, food is considered more "potent" since it is a whole package of synergistic nutrients and micronutrients. For extensive information on these nutrients, and the foods you can find them in, visit the World's Healthiest Foods at WHFoods.com. It is one of my favorite resources.

Absorb Some Vitamin D

In 2003, researchers at the Channing Laboratory of Harvard Medical School found vitamin D to be the true "healthy bone hero," reducing the risk for hip fracture by 37 percent. This massive eighteen-year prospective analysis followed over 72,000 postmenopausal women. Oddly enough, they found that neither a high-calcium diet nor milk was associated with a reduced risk for hip fracture.

Aside from mushrooms, fortified foods, and a small handful of other sources, it can be difficult to obtain enough vitamin D via our diets. Luckily, the best source of vitamin D is right above our heads. Approximately fifteen minutes of full sunlight per day is typically enough to meet vitamin D needs for those with fair skin; more time may be needed for those with darker skin. If you get little to no sun exposure, then your doctor might suggest vitamin D supplementation.

Drink Alcohol in Moderation

Alcohol is believed to weaken bones by reducing the body's ability to build new bone and replace normal losses. If you do indulge, it is recommended that you have no more than one or two servings of beer, wine, or liquor per day.

Cut the Caffeine

Several studies have shown a strong link between high caffeine intake and accelerated bone loss. If you still require that quick jolt, research suggests limiting yourself to one or two cups a day of caffeinated beverages.

Hide the Saltshaker

While some sodium is necessary, removing that little saltshaker from the table may be a wise move. Limiting sodium to 1,000 to 2,000 milligrams per day might encourage calcium retention. Sodium hides in processed foods, so stick to whole and natural foods whenever possible.

Don't Smoke

Just in case you needed one more reason to quit the habit, there is a strong link between smoking and a higher risk of fracture and calcium loss.

Understand Medical Conditions

Steroid medications, such as prednisone, and hormone imbalances have been indicated as potential causes of bone loss and fractures. These risk factors should be discussed with a doctor.

Consider Potential "Super-Bone" Foods

In recent years, scientists have pinpointed numerous unsuspecting foods that are showing great promise in the fight against osteoporosis:

Citrus

Superstars may soon be trading in their milk moustaches for pitchers of freshly squeezed orange juice. A 2006 study out of Texas A&M University cited citrus as a potential key to osteoporosis prevention. In the controlled study, they fed an abundance of orange and grapefruit juice to a group of lab rats. The results showed a surprising improvement in bone mineral density. The researchers believe this success was due to the high concentration of antioxidants in the juice, and have been confirming their findings with additional studies.

In 2017, a Chinese study was published that showed similar results in humans. The researchers found that a greater intake of citrus and several other fruits is associated with higher bone mineral density and lower osteoporosis risk in middle-aged and elderly adults. Some of the other fruits that exhibited the most positive effects include apples, peaches, pears, pineapple, and plums.

Dried Plums

My grandmother will be thrilled to know that her daily dose of prunes may be working overtime. Studies conducted at Oklahoma State University and Florida State University's College of Human Sciences indicated that postmenopausal women who consume moderate quantities of prunes (as few as five to six a day) present increased rates of markers of bone formation. If the beneficial results continue, dried plums may have the potential to produce clinically significant increases in bone mass. While this research has focused on the primary risk group for osteoporosis, women, it seems the opposite sex need not feel left out of the prune frenzy. Scientists at the University of Oklahoma believe dried plums may also help prevent skeletal deterioration in men.

Tea

A 2007 study published in the *American Journal of Clinical Nutrition* reported some potentially good news for tea drinkers. Australian researchers surveyed elderly women between the ages of 70 and 85 who were participating in a larger five-year study on osteoporosis about their green and black tea consumption. Bone density measurements were taken at the beginning and end of the five-year study, and the tea drinkers exhibited a higher bone mineral density in their hips and less bone loss than women who didn't drink tea. Interestingly enough, they found no correlation between the number of cups consumed per day and bone density.

The researchers took this as further confirmation of prior studies that have suggested a positive link between tea and osteoporosis prevention. Though they are not yet sure of the mechanism at work, the previous studies suggest that phytochemicals in tea, such as flavonoids, may be responsible for the protective effect against bone loss due to their estrogen-like properties.

HOW MUCH CALCIUM DO I REALLY NEED?

In 2010, the U.S. and Canadian governments requested that the Institute of Medicine (IOM) review the dietary reference intakes for calcium. It resulted in revisions that include some slight increases to the daily recommended dietary allowance (RDA) for certain life stages. The updated recommendations are reflected in the chart below. Note that for infants, an adequate intake (AI) level is given. Based on observed or experimental approximations, AI is used for those early life stages in which an RDA cannot be determined.

LIFE STAGE	CALCIUM RDA
0–6 months	200 mg (AI)
6–12 months	260 mg (AI)
1–3 years	700 mg
4–8 years	1,000 mg
9–18 years	1,300 mg
19–50 years	1,000 mg
Women 51+ years	1,200 mg
Men 51–70 years	1,000 mg
Men 71+ years	1,200 mg
Pregnant and lactating women 14–18 years	1,300 mg
Pregnant and lactating women 19–50 years	1,000 mg

Although some people may view these as an absolute minimum intake and be tempted to adopt a "more is better" approach, the IOM warns against this. Higher intake levels of calcium "have not been shown to confer greater benefits, and in fact, they have been linked to other health problems."

The IOM also provided tolerable upper levels (UL) that represent the safe limit for daily calcium consumption (as high as 3,000 milligrams for certain life stages; a UL could not be established for infants), but this isn't a number to strive for. On the contrary, the IOM determined that the "risk for harm" increases when calcium intake surpasses just 2,000 milligrams per day for healthy individuals. This may sound like an unrealistically high number, particularly in a diet void of dairy milk, but supplements and calcium-fortified foods make it quite easy to exceed.

It should also be noted that the RDA is set high enough to cover an adequate amount for almost all healthy people in the noted life stages, but many individuals might require less. Moreover, some medical experts think that these calcium consumption recommendations are in fact excessive. They are more concerned with nutrient balance and preventing calcium loss, and cite the bone health of other nations as examples.

In countries such as Japan, India, and Peru, the average daily calcium intake is as low as 300 milligrams per day (less than one-third of the U.S. recommendation for adults age 19 to 50), yet their incidence of bone fracture is quite low in comparison to that of the United States.

In another interesting comparison, the average daily calcium intake for African Americans is more than 1,000 milligrams, while it is only 196 milligrams for black South Africans. Oddly enough, the hip fracture rate for African Americans is nine times greater than the hip fracture rate for black South Africans.

Some speculate that the lower rates of fracture may be due in part to an increased level of vitamin D. It seems that excess calcium has a tendency to suppress circulating vitamin D. Others believe it may be a mix of cultural and dietary habits.

Calcium is essential for bone health, but what levels of calcium intake are optimal is still on trial in the scientific community. While the jury is out, you may wish to weigh your options in the next two sections on calcium-containing dietary choices and supplementation.

CALCIUM-RICH FOODS

Calcium is naturally abundant in a wide variety of foods, including most vegetables, fruits, and nuts. And many greens, such as broccoli, bok choy, and kale, have calcium absorption rates of 50 to 70 percent, much higher than the 32 percent calcium absorption rate of milk. As a quick guide, the following charts list the amount of calcium in numerous healthy, dairy-free foods.

Dairy-Free Calcium Charts

I've updated these charts with several calcium-rich foods that have become more readily available since the first edition of this book, and have also modified the serving sizes and corresponding calcium levels for several of the foods to better reflect reasonable consumption in one sitting or throughout the day.

As it so happens, all of the foods listed here are gluten free, and most are vegan. I've broken out a chart at the end for non-vegans, with eggs and seafood.

SOY FOODS	SERVING SIZE	CALCIUM (MG)
Edamame (cooked)	½ cup	49
Natto	1 cup	380
Soybeans (steamed or boiled)	1 cup	175
Soybeans (roasted)	1 cup	237
Soy Flour, Defatted	1 cup	253
Soymilk	1 cup	61
Soymilk, Calcium-Fortified	1 cup	340*
Tempeh	1 cup	184*
Tofu, Firm, Set with Calcium	½ cup	253*
Tofu, Raw, Firm, Set with Calcium	½ cup	861

NUTS & SEEDS	SERVING SIZE	CALCIUM (MG)
Almonds	¼ cup	96
Almond Butter	1 tablespoon	56
Brazil Nuts	¼ cup	53
Chia Seeds	1 ounce	179
Hazelnuts	¼ cup	32
Pistachios	¼ cup	32
Poppy Seeds	1 tablespoon	127
Sesame Seeds (hulled)	¼ cup	42
Tahini	1 tablespoon	64

VEGETABLES	SERVING SIZE	CALCIUM (MG)
Acorn Squash (cooked)	1 cup	90
Amaranth Leaves	1 cup	60
Artichoke, Globe	1 medium	56
Arugula	1 cup	32
Asparagus (cooked)	1 cup	36
Bok Choy (cooked)	1 cup	158
Borage	1 cup	83
Broccoli	1 cup	43
Broccoli Rabe	1 cup	43
Brussels Sprouts	1 cup	37
Burdock Root	1 cup	48
Butternut Squash (cooked)	1 cup	84
Cabbage, Chinese (Pak Choi)	1 cup (shredded)	74
Cabbage, Green	1 cup	36
Cabbage, Red	1 cup	40
Carrots	1 medium	20
Cassava	1 cup	33
Cauliflower	1 cup	24
Celeriac	1 cup	67
Celery	1 cup (chopped)	44
Chicory Greens	1 cup	29

VEGETABLES	SERVING SIZE	CALCIUM (MG)
Chinese Broccoli (cooked)	1 cup	88
Collard Greens	1 cup	84
Dandelion Greens	1 cup	103
French Beans (Haricots Verts) (cooked)	1 cup	111
Garlic	1 tablespoon	15
Grape Leaves	1 cup	51
Green Beans (cooked)	1 cup	58
Hearts of Palm (canned)	1 cup	85
Kale	1 cup	101
Kohlrabi	1 cup	32
Lamb's-Quarters (cooked)	½ cup	232
Leeks	1 medium	53
Mustard Greens	1 cup	64
Nopales (Cactus)	1 cup (sliced)	141
Okra	1 cup	82
Onion, Spring	1 medium	11
Parsley	1 cup	83
Parsnips	1 medium	59
Peas, Edible Pod (cooked)	1 cup	62
Pumpkin, Canned	1 cup	64
Radishes	1 cup (sliced)	29
Rutabaga	1 cup	60
Seaweed, Agar (dried)	½ ounce	87
Seaweed, Arame (dried)	½ cup	100**
Seaweed, Kelp	1 cup	137
Seaweed, Kelp Noodles	4 ounces	150**
Seaweed, Kombu (dried)	½ ounce	93
Seaweed, Wakame (dried)	½ cup	80**
Sweet Potato (cooked)	1 cup (cubed)	76
Tomatoes (canned)	½ cup	40
Turnips	1 cup (cubed)	39
Turnip Greens	1 cup	104
Watercress	1 cup	41

GRAINS	SERVING SIZE	CALCIUM (MG)
Amaranth (cooked)	1 cup	116
Amaranth Flour	¼ cup	40
Carob Flour	1 tablespoon	21
Corn Tortillas	2 small	100*
Oats	1 cup	84
Oatmeal (cooked)	1 cup	187
Potato Flour	¼ cup	26
Quinoa (cooked)	1 cup	31
Teff (cooked)	1 cup	123

FRUIT & JUICE	SERVING SIZE	CALCIUM (MG)
Blackberries	1 cup	42
Coconut Water	1 cup	58
Currants (dried)	¼ cup	31
Figs (dried)	1 cup	241
Goji Berries	¼ cup	41
Mulberries	1 cup	55
Orange	1 medium	56
Orange Juice, Calcium-Fortified	1 cup	300*
Papaya	1 medium	72
Prunes (dried)	1 cup	95
Raisins, Golden	⅔ cup	52

BEANS	SERVING SIZE	CALCIUM (MG)
Baked Beans (canned)	1 cup	126*
Black-Eyed Peas (Cowpeas) (cooked)	½ cup	105
Black Turtle Beans (cooked)	1 cup	102
Great Northern Beans (canned)	1 cup	139
Lima Beans (canned)	½ cup	35
Mung Beans (cooked)	1 cup	55
Navy Beans (canned)	1 cup	123

BEANS	SERVING SIZE	CALCIUM (MG)
Pinto Beans (canned)	1 cup	108
Refried Beans (cooked)	1 cup	88*
Snap Beans (cooked)	½ cup	32
White Beans (canned)	1 cup	191
Winged Beans (cooked)	1 cup	244
Yellow Beans (cooked)	1 cup	110

HERBS & SPICES	SERVING SIZE	CALCIUM (MG)
Allspice (ground)	1 teaspoon	13
Anise Seeds	1 teaspoon	14
Basil (dried)	1 teaspoon	16
Caraway Seeds	1 teaspoon	14
Celery Seeds	1 teaspoon	35
Cinnamon (ground)	1 teaspoon	26
Cloves (ground)	1 teaspoon	13
Coriander Seeds	1 teaspoon	13
Cumin Seeds	1 teaspoon	20
Dill Seeds	1 teaspoon	32
Dill Weed (dried)	1 teaspoon	18
Fennel Seeds	1 teaspoon	24
Marjoram (dried)	1 teaspoon	12
Mustard Seeds	1 teaspoon	19
Oregano (dried)	1 teaspoon	16
Poppy Seeds	1 teaspoon	40
Rosemary (dried)	1 teaspoon	15
Savory (dried)	1 teaspoon	30
Thyme (dried)	1 teaspoon	19

SWEETENERS	SERVING SIZE	CALCIUM (MG)
Maple Syrup	1 tablespoon	21
Molasses, Blackstrap	1 tablespoon	172*
Molasses, Light	1 tablespoon	33
Molasses, Medium	1 tablespoon	58

NON-VEGAN	SERVING SIZE	CALCIUM (MG)
Anchovies, Boneless (canned)	3 ounces	198
Blue Crab (canned)	3 ounces	86
Clams (cooked)	3 ounces	78
Cuttlefish (cooked)	3 ounces	153
Egg Yolk	1 large	22
Herring, Atlantic (cooked)	1 fillet	106
Herring, Pacific (cooked)	1 fillet	153
Mackerel, Boneless Jack (canned)	3 ounces	204
Ocean Perch, Atlantic (cooked)	3 ounces	116
Octopus (cooked)	3 ounces	90
Oyster, Dried	3 medium	45
Pike, Walleye (cooked)	1 fillet	175
Rainbow Trout, Wild (cooked)	1 fillet	123
Salmon, Chum with Bones (canned)	3 ounces	212
Salmon, Pink with Bones (canned)	3 ounces	241
Salmon, Sockeye with Bones (canned)	3 ounces	203
Sardines (canned)	3 ounces	317
Shrimp (fresh, cooked)	3 ounces	77
Shrimp (small, dried)	1 ounce	167

* Calcium content may vary by brand. For example, I have seen levels as high as 150 milligrams of calcium per corn tortilla and as low as 20 milligrams per tortilla.

** I had difficulty locating adequate numbers for these from the USDA, so brand packaging was used to ascertain.

A FEW NOTES ON THESE CALCIUM CHARTS:

- These numbers are intended for use as general information only. Actual calcium levels may vary.
- For comparison, 1 cup of 2 percent cow's milk has 297 milligrams of calcium.
- Most fruits, vegetables, seeds, and nuts contain some amount of calcium, but the above selections are limited to class leaders in each category.

- Spinach, rhubarb, beet greens, and Swiss chard are all very high in calcium. However, due to their very low absorption rates (approximately 5 percent), they have been excluded from the charts.

- With the exception of mung beans, dried beans do have a fairly low absorption rate (approximately 17 percent), so only those with over 100 milligrams of calcium have been included.

Homemade Broth/Stock

One more calcium-rich food worth mentioning is homemade broth that is prepared using beef or chicken bones. Since results can vary significantly, there is no hard and fast calculation for how much calcium is in a batch of homemade bone broth. Some speculate that it is as high as dairy milk, while new packaged brands show little mineral content. To help facilitate mineral extraction from the bones in your homemade broth, paleo experts suggest adding a little vinegar to the cooking water (1 tablespoon for every 8 cups of water should suffice).

It's in the Water

Depending on where you live, you may be getting quite a bit of calcium via your tap water. England, the prairies of Canada, some parts of Australia, and most of the United States (with the exceptions of New England, the South Atlantic Gulf, the Pacific Northwest, and Hawaii) have tap water that is quite high in minerals such as calcium, otherwise known as "hard water." It is important to know if you are already obtaining quite a bit of calcium from your drinking and cooking water, as too much of the mineral can have health drawbacks (see "How Much Calcium Do I Really Need?" on page 49).

How to Become Calcium Fortified

Still concerned? Have no fear . . . the food manufacturers are listening. They have been stocking grocery store shelves with calcium-fortified versions of your old favorites. So much so that doctors are now waving the red flag for calcium toxicity! These days you may find a good dose of calcium hiding in popular brands of frozen waffles, energy bars, dairy-free yogurts, "healthy" pastries, granola, cereal, beverages, crackers, and other snack foods.

If you choose to reach for calcium-fortified foods, stick to the healthier options. An 8-ounce glass of calcium-fortified orange juice or unsweetened fortified dairy-free milk beverage (almond, soy, coconut, rice, etc.) can supply you with roughly the same amount of calcium found in an 8-ounce glass of skim milk. As an added bonus, orange juice is typically fortified with calcium citrate, the most usable source of calcium.

Use caution if choosing ready-made hot and cold breakfast cereals as a calcium source, as some may be too heavily fortified. One name-brand cereal was packing each serving with 1,000 milligrams of calcium, which many doctors consider excessive for one meal.

What About Oxalates?

You may have wondered why health superstars like rhubarb and Swiss chard have such low calcium absorption rates. It's due to their higher oxalate content, which scientists believe reduces the bioavailability of calcium in certain plant foods. In beans, phytates are thought to be the calcium-reducing culprit. However, one notable exception is soybeans. Soy products are naturally high in both oxalates and phytates, yet they appear to have relatively high calcium bioavailability.

Though oxalates and phytates can reduce the available calcium in a food, they typically leave some behind for our use, and do not go out of their way to leach calcium from our bodies. Therefore, high-oxalate foods can be healthy additions to your diet, but aside from soy, they may not be great contributors to your personal calcium requirements.

CHOOSING THE BEST CALCIUM SUPPLEMENT

Although a well-balanced diet is believed to be the best way to consume vitamins and minerals, some people prefer to take out an "insurance policy" or two in the form of supplements. And one thing is for sure: there is no shortage of calcium supplements on the market. Here are some helpful consumer hints to narrow down your selections.

Understanding Elemental Calcium

Several different calcium compounds are utilized in supplements. The elemental calcium represents the actual amount or percentage of calcium in the compound. It is important that you read the labels of calcium supplements to verify the amount of elemental calcium available. On the nutrition/supplement facts, a percent of daily value is listed. This is based on a recommended daily value of 1,000 milligrams for calcium, so a supplement with a 25 percent daily value for calcium has 250 milligrams of elemental calcium. Also, be sure to note the serving size, or the number of tablets, pills, etc., you must take in order to obtain that level of elemental calcium.

Types of Calcium Supplements

It's usually best to ignore the sales pitches and consumer hype when purchasing calcium supplements. The cheapest, most basic brands of calcium carbonate or calcium citrate will typically do the trick:

Calcium carbonate is the most inexpensive and readily available option. It contains the highest level of elemental calcium (40 percent), so fewer pills may be required in order to reach your desired daily intake. However, a big pill typically accompanies this big amount of calcium. A chewable or liquid version may be preferred for those who find the tablets too large to swallow. Calcium carbonate should be taken with meals or with an acidic beverage such as orange juice since it is alkaline based and therefore requires extra stomach acid for maximum absorption. For some, intestinal distress in the form of gas or constipation is a possibility. If this happens to you, try upping your dietary fiber intake, and drink more water. If that doesn't help, switch to calcium citrate.

Calcium citrate usually costs a little more than calcium carbonate, and is not quite as easy to find, but overall it is an excellent option. Calcium citrate has less elemental calcium (21 percent), but it is better absorbed than calcium carbonate. It is acidic based and may be taken at any time in the day, even on an empty stomach. If you are taking acid blockers for indigestion, acid reflux, or other intestinal conditions, calcium citrate may be your best option from an absorption point of view.

Calcium phosphate is rarely recommended. Although some types of calcium phosphate contain high levels of elemental calcium, the average diet already contains too much phosphorus from processed foods.

Calcium lactate and calcium gluconate supplements are usually well absorbed, but they have a very low level of elemental calcium (13 percent and 9 percent, respectively). Calcium lactate is derived from lactic acid, but it isn't typically a problem for those with milk allergies or lactose intolerance (see page 27).

Coral and chelated calcium options are frequently overpriced and overhyped supplements. They supply no known advantages over any of the calcium compounds noted above. It is best to avoid supplements that contain dolomite, bone meal, or oyster shell, as these products may be contaminated with lead, mercury, and/or arsenic.

Most calcium supplements are dairy free because calcium is a mineral, not a dairy product or extract. However, some supplements do have lactose or other forms of dairy added, so be sure to read the label.

Isn't This Stuff Regulated?

Although the FDA does not currently regulate calcium supplements, you can check the label for the initials USP. This is a guarantee that the product meets with the U.S. Pharmacopeia's voluntary standards for quality, purity (lead content), and tablet disintegration.

Since the USP system is completely voluntary, it does omit some top brands. Sign up with Consumer Lab (**ConsumerLab.com**) for a broader selection of reputable vitamins and minerals. They test, and report on, various brands and types of supplements, utilizing the same basic markers as the USP.

Absorption Insurance

In reality, the body will easily absorb most brands of calcium products. However, if in doubt, check for the USP symbol, select an approved product from Consumer Lab, or try a simple at-home test. Place one tablet in a glass of warm water or clear vinegar. Stir occasionally. If the tablet dissolves within 30 minutes, then the supplement will most likely dissolve in your stomach as well. Chewable and liquid calcium supplements are a good alternative to ensure proper absorption. As a general rule of thumb, calcium from diet or supplements is best absorbed when consumed throughout the day, in increments of less than 500 milligrams.

Other Bone Builders to Consider

Adding to the confusion, calcium supplements can be found in varying combinations, often paired with other vitamins and minerals. Two of the most common calcium buddies you will find are magnesium and vitamin D—and for good reason.

Approximately half of the magnesium in our bodies is located in our bones, making it another important piece in the bone health puzzle. Many doctors argue that most healthy individuals do not need magnesium supplements, since magnesium is abundant in leafy greens, nuts, peas, beans, and whole grains. So those who consume a varied, well-balanced, whole food–oriented diet should be well covered. However, other medical professionals argue that magnesium is deficient in most modern diets due to high fat consumption, the tendency to cook vegetables, depleted minerals in the soil, and excessive use of medications that can block the absorption of magnesium.

Calcium and magnesium are synergistic, so if you do choose to supplement with magnesium, a combination of calcium and magnesium may simplify things. Those who believe they may have a magnesium deficiency due to illness should consult a physician.

Vitamin D is essential for promoting calcium absorption in the gut and maintaining adequate concentrations of calcium in the blood. It is also required for bone growth and remodeling. Most doctors seem to agree that sunscreen, age, and increasing indoor activities are depleting the levels of vitamin D we as humans are producing. This is prompting both Eastern and Western medical professionals to unite in the recommendation of vitamin D supplementation.

You may opt to take calcium supplements that contain vitamin D, which is great, but not an absolute must. Although vitamin D enhances calcium absorption, it is taken in and stored in a unique way and at a different rate than calcium. Therefore, it can be taken separately from calcium.

Will a Multivitamin Cover My Calcium Needs?

The multivitamin has become a convenient, one-stop vitamin and mineral insurance policy for today's hectic lifestyles. But not all multivitamins are created equal. Quality and dosages can vary greatly. Be sure to select a product verified by the USP or Consumer Lab and discuss the topic of a multivitamin with your physician.

Precautions

Always check with your doctor or pharmacist before adding calcium or any other vitamins or supplements into the mix. This is particularly important if you are taking any prescription or over-the-counter medications. Calcium has been shown to interfere with the absorption of iron supplements, Synthroid for hypothyroidism, bisphosphonate medication (such as Fosamax or Didrocal) for osteoporosis, and certain antibiotics such as tetracycline. A window of 2 hours or more between the medication and calcium supplementation is often recommended to prevent an interaction.

Also, if you choose to supplement, be careful not to go overboard. See the preceding section on "How Much Calcium Do I Really Need?" (page 49) for the current calcium recommendations and concerns.

CHAPTER 4
INFANT & CHILDHOOD MILK ALLERGIES

If a food allergy or intolerance is suspected in an infant, then the infant should be placed under close pediatric supervision. The following is merely baseline information for parents and parents-to-be. Always consult a physician before making any changes to a child's diet.

RECOGNIZING INFANT MILK ALLERGIES

According to the World Health Organization, based on studies from five European countries, the prevalence of infant cow's milk allergy is approximately 2 to 5 percent. This equates to as many as 1 in 20 babies who may suffer digestive, respiratory, and/or skin problems with dairy consumption. Unfortunately, milk allergy is often very difficult to recognize at such an early age, since infants are unable to put their discomfort into words. The following is a list of symptoms that may signal a potential milk allergy, and should be discussed with your pediatrician:

DIARRHEA: Diarrhea is a common occurrence in babies, but if it persists several times a day for more than a week, it could signal a milk allergy.

VOMITING: Babies often spit up bits of food, but a doctor should examine vomiting beyond the typical mealtime regurgitation. Reflux symptoms, such as excessive spit-up and difficulty swallowing, can also be symptoms of concern.

SKIN RASHES: There are many causes of red rashes, eczema, and hives, but any of these may signal an underlying milk allergy.

EXTREME FUSSINESS: Every baby cries, but crying continuously and inconsolably for long periods of time is abnormal. When there is no apparent reason, this is usually called colic. Sometimes this extreme fussiness is actually caused by the gastrointestinal pain resulting from an allergy to the proteins found in milk.

RESPIRATORY PROBLEMS: Colds are common for infants, but wheezing, struggling to breathe, and developing excess mucus in the nose and throat is not. In some instances, these respiratory problems could be the baby's reaction to the proteins found in milk.

FAILURE TO THRIVE: Babies with milk allergies often suffer from a lack of proper nutrition characterized by dehydration, loss of appetite, low weight gain, and lack of energy.

RECURRENT EAR INFECTIONS: It has been estimated that up to 79 percent of children with recurrent ear infections get them because of allergies. Signs of an ear infection may include a runny or stuffy nose, cough, fever, and/or irritability.

A few little-known facts are important to understand when dealing with a food allergic child:

FOOD ALLERGY SYMPTOMS VARY IN SEVERITY. Some children may experience dramatic respiratory symptoms, while others may develop a simple rash.

RAPID-ONSET SYMPTOMS SHOULD RECEIVE PROMPT MEDICAL ATTENTION. With an IgE-mediated milk allergy, an infant may experience allergic symptoms immediately upon feeding. These sudden symptoms can include irritability, vomiting, wheezing, swelling, hives, itchy bumps on the skin, and bloody diarrhea. In rare cases, potentially life-threatening anaphylaxis can occur and affect the baby's skin, stomach, breathing, and blood pressure.

FOOD ALLERGY SYMPTOMS MAY BE DELAYED. As discussed in chapter 2, symptoms of cell-mediated allergic reactions are typically delayed by at least a few hours. This can make diagnosis very difficult, and may require you to keep a journal of your baby's feeding schedule, your own diet (if you are breastfeeding), and when the symptoms occur. Delayed reactions may include loose stools (possibly containing blood), vomiting, gagging, refusing food, irritability or colic, and skin rashes.

THERE COULD BE MULTIPLE ALLERGENS. A child who is allergic to milk has a greater chance of being allergic to other foods, too. If a milk allergy has been confirmed but symptoms persist upon removal, consider having your child tested for other food allergies.

FOOD ALLERGIES SHOULD NOT INTERFERE WITH A CHILD'S DEVELOPMENT. Aside from mother's milk during infancy, there is no single food that is considered the Holy Grail for development. Children who are allergic to one food can certainly get the same nutrition from many other foods. However, if you continue to feed them a food that they are allergic to, it may hinder nutrient absorption, and consequently encourage a failure to thrive.

ALLERGY SYMPTOMS CAN CHANGE WITH AGE. Many children do "outgrow" milk allergies. However, when a food allergy or some level of sensitivity persists, it is very possible for the symptoms to alter over time. A skin rash may morph into wheezing later in life, for example.

FEEDING OPTIONS

When a milk allergy or intolerance is suspected or confirmed, it is essential to consult with a physician for feeding recommendations and to monitor your child's condition. The following is a list of the options that may be useful to know about when speaking with your pediatrician.

Breastfeeding

The primary benefit of breast milk is nutrition. Human milk contains just the right amount of fatty acids, lactose, water, and amino acids for human digestion, brain development, and growth. It also contains at least 100 beneficial ingredients not typically found in formula.

Breastfed babies tend to have fewer illnesses because human milk transfers a mother's antibodies for disease to the infant. About 80 percent of the cells in breast milk are macrophages, cells that kill bacteria, fungi, and viruses. Breastfed babies are protected, in varying degrees, from a number of illnesses, including pneumonia, botulism, bronchitis, staphylococcal infections, influenza, ear infections, and rubella (German measles). Mothers also produce antibodies to whatever disease is present in their environment, making their milk custom-designed to fight the diseases their babies are also exposed to. Furthermore, a breastfed baby's digestive tract contains large amounts of *Lactobacillus bifidus*, beneficial bacteria that prevent the growth of harmful organisms.

Babies are not allergic to their mother's milk, although they may have a reaction to something their mother eats. Babies with allergies or sensitivities may react adversely to proteins within these foods, as they find their way into the breast milk. In cases of milk-allergic infants, nursing mothers would most likely be advised to follow a dairy-free diet. A lactose-free diet would not be sufficient since it is the proteins in milk, not the lactose, that instigate allergic reactions.

In rare conditions, such as congenital lactose intolerance (page 29) or galactosemia (page 33), infants may be intolerant of their mother's milk. In these instances, a special formula and a strict lactose-free diet for the infant would be prescribed immediately. Unfortunately, it wouldn't matter if the nursing mother followed a lactose-free diet herself, as the infant would react to the lactose naturally occurring in her own breast milk.

Infant Formulas

Formulas available in the United States are approved by the FDA and have been created through a very specialized process that cannot be duplicated at home. Regular, commercially available soymilk, goat's milk, rice milk, and almond milk are not considered safe alternatives for infant formula. Here are a few types of infant formula to discuss with your pediatrician:

SOY PROTEIN-BASED FORMULA: Soy formulas are readily available; however, many doctors have differing opinions as to whether these are the best option. Some babies who are allergic to cow's milk also have a sensitivity or an allergy to soy. Do not confuse soy infant formula with soymilk; soymilk is not suitable for infants.

HYDROLYZED FORMULA: Hydrolyzed formulas are made from cow's milk, but the proteins have been broken down or "predigested" to be less allergenic. Partially hydrolyzed formulas have been shown to be of little to no benefit against milk allergies and related symptoms. Extensively hydrolyzed formulas may provide allergy symptom relief, and are frequently recommended by doctors as a first trial.

AMINO ACID-BASED FORMULA: Not all infants with cow's milk allergies respond to hydrolyzed formulas. For these babies, amino acid–based, or elemental, formula is often the next option. It contains protein in its simplest form (amino acids are the building blocks of proteins). Though it is derived from cow's milk, amino acid–based formulas have a high rate of success among dairy-allergic infants. However, this type of formula is extremely expensive and not always covered by health insurance.

LACTOSE-FREE FORMULA: In rare instances, babies may be born with congenital lactose intolerance (page 29). In this case, a lactose-free formula may be essential. Also, secondary lactose intolerance (page 28) can occur in babies suffering from acute diarrhea. In this case, a pediatrician may recommend the temporary use of a soy or lactose-free formula.

Once you switch your baby to another formula, the milk allergy symptoms should go away in two to four weeks if the new formula is successful.

Toddler Transition

After your child's first year, your pediatrician may have some other options to recommend:

MILK INTRODUCTION: Even in children who have been milk allergic, doctors may recommend the gradual introduction of cow's milk after one year of age. Some may have outgrown their allergy by this time, while others may not. Reintroduction of cow's milk should always be done under the strict supervision of a doctor. It is up to the parents and their pediatrician to decide the diet that their child should follow.

KID'S FORMULAS: Otherwise known as "nutritional drinks," these products are often dairy based, but rice-, oat-, and soy-based options have emerged for children from the age of thirteen months to five years. Some are ready-to-drink, but others are drink mixes that can be whisked into water or nondairy "milks" for a tasty toddler beverage with essential vitamins and minerals.

WATER OR MILK BEVERAGES: If your pediatrician feels your child will receive adequate nutrition through diet, then the pediatrician may simply recommend good hydration or perhaps a milk beverage fortified with certain vitamins and minerals. There are also milk beverages available with protein added to mimic the nutrient balance of milk.

Solid Foods

When you should introduce solids to your child, and what types of foods they should be, is up to the current medical guidelines, your pediatrician, and you. The following list includes suggestions to help spark some dairy-free ideas beyond baby food purees that may work for your infant or toddler.

FRESH, RIPE, PEELED, AND CUBED FRUITS: bananas, avocados, tomatoes, peaches, nectarines, melon, kiwi, mango, papaya, and pears

PEELED, SOFT-COOKED, AND CUBED OR MASHED STARCHY VEGETABLES: sweet potatoes, white potatoes, butternut squash, parsnips, and pumpkin

WELL-COOKED OR CANNED VEGETABLES: green peas, cut carrots, green beans, and broccoli florets

SOFT-COOKED GRAINS: oatmeal, baby cereals (rice, quinoa, etc.), rice, millet, teff, and pasta (various types, broken into bits)

COOKED PROTEINS: tofu cubes, ground beef or turkey, finely shredded chicken, cooked low-mercury fish chunks (deboned), beans and lentils (soft-cooked and whole or mashed), hard-boiled egg pieces, and scrambled eggs (cooked with water)

TEETHERS (most teething biscuits contain dairy): frozen cucumber or carrot strips; frozen dairy-free bagel pieces; and frozen bananas, strawberries, or grapes in a mesh feeder (to prevent choking)

CONVENIENT FOODS (dairy-free varieties only): freeze-dried fruit (the type that dissolves; not dried fruit); "O" cereals; graham, oyster, or soda crackers; yogurt alternative; soft bread or bagels, cubed; soft tortilla pieces; fruit and veggie squeeze packs; and cheese alternative shreds

For specific brand suggestions of pre-packaged, dairy-free infant and toddler foods, visit the following page on my website: **GoDairyFree.org/solid-foods**.

Easy Toddler Recipes

Many parents simply share bites of their own food with infants and toddlers who are making the solid food transition, but here are a few fast and easy dairy-free foods you can make specifically for your little one:

Banana Pancakes

Puree 1 ripe banana and 2 large eggs in a blender until smooth. Add a little of your preferred cooking oil to a skillet over medium heat. Pour a small amount of batter in, to create the size you want, and cook for 2 minutes, or until the edges look cooked. Flip and cook for another minute, or until both sides of the pancakes are golden. For an egg-free version, puree ½ cup oats, ½ cup dairy-free milk beverage, ½ ripe banana, and ½ teaspoon baking powder and cook as directed above.

Pumpkin Blender Muffins (by Emily Vallozzi)

Preheat your oven to 375°F. Puree ¾ cup canned pumpkin puree, ½ cup rolled oats, ¼ cup mashed banana, 1 large egg, 1 teaspoon ground cinnamon (optional), and ½ teaspoon baking soda in a blender until very smooth. Pour the batter into mini muffin tins and bake for 18 to 20 minutes. These also freeze very well. For an egg-free version, use 1 powdered egg replacer.

Frozen Yogurt Melts

Fill a small plastic bag with your dairy-free yogurt of choice. Snip off a small piece of a bottom corner and squeeze drops of yogurt onto a silicone baking mat or parchment paper. Transfer to the freezer and freeze until solid. Serve frozen and store leftover drops in an airtight container in the freezer.

Chicken "Noodle" Soup (by Emily Vallozzi)

Put 4 cups low-sodium chicken broth or stock in a large pot over medium heat. Add 1 or 2 carrots (peeled and shredded with a box grater), 1 celery rib (grated), 2 tablespoons frozen chopped spinach (thawed), and a pinch dried basil or oregano. Cook until the vegetables are soft. Shred or finely chop 1 small cooked chicken breast and add it to the pot with a few tablespoons of cooked pasta (such as pastina or acini di pepe) or quinoa. Pour leftovers into ice cube trays and freeze. Transfer the cubes to a plastic freezer bag. Thaw as many as you need in the refrigerator or microwave to serve.

Mama's Beef Stew (by Emily Vallozzi)

Put 4 cups low-sodium beef broth or stock in a large pot over medium heat. Add 1 or 2 carrots (peeled and shredded with a box grater), 1 celery rib (grated), 1 small potato or sweet potato (grated), and a pinch dried thyme or oregano. Cook until the vegetables are soft. Add about 2 tablespoons cooked ground beef. Pour leftovers into ice cube trays and freeze. Transfer the cubes to a plastic freezer bag. Thaw as many as you need in the refrigerator or microwave to serve.

Lentils and Brown Rice

Put 2 cups water (or a combination of water and low-sodium chicken or beef broth or stock), ½ cup dried red lentils, ½ cup uncooked brown rice, and ½ cup diced carrots in a medium saucepan. Stir and bring the soup to a boil over medium-high heat. Reduce the heat to a simmer, cover, and cook for about 20 minutes (add more liquid if needed), until the water is absorbed and all ingredients are soft.

Apple Pie Smoothies

Puree 1 cup ice, ½ cup dairy-free milk beverage, ½ cup unsweetened applesauce, ¼ cup apple juice, ¼ cup dairy-free yogurt (or ripe avocado), and ½ teaspoon ground cinnamon in a blender until smooth. For some sneaky greens, try the WILD BLUE SMOOTHIE on page 209.

Easy Teething Biscuits

Preheat your oven to 250°F. Cut the crusts from several slices of wholesome, dairy-free bread, and then cut each slice into thirds to make long pieces. Place the bread pieces on a baking sheet and bake for 1 hour. Let cool and harden further at room temperature. Leftover biscuits can be frozen.

Childhood Tips

Because milk allergies can persist through the growing years and even into adulthood, I wanted to include some more resources and friendly advice for making things a little easier in your dairy-free household:

DON'T IGNORE HEALTHY FATS. Many parents are concerned that their children may not be getting adequate fat for growth and weight gain in the early years. Soymilk and coconut milk beverage are the richest of the store-bought dairy-free milk alternatives, with fat levels similar to 2 percent milk. However, regular full-fat coconut milk (which can be used for pudding, soup, ice cream, sauces, and more), avocados, and the wide array of nut butters are even richer in plant-based fats. See page 73 for more information on gaining weight.

KEEP SNACKING SIMPLE. It is easier to prevent allergic reactions if the foods consumed contain few ingredients or are whole in nature. Try carrot sticks, celery, whole fruit (bananas, apples, pears, berries, melon, etc.), dried fruit, chunky applesauce, nuts, seeds, trail mix, olives, or popcorn. See the "Snack on This" recipe chapter (page 263) for more recipes and ideas.

GET THEM INVOLVED. Special diets can involve more made-from-scratch foods. Let children help with baking cookies, preparing snacks, measuring ingredients, and reading recipes. Not only will it be an excellent bonding experience, but it will also help them better understand and cope with their diet in the future. Plus, you will have better odds of getting your little ones to eat some broccoli if they were the ones to stir those steamed florets into the pasta salad! Visit **GoDairyFree.org/kids-can-cook** for family-friendly recipes and ideas.

ASK FOR HELP. Dealing with food allergies is no time to be shy. Ask questions, make requests, and, in return, help inform others. When you come across people or companies that are resistant or unhelpful, consider it a red flag warning that their foods may not be the best option anyway. However, you may be surprised by how many "safe" foods you discover, and which companies and restaurants are more than accommodating.

JOIN FORCES. Seek out or start a dairy-free support group in your local area or virtually. Food allergy moms around the world have united via meet-ups and international congregations online to offer one another help ranging from real-world discussions on food allergies in school to recipe exchanges. Facebook groups, Twitter hashtags, and Pinterest boards are great places to find like-minded individuals on the Web. I network and share on all major social networks via @godairyfree, use the hashtag #godairyfree, and have joined many fantastic groups through the interactions.

CHAPTER 5
OTHER DAIRY-FREE CONCERNS

Is a little dairy okay? How will I live without cheese? What if I need to gain weight? What about soy? This chapter addresses some top dairy-free FAQs to help alleviate a few more concerns.

CAN YOU BE ADDICTED TO DAIRY?

Whenever I mention to someone that I don't eat dairy (never even suggesting that they should follow suit), they often interrupt to profess their extreme passion for cheese and proclaim that they could never give it up! You may think this is an exaggeration, but in a study that placed 59 overweight postmenopausal women on a strict vegan diet, the food most missed was not milk, chicken, bacon, or even ice cream, it was cheese. For those of you with an obsession for curdled milk or any other dairy-rich food, I have a few tips that may help on your dairy-free journey.

KEEP AN EYE ON THE PRIZE. Odds are you are venturing into dairy-free territory with a purpose. It could be for weight loss, food allergies, social reasons, or general health. Every time cravings strike, make a conscious effort to remind yourself of that goal. Will dairy cause distress to the little one you are nursing? Will it cause your own allergies to flare? Will it threaten to derail your dieting efforts? Will it promote embarrassing GI troubles? Will it sap your energy or up your risk for certain diseases of concern? Does it conflict with your animal rights beliefs? Enough of these reminders will keep you motivated on your path and may even help those once sought-after foods seem rather unappealing.

LOOK FOR REPLACEMENTS BEFORE TAKING THE PLUNGE . . . Although there are no identical substitutes for dairy, there are many alternatives on the market that are pretty good. Delicious nondairy milk beverages and frozen desserts made from almonds, cashews, coconut, soy, rice, hemp seeds, and even grains are all the rage. Admittedly, cheese is the toughest dairy product to find a good substitute for, but the options are growing and improving each year. Test a few brands to find one or two that will suffice, or try a homemade "cheese" recipe (page 195) for a flavor boost.

. . . OR BREAK THE SPELL. Contrary to the above recommendation, you may need to cut ties completely from dairy and alternatives to rid yourself of cravings. For some people, teasing the taste buds with cheese alternatives that aren't quite "there" can actually increase their desire for the real thing. Rather than seeking out Cheddar and Brie substitutes, get cozy with recipes that are naturally cheese free.

CREATE A MENU. All too often I read about people diving headfirst into a new diet, only to find themselves eating apples and energy bars all day. A little forethought goes a long way toward making a successful free-from transition. Take a look at the foods you can eat, plan out two weeks' worth of menus, and make sure your refrigerator and pantry are adequately stocked. If you have some leeway in switching to a dairy-free diet (that is, if you're not dealing with a severe food allergy), you may even want to keep your diet as is for a few days while you take some time to lay a solid foundation of food ideas that you can build upon with time.

As an example, my husband and I decided to try the vegan diet for our health. I was a bit nervous about what we would eat, so I spent a weekend gathering recipe ideas before we took the plunge. With a prepared refrigerator and several meal ideas ready to go, it turned out to be a piece of cake, and my very omnivorous husband loved every entrée. Plus, the planned meals and snacks bought me some time to become comfortable with vegan cooking. I had no trouble coming up with delicious ideas even after my original menus had been exhausted.

Need some planning help? I've created a sample printable menu plan and shopping list for this book at **GoDairyFree.org/gdf-menus**.

CHOOSE YOUR METHOD WISELY. Sometimes weaning yourself off is easier, but other times quitting cold turkey is the only effective method. For me, transitioning to a strictly dairy-free diet happened overnight, and it worked very effectively. My vicious ice cream cravings stopped within three days, as did the food allergy symptoms I was experiencing. Still, sugar withdrawal has been a gradual process. I tried to toss all of the sweet stuff, but even after a completely sugar-free month I was still wrestling with jumbo cookie cravings. With sugar I have found that gradually changing my diet is helping me retrain my taste buds.

KEEP AN EYE OUT FOR SABOTEURS. You might switch to cheeseless pizza and tofu-ricotta lasagna, but if the premade pizza crust or bottled pasta sauce you are using has some sneaky cheese or milk in it, then your cravings may continue. For many people, even small amounts of an offending food can often keep those cravings going in full force. Scrutinize labels, no matter how simple the food.

DON'T ALLOW YOURSELF TO GET OVER-HUNGRY. When following a free-from diet, it is all too easy to find yourself in a ravenous state simply because you couldn't think of anything to eat. Make sure you always have a good supply of snacks on hand to keep hunger at bay while you are trying to figure out your next meal move. Otherwise, you might be more likely to succumb to those dairy cravings.

TURN YOUR ATTENTION AWAY FROM FOOD. Exercise can deter your attention from food, and it can even change which foods you desire. After a good workout, the last thing I crave is heavy foods, such as cheese. Refreshing salads and fruit smoothies make the menu instead. Too tired for fitness? Organize some ignored area of your home, catch up on emails, or relax with a good book. Eat when you are truly hungry, of course, but keep your mind busy so that your stomach is giving the cues.

MAKE YOUR HOUSE A DAIRY-FREE ZONE. It can be hard to cut out cheese, milk, or any other foods when temptation beckons from the other side of the refrigerator door. The support of your family—including sharing your special diet at home—will make the journey much easier. If your housemates are reluctant, remind them that it will help you significantly . . . and they can always sneak away for a slice of cheese pizza.

CHECK YOUR ADDICTION LEVEL. If you are absolutely sure that giving up cheese or other dairy products would be the biggest torture you could imagine, then you may actually have a "food addiction." No, I am not joking. Food addiction has been a heavily researched issue. Strong and consistent cravings for a particular food are not considered healthy, and are often compared to the behavior of drug addiction—but on a much smaller scale, of course.

Addictions to caffeine, sugar, and chocolate have been shown in studies, and now theories are circulating about milk addiction. A 2015 study at the University of Michigan examined food addiction tendencies in over 500 participants. Their goal was to show the addictive behavior stemming from processed foods, but they found that cheese was tops among the "unprocessed" foods for addiction.

Why cheese? Many believe it is due to the high concentration of milk protein in most types of cheeses. When casein, the primary protein in milk, is broken down in the digestive system, it produces casomorphins, otherwise known as opioid peptides. This part is well proven. The controversy comes with respect to what happens next. Some believe that the opiate effect is neutralized, while others state that these peptides can pass to the brain and various other organs to elicit an opiate effect. Some scientists believe that a mother's milk (cows are also mothers when they are producing milk) possesses this opiate effect in order to heighten the mother-baby bond and calm the baby enough to sleep following feeding.

Many people who have felt this strong "addiction" to certain milk products find that they actually have an allergy or a general heightened reaction to casein. Removal of the milk products for a certain length of time (which varies by individual) usually eliminates the cravings altogether, along with the symptoms or side effects, such as migraines and stomach pain. For some people it may be just a couple of weeks before the cravings and symptoms subside, but for others it may take a few months.

Am I suggesting that all cheese lovers are addicts who must give up milk? By all means no. But if you feel it is impossible to take a short break from any particular food, and have symptoms that could be the result of food sensitivities or a vitamin or mineral deficiency, it may be time to do a reality check and have a visit with your physician or dietician.

BEEF CROSS-REACTIVITY

Though meat allergies are relatively uncommon, research has shown that up to 20 percent of children with a milk allergy also have a beef allergy, while most children with a beef allergy (93 percent) are allergic to milk. Additional studies speculate that all red meat, including pork, could have cross-reactivity with milk.

If you do have a milk allergy, you may want to get tested for a beef allergy, and possibly a pork allergy, or discuss a red meat elimination diet with your physician to see if that aids in symptom relief.

MILK ALLERGIES & THE ROTATION DIET

If you do not experience severe allergic reactions to milk, some amount of dairy flexibility may be well tolerated in your diet, if you wish. In this type of situation, doctors often recommend a rotation diet.

Sometimes strict rotation diets are essential for people who have multiple food allergies, but they have been adapted in many ways to suit individual needs. The basic concept involves a four-day rotation cycle with three days on followed by one day off. In other words, keep your diet dairy free for three days, and the fourth day can be more relaxed. It is believed that this cycle allows your body to fully process a food, preventing a buildup of the offender in your body and thus minimizing any negative reactions. Many people rotate foods regularly for basic health, and to keep their diet varied.

Utilizing a dairy rotation diet can be quite simple if you keep your kitchen dairy free. By following a dairy-free diet at home (where it is assumed you do most of your eating and meal prep), you may not need to be as concerned about accidental milk ingredients slipping into your meal when eating away from home. It also allows you to schedule your "on" dairy days more efficiently.

A rotation diet will not work for lactose-intolerant individuals (lactase does not replenish, even on "off" days), but it may allow for better planning with those lactase enzymes.

IS SOY A GOOD OPTION?

Soy foods enjoyed heightened popularity in North America during the early 2000s, due to a rise in awareness of lactose intolerance, allergies, and chronic disease prevention. According to the United Soybean Board's 2006 annual report, 82 percent of Americans viewed soy foods as healthy (up from 67 percent in 1998). However, soy's fame has faded in recent years amid concerns from conflicting health reports and the emergence of other options for dairy alternatives.

I could write an entire book on the controversies of consuming soy; in fact, a few have already been written. However, those titles tend to be a bit sensationalized, while I like to take an objective approach and fully evaluate both sides of the equation. The following includes some of the facts that have helped me address the issue of soy in my own diet.

Scientific interest in soy emerged from observational studies of geographically based populations. Researchers noted that groups who consumed a lot of soy, particularly those in eastern Asia, experienced a significantly lower incidence of breast cancer, prostate cancer, age-related brain diseases, and cardiovascular disease, in addition to fewer bone fractures. The topic became more interesting as the researchers followed the health of Asians who immigrated to areas such as the United States. Those who altered their diets toward Westernized foods experienced an upward shift in disease rates. This indicated a strong tie to environmental and lifestyle influences, rather than ancestry.

Opponents to soy claim that the amount of soy consumed by Asians has been exaggerated. For the most part, this is true, yet the typical Asian diet is still significantly higher in soy than the standard American diet. A 2003 report from the UN Food and Agriculture Organization estimated the per-capita consumption of soy protein per day to be almost nine times higher in Japan than in most European and North American countries. Beyond the statistics, a sociable chat with a current or former resident of Japan, China, or most other East Asian countries will confirm that soy foods have been an integral part of their diet for generations.

Though many medical professionals view it as a very nutritious product, soymilk is relatively new throughout the world. It is now consumed in Asia and has been linked in several studies to reduced prostate cancer risk, but it is not typically considered a traditional food. Traditional soy foods primarily include tofu and fermented soy products, such as miso and tempeh.

It should be noted that the various methods of preparing soy (fermentation, boiling, etc.) for consumption have a dramatic effect on the health properties of the food. In other words, specific reports on health benefits and/or detriments should probably not be blanketed across "soy" as a whole. The portion of the bean that is utilized and the method by which it is prepared will have a dramatic effect on its composition and digestibility.

Much of the positive research to date has focused on dietary soy in the form of whole foods such as tofu and soymilk. The negative findings tend to focus on animal and human intervention studies that used soy concentrates or isolated isoflavones (plant compounds or phytoestrogens), rather than soy as a whole food. This implies that these isolated chemicals, which are sold in over-the-counter pills and powders and are sometimes used as ingredients in food products to increase the protein or isoflavone content, may be beneficial when a component of the whole food but harmful when extracted and consumed in high quantities.

The United States is one of the world's top soybean producers, in select years producing as much as 50 percent of the global soybean crop. This means that soy, like corn, is readily available and relatively inexpensive in the United States. Therefore, it is widely utilized in various forms throughout the processed food industry. In fact, it is believed that over half of all processed foods in the United States contain soy in some form or another. On food labels it may appear as soy flour, soy lecithin, soy protein isolate, hydrolyzed soy protein, protein concentrate, plant sterols, textured vegetable protein (TVP), soybean oil, or simply vegetable oil. With stats like these, it is easy to see how soy may be "overdone" in the United States.

Nonetheless, the research supports soy in moderation as a healthy addition to most diets, and some go so far as to add it to the list of highly respected "superfoods." Here are some soy suggestions that may be useful for nondairy consumers:

- Focus on whole soy foods (e.g., tofu, soymilk, and edamame) for disease prevention, and fermented soy products (e.g., miso, tempeh, and tamari) for digestive health. Try to limit or avoid processed foods with extracted types of soy, such as isolates, concentrates, and oil.

- Prioritize olive, coconut, and avocado oils in your cooking and baking. Grapeseed and rice bran oils can be good options when a neutral flavor is needed.

- Keep your diet well diversified. "Too much of a good thing" applies to just about any type of food, no matter how healthy it may be. Though your doctor may advise 5 to 10 servings of fruits and vegetables per day, it would sound ridiculous and unwise to simply recommend 5 to 10 servings of oranges per day. Soybeans qualify as a single food that can be an excellent contributor to a healthy diet but need not overwhelm it. To keep soy consumption moderate, rotate in a good selection of other foods (such as nuts, coconut, and avocado) when substituting dairy.

- Eat soy foods as a part of a balanced meal or snack, rather than on their own, when possible. The benefits with most foods are best recognized when consumed in combination with a wide variety of nutrients, vitamins, and minerals.

- If you like soymilk, but have trouble finding a pure brand, consider making your own from dried soybeans (page 180). This will ensure a high-quality product, without the additives or isolates that may be found in some commercial brands. You can purchase dried soybeans in bulk to produce quarts of homemade soymilk for pennies.

- Select organic products and/or those made with non-GMO soybeans whenever possible. Most soybeans grown in the United States are genetically modified. Genetically modified foods are still relatively new, so little is known about their safety. Organic soybeans should be non-GMO, and have been grown without the use of toxic pesticides or chemicals.

For most of us, moderation is the key, but soy can pose health problems that may supersede the great debate for some individuals:

Soy Allergies

Soy is one of the top eight allergens in the United States. Though it is not as common of an allergen as cow's milk, many people have found that they are in fact sensitive to soy protein. The only widely accepted treatment for any food allergy at this time is elimination from the diet. However, studies show that most individuals who are allergic to soy protein may be able to safely consume soybean oil (not cold pressed, expeller pressed, or extruded oil) and soy lecithin, as these products rarely contain soy protein. If you suspect a soy allergy, consult a physician.

Hypothyroidism

Evidence shows that excess consumption of the isoflavones found in soy may disrupt thyroid function in *some* individuals who already have a thyroid disorder or who consume insufficient levels of iodine (not a typical deficiency in North America). Fortunately, this does not occur with all hypothyroid individuals, and the studies have focused on high soy isoflavone consumption specifically via supplements and processed foods, not moderate intake of whole soy products. Nonetheless, if you have hypothyroidism, I would discuss the role of soy foods in your diet with your physician.

WHEN GAINING WEIGHT IS A GOOD THING

The topic of weight loss dominates our society, but for millions of people, weight gain is a more pressing issue. When it comes to growing toddlers in need of nutrition, athletes, and anyone who can't afford to shed another pound, too little fat and protein can be a concern with dairy-free diets, especially since Western societies do tend to use consumption of cow's milk products as a shortcut to weight gain. Intended for rapid growth of calves, the milk from dairy cows is rich in fat, protein, and hormones that can easily pack the pounds on our significantly smaller species. In fact, most people do not realize that cow's milk contains three times the protein of human breast milk.

Of course, eggs, fish, and meat can easily fill the fat and protein void, but there are many other options for those who forsake these animal products, whether for religious, social, health, or taste preferences.

Sources of Plant-Based Dietary Fat

Many argue that the fatty acids from plant sources (such as the monounsaturated fat in olive oil and the omega-3s in nuts) are not only less harmful to our bodies than the saturated fat from animal sources but could also be a healthy addition to most diets.

Coconut "Meat" and Milk

Dried coconut "meat" contains 18 grams of fat per ounce, while regular coconut milk (in cans or small packages, not milk beverage) contains 25 grams of fat per ½ cup.

Coconut is quite high in saturated fat; however, some experts maintain that the saturated fat in plants (most foods have some amount of saturated fat, no matter how little) is quite different from the saturated fat found in meat and dairy products. In fact, some even tout the fatty acids in coconut as possessing antiviral, antibacterial, and antifungal health benefits.

Let the truth be told that I am on the pro-coconut side, but partially because I love the stuff. Coconut milk is a fantastic natural stand-in for cream, shredded coconut offers tropical flair to smoothies and baked goods, and coconut oil (fat content discussed next) provides a rich, almost buttery flavor to whatever it touches. For those who have an aversion to coconut, do not immediately shy away from the milk and oil. When used in recipes, the coconut flavor often fades or even vanishes.

Food-Grade Oils

Pretty much all oils possess 14 grams of fat per tablespoon.

Before cooking entered my personal repertoire (beyond the reheat and serve method, that is), I thought oil was oil. I grew up with that big jug of multipurpose vegetable oil, always ready to report for duty. Of course, using any oil will help ensure adequate fat in the diet, but there are many flavorful oils to choose from, and each has a different ratio of fatty acids. A few that I always keep on hand are grapeseed oil or rice bran oil (for neutral flavor in baking and cooking), avocado oil (for rich, savory cooking and chocolate desserts), coconut oil (for spreads, popcorn, and specialty recipes), extra-virgin olive oil (for dressings and drizzling), peanut oil (for stir-fries and Asian dishes), and sesame oil (for drizzling on Asian dishes). See the chapter on butter alternatives (page 143) for more information on the various types of oil available, and how to use them.

Avocados

One medium-size avocado contains approximately 30 grams of fat.

It's a vegetable . . . no, it's a fruit . . . who cares? Avocados are nutritious and delicious, and that is really all that matters to me. They are loaded with monounsaturated fat (the kind that shot olive oil to world-class health fame) and very versatile. Chop up the flesh and enjoy it on salads and in sandwiches, or blend it up to create a creamy base for dips. Avocados can even be snuck into both sweet and savory recipes as a thick cream or binder.

Tree Nuts and Peanuts

Nuts range from 13 grams of fat per ounce (cashews) to 21 grams of fat per ounce (macadamia nuts).

For those who don't have a peanut or tree nut allergy, nuts are excellent options for supplying "healthy" fats. Plus, the flavorful selection is vast, with walnuts, almonds, Brazil nuts, hazelnuts, pecans, pistachios, pine nuts, and more. For snacks, peanuts and tree nuts can be enjoyed on their own or tossed into a homemade trail mix blend. In recipes, add some chopped nuts to baked goods; stir them into rice or other grain dishes; grind them to use as coatings for meat, fish, or vegetables; use them for structure and flavor in veggie burgers; or simply sprinkle them atop a salad. You can also find most nuts in nut butter form, but if not, you can make your own by grinding the nuts in a food processor until a paste forms, adding oil to thin if needed. Yes, it is that easy.

Seeds

Seeds range from 9 grams of fat per ounce (chia seeds) to just over 13 grams of fat per ounce (sunflower seeds).

This often-overlooked food category can jump right into any nut's role. You can choose from sunflower seeds, pumpkin seeds, hemp seeds, chia seeds, flax seeds, and sesame seeds. Sunflower and pumpkin seeds are sizable enough for snacking, but the other varieties are best used in recipes, either whole or ground. Both chia seeds and flax seeds make great egg replacers in baked goods when blended with water (1 tablespoon seeds + 3 tablespoons water = 1 egg replacer). And though slightly harder to find than nut butters, seed butters are gaining in popularity. Sunflower seed butter is becoming a staple at many grocers, and sesame seed butter, otherwise known as tahini, is relatively easy to find due to its important role in hummus. Pumpkin seed butter and hemp seed butter are a bit more elusive, but both can typically be found in natural food stores. Seeds and seed butters may be safe alternatives for some individuals with nut allergies, but use caution as they are often processed on shared lines with peanuts and tree nuts.

Olives

Kalamata olives have about 7 grams of fat per ounce, while black olives are lighter, with about 3 grams of fat per ounce.

Just like its oil, this finger food packs in a good dose of those "healthy" fats. Olives are a fun food for kids, too. Well into adulthood, my grandfather would comment every time I saw him about how when I was very little I used to head straight to the olive appetizer each time we visited, popping an olive onto each fingertip, and enjoying them one by one. Beyond straight snacking, olives add wonderful flavor to savory recipes. I often dice olives (green, black, or kalamata) and use them as a flavorful Parmesan stand-in atop pasta dishes.

Chocolate

Chocolate ranges from 9 grams of fat per ounce (semi-sweet) to 15 grams of fat per ounce (unsweetened).

Last time I checked, chocolate ranked as a health food. (Well, that's my story and I'm sticking to it!) Rich in cocoa butter, good-quality chocolate is an excellent source of fat and indulgence, in my opinion. But do use caution. Many brands of chocolate are made on shared equipment with milk chocolate. For most dairy-free dieters, trace quantities of milk will not be a problem (many companies do a thorough cleaning of equipment between milk and non-milk chocolate batches), but for some who are highly sensitive or allergic, even the minute amount of "parts per million" could spell disaster.

Sources of Plant-Based Protein

Technically, humans have a biological requirement for amino acids, the "building blocks" of protein, rather than protein itself. We are unable to internally produce certain amino acids, known as essential amino acids, so we must obtain them from our diets. How many of these essential amino acids a food contains determines whether it is classified as a complete or an incomplete protein—an important issue when discussing a heavily plant-based diet.

Complete Versus Incomplete Proteins

Meat, fish, eggs, and milk are often referred to as "complete proteins" because they contain all the essential amino acids in sufficient quantities. Plant foods that are frequently labeled as complete proteins include spirulina, quinoa, soy (soymilk, tofu, tempeh, etc.), buckwheat, hemp seed, and amaranth.

Most plant-based foods are considered "incomplete proteins" because they are low in one or more of the essential amino acids. Yet, as one might expect, the incomplete protein sources do add up. A varied diet will allow certain foods to fill in with an essential amino acid that another food may be lacking. And contrary to prior beliefs, these complementary foods need not be eaten together. The various essential amino acids will jump into their role whether or not their companions have yet to arrive. Thus, a food can be a good source of protein even if it is not "complete."

Various grains, legumes, nuts, and several vegetables can provide our bodies with a good dose of incomplete proteins and assist in meeting those essential amino acid requirements. Foods like broccoli, peas, lentils, and beans are relatively high in protein, while most nuts (almonds, walnuts, cashews), seeds (sesame, sunflower), and grains (brown rice, bulgur, wheat bread) contain at least 2 grams of incomplete protein per reasonable serving size.

Protein Powders

The protein powder world was once dominated by dairy, in forms such as whey, but thanks to the sizable vegan and paleo movements, dairy-free options now abound. Soy protein powder is a longtime contender that is readily available, but one need not feel limited to the bean alone.

Brown rice protein is a popular powder that is made by several brands and also used widely in other food products. It can be a bit dry and sandy, which is why I prefer pea protein. Pea protein powder produces thick, very creamy smoothies and is being used increasingly in protein powder blends. Other plant protein powders, which you might see alone or in products, include hemp seed, chia seed, pumpkin seed, sunflower seed, sacha inchi, cranberry, and even protein from greens. The various types are often combined into protein powder blends with a goal to create a complete protein product with all the essential amino acids. For a guide to dairy-free protein powder brands, see GoDairyFree.org/protein-powders.

As noted, protein powders are frequently purchased by food manufacturers to be used as ingredients in their products. Due to an increasing demand for "functional foods," you may find energy bars, cereals, beverages, mixes, and even cookies that are fortified with one of the above-mentioned protein powders or concentrates. However, be vigilant when considering packaged foods that boast a good dose of protein. Though nondairy sources are growing in popularity, many of these products still use milk in some form as the primary protein source.

FINDING SAFE SKINCARE

Lotions, sunscreen, soaps, makeup, and other skincare items frequently contain food-based ingredients, including milk in various forms. Since topical applications of food allergens are of less concern than their ingestion, labeling isn't quite as stringent. Yet some people do have reactions to these products when applied, and others prefer not to support the dairy industry for environmental or social reasons. In the United States, the FDA does require cosmetic manufacturers to list the ingredients on the product label, but "trade secrets" (including certain fragrances) do not have to be specifically listed.

Since it is odd to see skincare products that are labeled as dairy free, I look for those that are touted as vegan. Not only are vegan products made without milk, but they also tend to contain "natural" ingredients that are easier to decode. Otherwise, be prepared to translate the chemically worded ingredient labels into plain English, and contact the manufacturer to verify ingredients and processes. A customer service phone number is typically listed on each package. Even if you feel "safe" with the product, do a mini patch test on your elbow, and wait 24 hours to see if a reaction occurs before liberally applying it.

When considering skincare options, also keep in mind that small amounts of the product could still be incidentally ingested, particularly with lip products or hand lotion, which could pose a risk for those with a severe food allergy.

For a list of some dairy-free skincare products, visit **GoDairyFree.org/skincare**. For natural makeup brands with dairy-free offerings, visit **GoDairyFree.org/makeup**.

SNEAKY SUPPLEMENTS AND MEDICATION

Since they are ingested but relatively unregulated in terms of food allergen labeling, supplements and medications can be a small minefield for those with severe allergies or intolerance. Lactose and other milk-based ingredients are often added to those little pills as fillers without warning. In fact, lactose is used as the base for more than 20 percent of prescription drugs and about 6 percent of over-the-counter medicines and vitamins.

For most people, the small amount of lactose in pills may not be a problem, but it is wise to use caution, since it can be for some. If you have a milk allergy, consult your physician to discuss whether a lactose-containing medication may be safe for you since your nemesis is milk protein rather than lactose, and such a small amount might not pose a risk. If you have severe lactose intolerance and the small amount of lactose in a particular medication causes discomfort, seek another brand. If this isn't possible, ask your physician whether it would be safe to take a lactase enzyme with the medication.

Keep in mind that while lactose is the most commonly used milk ingredient in medications, some medications may contain milk protein or other milk-based ingredients. When ordering a prescription, be sure to ask your pharmacist whether the medication is milk free before they fill it. They should have a list of ingredients for each medication on hand. With over-the-counter medications, all inactive ingredients should be listed on the packaging to alert you to any dairy-containing filler.

Allergy sufferers may have a particularly hard time locating dairy-free antihistamines, as many of the brands and generics do harbor lactose. While ingredients in medications can change at any time, at the time of writing, I found lactose-free options with Allegra (fexofenadine) and several antihistamines in liquid form.

Another milk-free challenge is oral contraceptives. At the time of writing, there were still no completely dairy-free birth control pills. Most contain lactose, so other forms of contraception may need to be considered if you are concerned about this ingredient.

As with food and cosmetics, the ingredients in supplements should be listed on the label, but may change without warning. Once again, seeking out vegan brands of supplements is a good way to identify potential options, but scouring the label and contacting the manufacturer may still be necessary steps. I would like to briefly address two of the most common supplements taken by dairy-free consumers: calcium and probiotics.

Calcium itself, whether in the form of carbonate, citrate, phosphate, etc., is not a dairy product; it's a very abundant mineral found all over the earth. While calcium is found in milk, calcium pills should not be derived from milk, as that would be a rather laborious and expensive process. However, like other supplements, it is possible to find brands with milk ingredients used as fillers, so double-check the ingredient statements. See page 58 for more information on calcium supplements.

As for probiotics, I have spoken with the customer service lines of many manufacturers and, unfortunately, the staff members are frequently underinformed regarding the source of their company's probiotics. In their purest form, probiotics are simply bacteria, but many are cultured or "produced" on dairy. The result is a product that may contain trace amounts of casein, whey, or other milk allergy aggravators. This may not be a problem for those with less severe allergies or lactose intolerance, but you might not choose to take this risk. I seek out probiotics specifically touted as dairy free and/or vegan. When a severe milk allergy is of concern, I would take it a step further and contact the manufacturer to verify their dairy-free claim.

You will see several types of probiotic strains that begin with the term *Lactobacillus*. They are named as such for their ability to convert lactose and other sugars into lactic acid, not because they are derived from dairy. This does not give the green light to all bacteria in the Lactobacillus group—as mentioned, some may be cultured on dairy—but it also means that you may find these types of bacteria in a "safe" dairy-free probiotic.

For a list of supplement brands that are represented as vegan and/or dairy free, visit **GoDairyFree.org/supplements**.

SECTION 2

EATING AWAY FROM HOME

CHAPTER 6
RESTAURANT DINING

Though home-cooked meals have made a comeback, who doesn't crave a night out once in a while? Going to a restaurant can be a fun social outing, offer a much-needed break from the kitchen, and provide sustenance when traveling or in a rush. With some helpful tips and an open mind, you can easily indulge in a night (or two) on the town without sacrificing your health or nondairy lifestyle.

SEVERE FOOD ALLERGY CONCERNS

Before moving on, I must include an upfront disclaimer: several tips in this chapter are geared toward those who need not fear potential cross-contamination. Restaurant kitchens are notorious for shared knives and equipment that are not always properly cleaned. For example, while your meal may be made without milk, the utensils used to serve it may have come in contact at some point in the process with your friend's lasagna. If you are dealing with a severe food allergy, then you must exercise extreme diligence when dining in restaurants. You can never be too careful.

When it comes to coping with severe food allergies away from home, my idol is Sloane Miller, aka "Allergic Girl." Sloane has life-threatening food allergies (epinephrine auto-injector and all), but she refuses to let them get in her way of living. In fact, she eats out in New York City most days of the week. Sloane shares food allergy advice and restaurant stories on her blog (**AllergicGirl.blogspot.com**), and she was kind enough to offer a checklist of "to do's" for managing severe food allergies in restaurants:

- ✓ Call ahead and speak with the manager.
- ✓ Bring your medications.
- ✓ Bring allergy cards.
- ✓ Make sure someone at the table knows you have allergies and how to help you in case of an emergency.
- ✓ When ordering, talk slowly, calmly, and clearly.
- ✓ Make eye contact.
- ✓ Relax.
- ✓ Be assertive and clear, not aggressive and scary.
- ✓ Talk with the highest-level person you can, such as the manager and/or chef.
- ✓ Ask the kitchen's comfort level with your allergies; if they hesitate, go elsewhere.
- ✓ Repeat your needs after every course.
- ✓ Thank your server.
- ✓ Tip well.

✓ Thank the manager.

✓ Go back; re-patronize a restaurant that is able to deal with your needs.

If you are dealing with a child with severe food allergies, I also recommend picking up a copy of *How to Manage Your Child's Life-Threatening Food Allergies* by Linda Coss. She touches on many different challenges and solutions for facing the "real world" with severe food allergies.

ORDERING OFF THE MENU

While jotting down tips for choosing potential dairy-free menu items, I stumbled across a strange coincidence. My advice for dining dairy free has many overlaps with healthy eating words of wisdom. What fantastic news! Diners who choose dairy-free options also open themselves up to healthier restaurant habits, perhaps freeing themselves (at least a bit) from that post-meal sluggishness and belly bulge.

Remember, these suggestions are most applicable to those who can tangle with a stray cheese shred or two without a trip to the ER, but should offer general guidance to anyone seeking dairy-free menu items. As always, use your best judgment, and take all necessary precautions.

ASK QUESTIONS. This is by far the most important tip. Don't be afraid to inquire about the ingredients of a dish or to ask for changes to a menu item. Any good server will be able to help or will not hesitate to go ask the chef. Food allergy incidence is growing at a rapid pace, the paleo community is demanding bun-less burgers, and people waging a war on weight are requesting smaller portions. The hospitality industry recognizes the need to respect those with special diets as a key to success. In fact, research shows that an increasing number of restaurants are providing flexibility in food preparation methods, varied portion sizes, and expanded menu offerings. Your requests are what make this happen.

BE CLEAR. You don't want the staff to be lackadaisical about your food concerns, but you also don't want them to go into an unnecessary panic about serving you. If you have a milk allergy, calmly let the server know the severity of your allergy. It's important that they understand whether or not cross-contamination is a concern and that you are managing your food allergy. Likewise, if you are dairy free for lactose intolerance or for other reasons, a full allergen protocol may not be required in your food preparation—this is important for the restaurant staff to know.

AVOID FRIED FOODS. If general health isn't reason enough for you to stay away from the deep fryer, then keep in mind that milk (and egg) products may linger within coatings, and deep fryers are often a major source of food allergen cross-contamination.

CHOOSE HEART-HEALTHY OILS. The menu will usually specify whether a dish is cooked in oil or butter, but if in doubt, just ask. Most kitchens have vegetable and olive oils on hand. Also, when ordering meat, fish, pasta, or vegetables, request that butter not be added. Some chefs add a pat to grilled, boiled, or steamed foods for flavor.

GO MEDITERRANEAN. When ordering pasta dishes, look for tomato- and olive oil–based sauces rather than cream sauces. You will save yourself loads of saturated fat, and the tomato sauce can even be counted as a serving of vegetables. Just be sure to verify that the sauce is truly dairy free.

DRESS LIGHTLY. Oil and vinegar, honey mustard, French, Thousand Island (contains eggs), and vinaigrettes are often suitable dairy-free salad toppers (always check!), but you'll want to avoid the heavy ranch and blue cheese choices. Mustard, ketchup, barbecue sauce, and mayonnaise (contains eggs) are usually dairy free, but use a light hand to limit your sugar and fat load.

GET EVERYTHING ON THE SIDE. Ask that your condiments and salad dressings come on the side. This is a very common request that many diners have made more than a few times. Benefits include portion control and the ability to give the condiment a once-over before it comes in contact with your entire meal.

PICK SOUP OR SALAD. Salads are an excellent way to get your greens. Mind the salad dressing tips above, order it without cheese, and you will usually be good to go. Although several soups appear obviously dairy free (chicken noodle, vegetable, chili, split pea), your best option is to ask what dairy-free soups are available. Many restaurants even serve up vegan "cream" soups.

TAKE A MEAT BREAK. Many restaurants have added a vegan option or two to their menus over the past few years. Although the entrées may be noted as "vegetarian" (meatless), the growing trend in cutting out all animal products has turned many vegetarian dishes into vegan ones (meat, egg, and dairy free).

UNLOAD THAT POTATO. Skip the sour cream, butter, and cheese customarily found on a "loaded" baked potato or blended into your typical mashed potatoes. Salsa, nondairy salad dressings, oil and vinegar, or a touch of salt and pepper can add ample flavor to a baked potato. Better yet, choose roasted, steamed, or boiled potatoes.

GET OUT OF THE BUTTER RUT. Many restaurants offer fantastic dips and spreads for your dairy-free bread, appetizers, and meal. Some are loaded with dairy, but others, like flavored oils, sweet and savory salsas, tapenades, fresh guacamole (check to make sure that sour cream has not been added), or hummus, could be your gateway to dairy-free flavor.

COOK IT RIGHT. Selecting menu items that are baked, grilled, dry-sautéed, broiled, poached, or steamed will yield the healthiest food as well as better odds at a dairy-free plate.

KEEP RECIPES IN MIND. Think about the traditional recipes for foods when scanning the menu. It can help to quickly identify potential options that are typically dairy free and give you a quick list of specific questions to ask, like "Do you use milk or buttermilk in the pancakes?"

WATCH FOR DIET TRENDS. Many of the new diet and health options listed on menus are cream-, butter-, and cheese-less. When at a restaurant with a large menu, I often jump right to the "light menu," which is usually filled with options that are either dairy free or can easily be made dairy free with very few modifications.

TAKE IT BLACK. Have your coffee and tea sans milk and cream. Ask if they have almond, coconut, or soymilk; you will be surprised how many places do.

SAVE DESSERT FOR LATER. Still craving something sweet? Head home for one of your own dazzling recipes or store-bought treats. Restaurant desserts are typically quite heavy (translation: full of cream and butter), but if you must, fruit and sorbet are usually safe options.

READ THE MENU. No, I mean *really* read the menu. Most restaurants provide a description of the entrées, often in detail. This will allow you to narrow down your options and ask specific questions about the remaining choices.

INSPECT THE DISH UPON ARRIVAL. This doesn't have much to do with the actual ordering process, but make sure that the meal arrives as you requested. I have ordered many entrées without cheese, only to find a slice or two lurking within by mistake.

And my absolute favorite tip . . . drum roll, please:

GO ETHNIC. That's right, we dairy-free consumers eat like well-traveled food connoisseurs, even if we have never left the continent. The following pages include some general guidelines for international cuisine.

NAVIGATING CULTURAL RESTAURANT CUISINE

Expand your menu of options with tastes from around the world, but remember that no restaurant follows exactly the same recipe. In fact, many "Americanize" their dishes to reduce costs and to make them more appealing to less adventurous taste buds. There are no guarantees of authenticity; you must always ask the chef! For example, while a traditional Thai curry would be made with coconut milk, some restaurateurs might use cow's milk or cream (yuck!).

With that said, the following are baseline suggestions to help get you started. Conduct your own due diligence, and perhaps some of these ideas will translate into deliciously "safe" restaurants that you can enjoy frequenting.

Green Light Cuisine: Many Dairy-Free Options

Most Asian restaurants provide an abundance of dairy-free menu items, but always double-check with each restaurant and exercise precaution whenever there is cause for concern.

Chinese

Chinese menus can be expansive, and the majority of items listed qualify as dairy free. Indulge in egg rolls, hot and sour soup, chicken in black bean sauce, moo shu pork, fried rice, beef and broccoli, shrimp in lobster sauce, or Buddha's (vegetarian) feast. Don't forget about dim sum, too. This appetizer-size assortment of dumplings, rice rolls, and steamed buns makes for a fun and delicious meal.

KEY WARNINGS:

- Crab rangoon is made with cream cheese.
- The batter used to deep-fry certain dishes (such as sweet and sour chicken) should be free of milk ingredients, but use caution. If in doubt, take the healthy route and avoid the deep-fried entrées.
- Vegans and those with multiple food allergies should take note that the batter used to deep-fry is usually made with eggs. Eggs may also be found in won ton or egg-roll wrappers and select dishes, such as fried rice.
- I have spotted a few store-bought Chinese sauces that contain a very small amount of dairy. If concerned, ask to verify the ingredients with the chef.
- Aside from fresh fruit, the dessert menu generally contains dairy-rich items.

Japanese

Thank goodness for sushi! Okay, not everyone is a fan, but there is much more to Japanese cuisine than raw fish and seaweed wrappers. Virtually the entire menu, including teriyaki bowls and noodle dishes, is abundant with dairy-free options.

KEY WARNINGS:

- Vegans and those with egg allergies should be aware that the batter used in tempura is usually made with eggs, though rarely with milk. And egg-based mayonnaise is often used in the spicy sauce or to add richness to some of the vegetarian sushi.
- Some "American-style" sushi rolls (such as Philly or Boston rolls) may contain cream cheese.
- Some brands of imitation crab (frequently used in California and other "American-style" sushi rolls) do contain a dairy ingredient or two, as well as other top allergens.
- Aside from fresh fruit, the dessert menu generally contains dairy-rich items.

Thai

Thai food is an excellent indulgence. The generous use of coconut milk creates many rich, creamy, dairy-free meals. You can enjoy curry, basil, and ginger-flavored dishes, and as an added bonus there may be a few items on the dessert menu, such as sticky coconut rice, that get the go-ahead.

KEY WARNINGS:

- As noted, there are no coconut milk guarantees. Verify that the chef is not using milk or other dairy-based products.
- As a warning to vegans and the egg allergic, fish sauce is a very common ingredient in Thai cuisine, as are eggs, but many Thai restaurants offer several vegetarian options.

Vietnamese

Aside from the desserts, it would be difficult to find any dairy-containing items on a Vietnamese menu. The cuisine includes numerous noodle and broth dishes, as well as uniquely seasoned meats and vegetables served atop rice. The appetizers can also make a filling meal; sample the various spring rolls, summer rolls, and skewers.

KEY WARNINGS:

- Vegans take note: though vegetarian items are readily available, fish sauce is frequently used. Request seasonings utilizing soy sauce, lemongrass, and lime.
- Vietnamese desserts typically contain dairy.

Yellow Light Cuisine: Proceed with Caution

Since dairy products are quite prevalent in these establishments, there is a higher probability of cross-contamination. As always, ask to verify that a menu item is safe for you before ordering.

Mexican

Mexican restaurant chefs do tend to love cheese and sour cream, but the more authentic establishments are generous with meat, fish, and vegetables and lighter on the fatty dairy-based additions. Also, Mexican food is frequently assembled rather than prepared. Sour cream and cheese are often added as condiments, but rarely constitute the base of the meal. So they can usually be omitted on request.

SUGGESTIONS:

- Choose the green and red sauces, and ask to make sure they are not prepared with cream or butter. These are usually tomato and pepper blends that are free of milk ingredients.
- Try fajitas, burritos, tamales, wraps, or tacos, but "hold the cheese and sour cream, please." Any Mexican restaurant should easily be able to accommodate this, and almost all of the dishes can hold their own without the added fat. If you are craving some richness, ask to substitute avocado slices or nondairy guacamole.
- Ask for "Mexican guacamole," which is almost always dairy free. "American guacamole," which is often served at Mexican establishments along with or in place of the authentic variety, may be blended with sour cream.
- Tortilla soup is delicious and may be dairy free. Confirm that it is made without cream, and request chopped avocado instead of the usual cheese topping.
- Enjoy some seafood Veracruz. This delightful fish preparation is loaded with tomatoes, olives, and capers. Try other grilled seafood and meat entrées (such as carne asada), and request that they be cooked in oil rather than butter.
- Skip the horchata. Though it is traditionally a rice milk drink, horchata is often made with cow's milk in North America.
- House-made chips and salsa almost always get the go-ahead.
- Skip dishes like taquitos and smothered burritos, which are typically prepared ahead and contain cheese.
- Pass on the custard- and cream-based desserts.

Spanish

The bold, fresh flavors of Spanish cuisine are gaining popularity at tapas bars all over North America. Fortunately, many of Spain's cheese-less dishes are prepared without any milk ingredients. And, as with most Mediterranean cuisines, olive oil, not butter, is the primary fat used.

SUGGESTIONS:

- Cheese is typically served as a stand-alone tapa or added as a topping, rather than baked into dishes. So you can often simply request that it be omitted on your order.

- Egg-based dishes, such as the famous Spanish tortilla (a potato omelet), are traditionally dairy free, but be sure to ask. In North America, milk, cream, or cheese may be added.

- Don't shy away from the sauces. Most of the rich toppers, like romesco and sofrito, are traditionally made without dairy—just double-check to be sure.

- Warm up to Spanish soups and stews, which are usually dairy free and tend to be hearty enough for a full meal.

- If you do eat meat, this may be the time to indulge. Spanish meat and seafood dishes (including paella) are typically made without any milk ingredients.

- Ask about bread and bread-based desserts like churros, biscuits, and tortas (without fillings). They're traditionally made simply with olive oil, rather than butter.

Greek

Greece is at the heart of the Mediterranean diet, which means olive oil is used abundantly. However, yogurt, feta cheese, and béchamel (white sauce) are ever-present dairy concerns at Greek restaurants.

SUGGESTIONS:

- Hold the tzatziki. This yogurt and cucumber sauce is a common topping for gyros and a dip for other traditional dishes. Ask if they have a dairy-free tahini sauce or hummus instead.

- The flatbreads used in Greek cuisine are usually quite simple and rarely contain dairy derivatives. This means that gyros, sans feta and tzatziki, might serve as delicious and hearty wrap alternatives.

- Try an authentic Greek salad; the dressing is typically made with a blend of olive oil, vinegar, lemon juice, and oregano or other fresh herbs. Eggplant (aubergine) salad and beet salad are two great selections. Some salads may contain fresh mozzarella or feta, so be sure to ask.

- Chickpea, lentil, bean, and vegetable soups are very popular at Greek restaurants. Most are prepared with olive oil and vegetables as the base. Just a few may incorporate butter or cheese, though cream is rarely used.

- Ask about the filo-wrapped items. Though many may be stuffed with only spinach, chicken, or ground meat, feta could lurk within.

- Enjoy some traditional dishes, including hummus, souvlaki (meat or fish grilled on a skewer, hold the sauce), dolmades (stuffed grape leaves), and falafel (deep-fried croquettes of ground chickpeas or fava beans). Moussaka (eggplant casserole) is sometimes dairy free, but it may be made with a cream sauce and topped with cheese.

- In traditional Greek cuisine, the meat sauce is tomato based, and the garlic sauce is rich in olive oil. Check with your server, but these should be free of milk ingredients—and make good alternatives to béchamel.

- Many Greek meat dishes and even some casseroles are free of milk ingredients. Since the recipes tend to be simple in terms of the number of ingredients, the restaurant should be well aware of which entrées contain butter or cheese.

- Greek desserts (butter cookies, cakes, baklava, and custards) are typically off-limits, as they are usually rich in butter. Halva is one option that should be dairy free. Also, if they have loukoumades (Greek-style donuts), ask whether they are made with butter or oil; you may just get lucky on this one.

African

Africa is an enormous continent, and the cuisine can vary widely by region. While traditional African food tends to be rich in milk, curd, and whey, dishes that hail from the more tropical regions are often dairy free. These nondairy options are typically abundant in grains, vegetables, and flavor. Don't hesitate to call around and ask about the cuisine; you may find a unique new restaurant to frequent.

Caribbean

Because many small islands have limited access to dairy products, their cuisines have adapted to the use of local spices, herbs, oils, and flavors. This is region dependent, but worth calling around. One of my favorite restaurants in San Francisco was French Caribbean; the entire menu was fragrant, delicious, and completely open to my special diet.

Red Light Cuisine: Be on High Alert

Extra diligence may be required to unearth nondairy dishes in the following types of restaurants, though it is usually possible to find items that will fit your diet.

American

Butter, cream, and cheese are staples in most American-style restaurants, from casual diners to continental fine dining. Mashed potatoes are whipped with butter and milk, sauces are indulged with cream, pastas are coated in cheese, eggs are scrambled with milk, and even a basic steak may be grilled with butter.

SUGGESTIONS:

- Order salads, hold the cheese, and get the dressing on the side. Ask the server if there are any nondairy dressing options.

- If you can, avoid breakfasts out. Most omelets, scrambled eggs, French toast, and pancakes are made with milk. If you must, ask for your eggs poached, hard-boiled, or soft-boiled, or see if they can scramble them without milk. Meats like ham, breakfast sausage, and bacon are usually nondairy, but not always. Plain bagels topped with peanut butter, jam, or honey may be another option, but use extra caution with toast. Sourdough is typically dairy free, but other loaves are often made with milk ingredients. And, of course, fresh fruit is always a good selection.

- Order steamed vegetables, herbed potatoes without butter, or a plain baked potato. Request seasonings like salsa, salt and pepper, or oil and vinegar for adding flavor at the table.

- Stick to grilled meats and fish. Request that they be prepared with oil rather than butter.

- If you are not super-sensitive to milk, then hamburgers, chicken burgers, and other sandwiches, hold the cheese, may be good options. But verify that the protein is not cooked in butter and that the bun or bread doesn't contain any milk-based ingredients. And make sure to request a dry bun, as most restaurants give it a quick toasting with butter for added flavor. Another option is to skip the bun altogether and order a low-carb burger lettuce wrap or salad.

- Look for a good international option. Many fast-casual bar and grills have a good selection of not-so-traditional entrées. I can nearly always find Italian pasta dressed with a tomato-based sauce or a Chinese-style stir-fry.

- Skip dessert. Unless you spot sorbet or fresh fruit, American-style restaurants tend to hide milk ingredients in what would appear to be dairy-free desserts. Cobblers and crumbles most certainly harbor loads of butter, while cakes and pies are typically made with cream and milk. A homemade brownie may be made with oil, but in the restaurant world, it likely contains some creamy ingredients to up the indulgence factor.

Irish/English Pubs

In general, the above suggestions for "American" cuisine carry over quite well to Irish and English pubs. Cream, butter, and cheese are mainstays on their menus, so care needs to be taken when ordering, and substitutions or changes to the entrée may need to be requested. It's also best to avoid the fried foods, as the batter is usually a mix of dairy and eggs. However, Irish pubs frequently offer a few hearty stews, such as the traditional corned beef and cabbage, which are typically dairy free.

Indian

If you are craving a curry, then Thai food is certainly a better option than Indian cuisine. Nonetheless, there are a few potential selections from Indian menus, particularly if you are willing to ask questions.

SUGGESTIONS:

- Most Northern Indian curries are made with cream and/or ghee (clarified butter; see page 144). However, chana masala (chickpeas in a tomato curry); gosht vindaloo (spicy lamb curry), and jhinga masala (shrimp in coconut curry) are usually made without cream, and might be free of ghee, too. Be sure to ask specifically about the ingredients as some Indian restaurants don't label ghee as dairy.

- Skip the tandoor and kabob entrées. Though they may look completely dairy free, these specialties are typically marinated in yogurt.

- Try some Southern Indian cuisine. Dosas are vegetable-filled crepes that are frequently free of milk ingredients, and may also be gluten free (always check). They may be prepared using ghee or oil, so be sure to ask.

- Steer clear of any entrée with the word *paneer*. Paneer is an Indian cheese that is the highlight of many well-known dishes.

- Inquire about the samosas. They are deep-fried little triangles with a stuffing of meat, potatoes, or other vegetables. A small amount of ghee may be used, and the occasional variety stuffed with cheese is always a possibility.

- Sorry, but Indian desserts are definitely off-limits. (Somehow I think cheese balls in sweet cream may be dairy loaded!)

Italian

When I think of the Italian food of days gone past, it brings to mind rich lasagna and manicotti stuffed and topped with mounds of cheese. Sad, but true, these dishes will be a no-go, unless you find one specifically labeled "vegan." Cream, vodka, and pesto sauces are also best to avoid. Though some pesto sauces may be free of milk ingredients, most include Parmesan, and may also be thickened with cream.

Suggestions:

- Pizzas are becoming such elaborate creations. Pepperoni is out; Thai peanut chicken and sun-dried tomato with basil are in! If the toppings sound bold enough to stand on their own, order the pizza without cheese. Just ensure that the sauce they are using is dairy free and that the crust does not harbor milk or cheese.

- Most plain pasta varieties are safe, though raviolis are more often than not stuffed with cheese. Check on the gnocchi; some may be made with Parmesan, though the plain varieties are often dairy free.

- Peruse the menu for fresh tomato sauce, arrabiata (a spicy tomato sauce), or pasta dressed simply with olive oil.

- Try an upscale Italian restaurant; many use flavorful vegetables and grains in place of cheese for a more "impressive" creation. After all, anyone can throw cheese on a dish to make it taste good.

- Order a chicken, meat, or fish entrée, and request that it be cooked in olive oil, not butter. This should be an easy request, as any good Italian restaurant will have an abundance of olive oil on hand.

- Try one of the many green salads and request a dairy-free dressing on the side.

- Most Italian desserts are loaded with dairy—think tiramisu, cannoli, and panna cotta. But the Italians do make a mean sorbetto, which is usually dairy free and vegan.

French

When I think of French restaurants, I envision stylish Parisian women nibbling on billowing salads at an outdoor café. In reality, French cuisine can be very heavy—after all, the French love cheese and cream and butter and . . . well, you get the point.

SUGGESTIONS:

- Ask about the regional influence. While cuisine from the northwest of France uses a lot of butter and cream, in the southeast they favor olive oil and fresh herbs and vegetables. Most other regions rely more heavily on animal fat for cooking and flavoring.
- On the appetizer menu, forgo the escargot, but you may be able to enjoy the salmon or beef tartare if not following a vegan diet.
- Order the "whole food" items, such as herbed potatoes rather than mashed, steamed vegetables rather than purees, and fresh fish. Request that the items be cooked in oil or other nondairy fat if you prefer.
- Enjoy French salads. Salade niçoise, mixed greens, and the various vinegar-based vegetable salads are relatively light and often dairy free.
- Avoid French soups, as they are primarily cream based.
- For a touch of indulgence, consider aioli. It is a garlicky mayonnaise, and thus typically dairy free (but not egg free or vegan).
- On the dessert menu, it is best to stick to sorbet. Though mousses, custards, and fruits à la crème may be tempting, they are most certainly dairy rich.

German/Swiss

Cream, butter, and cheese, oh my! My last dining experience at a German restaurant left me with one item on the menu to order. It was delicious, but limiting nonetheless.

SUGGESTIONS:

- Though schnitzel (breaded cutlet) itself may be dairy free, it is often cooked in butter. Inquire about the ingredients and request that your entrée be cooked in oil.
- Fondue is the most popular way to enjoy Swiss food in the United States. Although cheese fondue is obviously off-limits, meat and vegetable fondues are typically cooked in a mixture of broth and oil. Also, ask if the chocolate fondue is milk based. Finer restaurants often prepare a rich dark chocolate version, which might be dairy free.

Use Caution

Remember, the above tips are general guidelines, but there are no dairy-free guarantees when dining out. Ask questions, survey your meal, and, when in doubt, move on.

For restaurants (worldwide) with dairy-free options that have been recommended by others, see the restaurant listings at **GoDairyFree.org/restaurants**.

FAST FOOD

We all have those moments when sustenance is essential, but we find ourselves trapped in an airport food court, in a late-night conundrum looking for food, or simply "allergic" to the kitchen. When easy and inexpensive is the only way to go, utilize these tips to navigate the fast food maze:

GO GREEN. Opt for salad, sans cheese, and consider the vinaigrette, honey mustard, Thousand Island, or French dressing. With fast food, dressing almost always comes on the side. Ask what your options are, check the ingredients where readily available, or go without!

EAT REAL FOOD. Choose the most "whole" looking options. If it is fried, and thus unrecognizable, it is probably coated with numerous unknown ingredients.

HEAD EAST. Asian fast food eateries, as well as Asian menu options, are everywhere. Avoid the fried dishes if you can; this should still leave you with myriad choices.

THINK SOUTH OF THE BORDER. The "Fresh Mex" trend grew rapidly in the '90s and may still benefit you today. Enjoy homemade salsas and tortillas stuffed with a mix of creations, but hold the cheese, sour cream, and special sauce, please. Ask about the guacamole; it may, in fact, be free of dairy ingredients.

PICK THE BEST. Sandwich shops and delis vary in quality, but a good sandwich needs no cheese. Though you may want them to use a light hand, mayonnaise is almost always dairy free (but not egg free or vegan). Make sure the bread is dairy free and avoid the croissants; there is enough butter in these to make anyone's stomach churn.

KEEP KOSHER. Jewish dietary rules forbid mixing milk and meat, making kosher delis an excellent lunchtime resource for dairy-free dieters. Plus, the staff should be fairly knowledgeable on nondairy offerings.

CHECK THE SOUP BOARD. Most fast food places have daily soup specials, but you may have to look around to spot them. Bean, tomato, vegetable, Mexican tortilla, split pea, and the ever-popular chili are often excellent options.

SPLURGE ON A SLIGHT UPGRADE. Thank goodness for the growing trend of "fast-casual" chains. They work to offer the quality foods of nicer sit-down restaurants in a fast food atmosphere.

ALWAYS ASK. Never hesitate to inquire whether a particular menu item contains dairy. If you make such a request at the golden arches, you are likely to get a blank stare, but many emerging fast food eateries are targeted more specifically at the health-conscious consumer and the special dieter. If the staff doesn't know, most fast food eateries (including the golden arches) have a handy book or poster of ingredients.

EDUCATE YOURSELF IN ADVANCE. Many fast food eateries post their ingredients and allergen charts online, so that you can have a little advance notice on your best menu options. For some quick snapshots of menu items, see the fast food listings at **GoDairyFree.org/fast-food.**

TAKE A LOOK. Never assume there are no dairy-free options. Even my local smoothie shop offers soymilk upon request and pure fruit smoothies.

Use Caution

If you are severely allergic or intolerant, very few fast food joints will be accommodating. Though they may have nondairy dishes, they are typically prepared in the same kitchen and using the same equipment as dairy-based products. Restaurants that receive "pre-prepared" and packaged foods run a slightly lower risk of cross-contamination. Nonetheless, more vigilant measures must be taken for severe food allergies. Furthermore, ingredients and processes change very often at fast food eateries. A "safe" item last month may contain milk this month. Again, when in doubt, move on.

CHAPTER 7
SOCIAL EVENTS & TRAVEL

Restaurants aren't the only places where tricky situations can present for those with special diet needs. Parties, holidays, everyday functions (both formal and informal), and out-of-town trips typically require some food navigation, too.

FRIENDLY GATHERINGS

Whether you're invited to a fancy dinner party, a holiday get-together, or a potluck, I have some simple suggestions for making social outings more enjoyable:

GIVE THE HOST ADVANCE NOTICE OF YOUR DIETARY NEEDS. They may easily be able to put cheese or salad dressings on the side for guests to add on their own, avoiding the need to prepare additional menu items. And by notifying them as early as possible, it may help them make that final decision between lasagna or chicken cacciatore.

ALWAYS LET THE HOST KNOW, REGARDLESS. If advance notice wasn't possible, politely tell them once you arrive that certain foods are off-limits. Even at larger events, the person greeting guests is usually running the show or can point you to the overall host. Most will be happy to check on the dishes to let you know which will be safe, allowing everyone to relax as the party proceeds.

TAKE ALL NECESSARY PRECAUTIONS. If lactose intolerance is your nemesis, be sure to have some lactase enzymes stashed in your purse or pocket. If milk allergies are a concern, double-check that your medicine is in tow. Just because it's a more personal event doesn't mean that you should let your guard down.

SCHEDULE YOUR PERSONAL MENUS. If you are able to follow a rotation-style diet, where a little dairy is okay, be sure to plan your "on" day for the day of the get-together. It doesn't mean you should necessarily eat dairy, but it will offer you more flexibility.

BRING AN ENTRÉE AND PREFERABLY A DESSERT TO SHARE WITH EVERYONE. Even if it isn't a potluck, ask the host if you may bring something that accommodates your needs and may be enjoyed by others. This could actually take some burden off the host. Also, if the guests are eating some of the same foods as you, then you won't feel so out of place.

LOAD UP ON THE NONDAIRY OFFERINGS. Most dinners or potlucks will have some salads, vegetables, or breads that are likely dairy free. Ask the person who made the dish to double-check on the ingredients. If you can't eat it, they will be less offended knowing that you weren't simply snubbing their dish, and they may be more inclined to accommodate your needs at a future event.

ENSURE AMPLE SERVING UTENSILS. I can't count the number of times that I have spotted the serving spoon for something like macaroni and cheese double-dipped into a nice bowl of dairy-free pasta salad. Help the host by putting a proper serving utensil in each dish to prevent cross-contamination. If you know the host well, you may even offer to bring some matching bowl and server sets (color-coding helps tremendously!), giving guests a visual cue for which spoon goes where.

BRING SOME BACK-UP FOOD. It is possible that not a single item will be dairy free at the party. And if you have a severe milk allergy, you may be too concerned about how the foods were prepared to enjoy yourself. Bring a back-up meal or packaged snacks, just in case.

FOCUS ON THE PARTY. Most events are about the people, not the food. If the dining situation is causing excessive angst, eat enough "safe" food at home to satiate before you leave, and simply go to enjoy the company.

DON'T FORGET ABOUT THE DRINKS. Specialty cocktails, particularly around the holidays, can be made with dairy. Check the ingredients on the bottle for any that arouse suspicion. You will want to avoid outright creamy blends (like Baileys Irish Cream) or milky mixers (skip the White Russians, for example), but may be pleasantly surprised to find that indulgent liqueurs like crème de menthe are actually dairy free. For the highly sensitive, it's important to note that milk protein is occasionally used in the fining process of wine (as are other top allergens like eggs). If this raises concern for you, pick up a vegan wine to bring along. Hard cider and beer are usually safe bets, but strange combinations like milk stout do exist. For additional help, see my Guide to Dairy-Free Alcohol at **GoDairyFree.org/dairy-free-alcohol.**

BE GRATEFUL. Send a thank-you card or even a gift to an accommodating host. Whether they show it or not, catering to special diet guests does add some stress. Letting them know how appreciative you are of their efforts will help ensure an invite to their next party.

AVOIDING FAMILY FEUDS

Let's face it—we're all more critical with family. We love one another, but we're so close that we subconsciously expect one another to think and act just like we do. And when one person makes a change, it can make us feel like we should, too. After all, we're related.

So when you spring it on Aunt Martha that you or your loved one can't eat dairy, don't be surprised if she takes it personally and even insists, with words or actions, that it isn't true. And be warned that dairy free seems to elicit some of the most resistant special diet responses.

For holidays and extended family dinners, most of the tips in the preceding section carry over, but siblings, parents, grandparents, cousins, aunts, and uncles often require some extra attention:

START A CONSTRUCTIVE DIALOGUE. Unlike the friend who simply hosts an annual New Year's Eve party, your family probably gets together several times throughout the year. This means it is essential that they understand your dietary needs. Sit down with them and explain the reasons behind the dietary shift, why it's important, and if your needs are somewhat relaxed or stringent. In the case of a severe allergy, it's essential to relay to them the potential consequences and how this came about. Be very open and encourage them to ask questions. Letting them be a part of your journey without expecting them to follow suit can not only encourage empathy, but it may also help them feel closer to you and more willing to help. And try not to spring this on them as everyone sits down to Thanksgiving dinner. Drop by for a friendly visit or pick up the phone in advance rather than putting them on the spot.

DON'T EXPECT THEM TO UNDERSTAND. It's possible that they still won't get it. To be fair, there are so many fad diets that it can be hard for people to discern a passing food phase that is just an inconvenience from a true life concern that should be taken quite seriously. Or perhaps allergies just "didn't exist" in the area where they grew up, so they can't fathom such a rarity would occur in their family. In this case, use extra caution when food is involved, as they may even try to sabotage your needs, and just give them some time. Diet trends and fads are fleeting and can irritate accommodating loved ones. If you are rock solid and consistent with your diet and requests, then they will usually come around.

MAKE IT A FAMILY AFFAIR. Most relatives cherish bonding time above all else. Bring them into your world by offering to prepare the meals with them. Go shopping together and show them exactly which foods are safe. As you cook together, share some of your favorite new food combinations and use the opportunity to demonstrate how to avoid cross-contamination, if needed. Initially, don't suggest that they change any of their own dishes or try to make an exact duplicate. (Mom may feel slighted if your dairy-free sweet potato casserole gets gobbled up before hers.) Instead, start by augmenting the meal with one or two of your dairy-free dishes for everyone to sample. Soon your recipes could become a part of the tradition.

BE APPRECIATIVE. I know this was covered previously, but with family, that warm hug and heartfelt thank-you is even more important.

ON THE ROAD

Whether you are running errands around town or heading out on a cross-country road trip, keeping adequate supplies of snacks on hand can be a lifesaver. At home, several safe meal options may be within arm's reach, but when in transit, good options may not always be available when hunger strikes. The following foods are some of my favorite suggestions for quick, easy foods to pack along. As always, be sure to purchase dairy-free versions that are safe for your needs.

- Small boxes or baggies of cereal or granola
- Trail mix (avoid chocolate in warm weather)
- Energy, granola, snack, or cereal bars
- Dried fruit, fruit leather, or fruit snacks
- Popcorn
- Single-serve packages of cookies, crackers, or chips

- Bagels, muffins, or other homemade baked goods
- Whole fruit, such as apples, oranges, bananas, grapes, berries, or peaches
- Carrot or celery sticks with shelf-stable, single-serve hummus
- Single-serve applesauce
- Packets of peanut butter or nut butter (great for spreading on bagels or fruit)
- Jerky, regular or vegan
- Bottled water, single-serve dairy-free milk beverages or protein drinks, or juice boxes

For reviews of several dairy-free snacks, see my product reviews by category at **GoDairyFree.org/reviews**. For a printable list of dairy-free and nut-free snacks (great for school food allergy policies), visit **GoDairyFree.org/snack-list**.

SAFE TRAVELS

If dairy-free, vegan, or even GFCF living is your concern, then it may help to investigate the dining options at your destination before you head out. Many cities, particularly large ones, have restaurants that cater to a variety of special diets. A quick search online may reveal some delicious raw eateries (typically dairy free, vegan, and gluten free), vegan restaurants, or other dining spots that go to extra lengths to accommodate special diets.

However, if you are dealing with severe food allergies or simply can't find suitable restaurant options for your upcoming journey, then a little creativity may be in order. For suggestions on traveling with dietary restrictions I went straight to the expert, Loretta Jay, the president of Parasol (**ParasolServices.com**), a consulting organization that specializes in the management of food allergies and celiac disease.

In Loretta's family of four, three live with celiac disease and both kids have extensive food allergies. Yet even with these dietary challenges, they travel and experience the culture of wherever they visit, thanks to some special planning by Loretta. She shared with me her travel tips, which were originally published in *Foods Matter* magazine:

HOTEL: For weekend trips, ensure that your room has at least a microwave and a mini-fridge. For longer trips, book a room with a kitchen or kitchenette.

PACKING: Consider shipping a box of food ahead to your hotel for emergencies, rather than risking your food in the maze of lost luggage. The box should include a two- to three-day supply of nonperishable "must haves" that may be difficult to find at your destination. If perishable items are needed, pack these last, in an insulated bag, which you should then pack in a hard-sided suitcase for your checked baggage. The bag should also include a signed letter from your physician explaining any allergies, just in case the contents of the bag come under question. When traveling abroad, don't forget to check on international customs regulations, as certain types of foods may not be permitted to cross borders.

AIR TRAVEL: Since quick five-hour flights can easily turn into two-day adventures with delays, cancelations, and rerouting of flights, carrying on an ample supply of snacks to cover a full day of meals can be worth its weight. Be sure to check the current airline restrictions for carry-on baggage, though. You may be limited on the types of foods you can pack, or a note from a physician may be needed. Food allergies are considered a hidden disability, so accommodations can often be made with some planning. And this is my own tip: Call ahead to the airline, as they might be able to accommodate you with a special meal, should they serve food. Many airlines offer vegan/vegetarian, kosher (often dairy free), and other special meals for dietary restrictions.

SHOPPING: Markets in most regions of the world carry basic foods such as potatoes, rice, onions, legumes, salt, and olive oil. In addition, roadside vendors and local markets can be great places to learn more about the culture while stocking up on local whole foods. While shopping, don't be afraid to strike up a conversation and ask about favorite recipes. You may discover some popular local fare that you can easily prepare and customize to your diet.

COOKING: Loretta's family doesn't eat in restaurants when traveling, but she still wants her family to experience the culture of the land they are visiting, including the food. Before leaving home she does some pre-travel homework (online or at the local library) to learn the types of food and mode of cooking indigenous to the region they will be visiting. For example, in the Caribbean she might add a tropical twist to plain old pancakes by preparing them with coconut milk and serving with plantains; in Spain some homemade tapas are perfect for a take-along lunch, while a Spanish tortilla can serve as a native dinner. To avoid getting too overwhelmed with cooking, Loretta also suggests creating simple side dishes (rice, local vegetables, etc.) and going with basic desserts, like dairy-free chocolate brought from home, melted, and served with native fruit for dipping.

KIDS: BACK TO SCHOOL & CELEBRATIONS

Caring for your own special diet needs is one thing, but having to watch out for what children eat when you may not be there to help them brings a whole new level of challenges. Here are a few tips and considerations for navigating the food aspect of general life situations with kids who don't consume dairy.

School Lunch and Activities

This section contains excerpts from a feature article that I wrote for *Allergic Living* magazine.

While we are hearing more about "peanut-free policies" and "nut-free classrooms," a ban on milk simply isn't feasible in most schools. Milk is the only food singled out in the National School Lunch Act, the U.S. federal law that governs the National School Lunch Program (NSLP), as one that cannot be prohibited on participating school premises or at any school-sponsored event. Dairy-based foods are also offered in the National School Breakfast Program, which has been expanding in recent years through the Breakfast in the Classroom initiative. To further guarantee its presence, the U.S. Department of Agriculture's Special Milk Program provides subsidies to supply milk to kids in nonprofit private schools and half-day kindergarten programs, and to other students who may not have access to school meal programs. In our educational system, milk is not just a beverage—it's considered a personal right.

In fact, if you opt to have your child participate in the NSLP, they may actually be *required* to take milk if you have not supplied the school with a note from a physician stating that they have a milk allergy. Your child or teen can discard the milk, but they may not be given another drink option. In 2009, the USDA issued an addendum on the topic of milk substitutes for schools that participate in the NSLP as well as the Breakfast and Milk Programs. Under the new policy, schools are *permitted* (but not required) to provide a nondairy beverage that meets the USDA nutrition standards for milk substitutes to students who wish to forgo fluid milk for any reason, including "non-disabling" allergies, culture, religion, or ethical beliefs. Currently, the only nondairy beverages that qualify under these guidelines are certain brands of soymilk.

Even if your child avoids the school meal and milk programs, reducing the presence of milk in schools is beyond controversial. Milk is one of the most revered and protected foods in Westernized diets and is ubiquitous in our food supply. From the "good for you" image of milk and yogurt to festivities centered on pizza and ice cream, the mere suggestion of an event without dairy can result in dramatic backlash from other parents and teachers.

Dairy also poses a high exposure risk. It is conveniently packaged in a multitude of ways for kid-friendly lunch boxes, but once opened, the residues are far from contained. Spilled liquids can easily spread and may not be properly cleaned up; powdered milk or cheese from snack foods can float through the air and settle like dust; and yogurt is often smeared onto clothes and tables by little hands.

Finally, there is the issue of confusion. Few understand the wide range of medical effects dairy can have, from simple ingestion issues like lactose intolerance, to contact reactions such as hives, to severe life-threatening allergic responses. All of this can impede your child's ability to learn and enjoy school.

Fortunately, understanding what you are up against is a good first step that can help you create a safe and inclusive environment for your child at school. The following suggestions offer further steps you can take to potentially address the above issues:

- Walk through scenarios with your child on how to handle everyday situations that they may run into at school. They should understand how to politely say "no" to foods offered, speak up when they feel at risk or uncomfortable, and practice excellent hygiene, with frequent hand-washing if severe allergies are a concern.

- Arrange a meeting with the school staff before school begins and establish credibility by remaining calm, keeping your requests reasonable, and providing solutions that can be easily implemented. Make sure they understand why your child avoids dairy, and why it is important to your family. If you are dealing with a life-threatening food allergy, be sure to address creating a dairy-free zone for your child when food is present.

- Shift the focus to food-free fun. When a celebration or reward centers on food, such as ice cream socials or pizza parties, milk-allergic kids can feel excluded. Encourage a transition in traditions by offering ideas that take food out of the equation. This can allow your child the satisfaction of working toward a goal or enjoying a special day while taking the pressure off teachers and custodians.

- Consider setting up a 504 plan if your child has a medically diagnosed food allergy that qualifies as a disability. This is an individualized plan set up by you and the school staff, with accommodations that should allow your child to fully participate in school activities. The modifications are completely customizable and may include things like setting up a milk-free table in the lunchroom, implementing proper cleanup and mandatory hand-washing for all kids, extra precautions on field trips, and more. 504 plans are available to all special-needs children enrolled in the U.S. public school system. However, many U.S. private schools and school systems worldwide have their own programs set up for accommodating food allergies. Contact the school administration directly to find out your rights and options.

Birthday Parties

Allergen safety may be the number one priority, but no parent wants their child to feel left out during a celebration. To keep the festivities cheerful, Sarah Hatfield (associate editor for GoDairyFree.org and busy mom behind NoWheyMama.com) recommends stocking an arsenal of dairy-free cookies, cupcakes, and ice cream sandwiches in the freezer.

Sarah keeps sugar cookies and chocolate chip cookies unfrosted, but she has a special trick for cupcakes: After baking, let the cupcakes cool completely and then peel back one side of the cupcake wrappers. Slice the cupcakes almost in half horizontally (as you would a hamburger bun) and spread frosting in the middle of the cupcakes, so they are technically frosted, yet easy to freeze and ready for the road. To store, she rewraps the cupcakes individually and stores them together in a freezer bag. When her daughter attends a birthday party, Sarah sends her off with one ice cream sandwich and one cupcake, so that she can join in the food fun.

Since school birthdays and celebrations can come up without warning, Sarah suggests asking your child's school if you can store "safe" treats with them. Her daughter's school permits them to keep cookies and cupcakes in a freezer in the nurse's office for class parties.

Day Care and Play Dates

Beyond any allergy "safety" equipment you may need (such as epinephrine auto-injectors and antihistamines), always keep a stash of snacks on hand. See the "On the Road" suggestions on page 95 for some ideas. Sarah once again has a nice tip for food and snack storage when away from home: plaster "dairy-free" and "wheat-free" stickers all over the containers to keep food thieves away. Many people view the special diet labels as unappealing and will seek sustenance elsewhere. For dairy-free adults, this advice carries over quite well into the workplace, where lunches can magically disappear from communal refrigerators.

Don't forget about project-related sources of dairy in a child's environment. In preschool, day care, or early school settings, M&Ms or similar foods may be used for counting and learning activities, and empty milk, cream, or yogurt cartons are popular for projects. Dairy can even lurk in unsuspecting inedible products, such as finger paints, shaving cream (often used for craft projects), and general hygiene products for cleanup time, like soaps and lotions.

Since your young child may feel shy about their diet, or may even be unable to properly communicate, make sure to tell any adults who will be at a particular event about your child's needs.

SECTION 3

GROCERY SHOPPING & PREPARING YOUR KITCHEN

CHAPTER 8

DECODING FOOD LABELS

I used to spend so much time worrying about fat and calories that I would completely bypass the ingredient statements—you know, what is actually *in* the food. After scanning thousands (no exaggeration) of food labels, I was amazed to discover countless products that utilize dairy in one strange form or another. Though deciphering the "secret code" used on ingredient statements was a mind-boggling experience, it allowed me to collect some excellent information to help simplify the process for you.

DAIRY FREE VERSUS NONDAIRY

As you will note throughout this guide, I use the terms *nondairy* and *dairy free* interchangeably. According to my definition, both equate to "made without dairy ingredients," including lactose, casein, whey, and any of their constituents. However, in the food labeling business, they can take on very different meanings.

Nondairy (or Non-Dairy)

The FDA has created a regulatory definition for the term *nondairy* that, amazingly, does not equate to milk free. A product labeled as nondairy can contain 0.5 percent or less milk by weight, in the form of casein/caseinates (milk protein). This is why you may spot nondairy creamers, nondairy whipped toppings, and other nondairy products that note milk on the ingredient statement. This does not mean that all products labeled as nondairy contain milk, but it is a word of warning to always read the ingredient statement.

Dairy Free

On the other hand, there is no regulatory definition for the term *dairy free*, yet I find it to be a much more accurate indicator of milk-free products. Even though the FDA has not established guidelines for this term, there is a blanket policy that forbids the use of false and/or misleading terminology in general on food labels. This seems to be enough of a fear tactic, as I have yet to stumble across a food item that is promoted as dairy free but contains milk ingredients. That being said, the misleading use of the term *dairy free* could easily exist, so always read the label, and contact the manufacturer when cross-contamination may also be a concern. Even if a product is free from milk ingredients, it could contain trace amounts of milk from the manufacturing processes.

FOOD ALLERGEN LABELING LAWS

Otherwise known as the "plain language" labeling law, the Food Allergen Labeling and Consumer Protection Act (FALCPA) went into effect for food and supplements manufactured on or after January 1, 2006, that are intended for sale within the United States. FALCPA is governed by the FDA, and requires that the top 8 allergens (including milk) be declared on food labels using easily recognizable names. This can be done either with an allergen notation in parentheses within the ingredient listing or in a statement immediately following the ingredients. I will use a dairy-based protein powder ingredient statement to demonstrate:

WITHIN THE INGREDIENTS: whey protein concentrate (**milk**), cocoa powder, stevia leaf extract, soy lecithin.

FOLLOWING THE INGREDIENTS: whey protein concentrate, cocoa powder, stevia leaf extract, soy lecithin. **Contains: Milk, Soy**

In the first example, soy doesn't need to be called out since it is written in recognizable language within the ingredients.

The government has made it clear that even a seven-year-old should be able to read and understand the food labels, but the allergen labeling law certainly isn't foolproof. While there are penalties for noncompliance, the FDA is not reviewing all the food labels that go out the door. I've seen numerous allergen errors and omissions on ingredient statements, particularly with dairy, and it is up to the company or consumers to catch them.

It's also important to understand that certain types of food and beverages do not fall under the FDA's jurisdiction in the United States. Meat, poultry, and egg products are regulated by the USDA's Food Safety and Inspection Service (FSIS). FSIS heavily encourages the use of allergen statements, and will consider legislation if they do not see widespread voluntary compliance. Alcoholic beverage labeling is regulated by the Federal Alcohol Administration (FAA). The FAA does not currently have any policies requiring food allergen labeling, but rules are under consideration.

Canada has since enacted similar legislation to FALCPA, but their allergen labeling covers the top 11 food allergens (including milk). Likewise, the European Union has adopted regulations on the disclosure of top food allergens for pre-packed foods. On their food labels, ingredients derived from milk must be adequately identified (along with 13 other top food allergy and sensitivity offenders) in all cases, with the following exceptions: whey used for making distillates or ethyl alcohol of agricultural origin for spirit drinks and other alcoholic beverages and lactitol. These ingredients are believed to be so far removed from milk that they are not at risk for eliciting a reaction.

In a perfect world, with all companies printing accurate allergen notations on their ingredient statements, we would expect that reading allergen statements would be a straightforward solution for anyone with a top food allergy or intolerance. Unfortunately, due to manufacturing processes, unregulated "may contain" labeling practices in all of the aforementioned countries has led to mass uncertainty.

MAY CONTAIN: CONFUSION

Food production is much more complex than the average consumer can fathom. It includes supply chains where ingredients may pass through multiple plants, manufacturing lines on which varying batches of food may be mixed, and even separate packaging facilities handling a broad range of raw or finished goods.

As you can imagine, there are often numerous places where a product could be cross-contaminated with small amounts of ingredients from another product. Most companies do follow good manufacturing processes, and many have special allergen protocols that require them to thoroughly wash lines between batches and even rotate foods on an "allergen schedule." But others don't want the liability of someone with a severe food allergy simply looking at a label, seeing that their allergen isn't in the ingredients, and eating it, when there could be a risk that the product was cross-contaminated with small amounts of the allergen somewhere in the process.

And thus, a varying array of statements began to emerge on food labels: "may contain," "made on equipment with," "produced in the same facility with," "may contain traces of," and so on.

These Statements Are Voluntary

"May contain" and similar disclaimers are not required or regulated, and they are not defined by set guidelines in FALCPA. They are just statements that some companies opt to add. This is a hotly contested issue because it has led to great consumer confusion over the years.

One company might include a "may contain" warning merely out of fear, even if they follow heavy allergen protocols, while another running high-risk operations for cross-contamination might choose not to note anything at all. Some products with "may contain" statements have been tested and shown to be completely free of the allergen, whereas others without warnings have been tested and shown to have high levels of certain allergens. There are even some nervous chocolate companies that put "Contains: Milk" right on the ingredient statement when milk isn't used in the product, just because they are concerned about cross-contamination with milk ingredients.

Manufacturers also often fail to take into consideration the risk of the actual ingredients being used. Powdered milk or cheese used on snack foods can take to the air with ease, landing on once-clean lines. Liquid milk, on the other hand, is relatively easy to contain and wash away.

The Bottom Line

For most people who are dairy free, simply reading the ingredients to see if milk is a part of the product is enough. The "may contain" warnings typically indicate the potential of trace or very minute amounts of the allergen, which is of little concern in many situations. However, if you have a severe, life-threatening food allergy, it's essential that you *never* rely on just the ingredient statement and the presence or omission of "may contain" warnings. You *must* call the manufacturer to personally assess a product's safety for your consumption.

In other words, the only notable purpose of "may contain" warnings is to provide extra cushion against liability issues for food producers. As I write, I feel that these statements are practically worthless for consumers and, quite frankly, lead to more problems and allergen confusion. Hopefully, in the near future, the FDA will step in to either provide strict guidelines for allergen testing or make across-the-board amendments for products that may be at high risk for cross-contamination with top allergens.

UTILIZING KOSHER CERTIFICATION

Kosher certification is a system of labeling that was originally created for spiritual purposes. However, over the years many individuals have also found it to be a handy way of identifying foods for special diets.

First, I believe it is important to address an ongoing debate regarding the safety of certified kosher pareve products for those with milk allergies. Based on policies of the Orthodox Union, the world's "superpower" of kosher certification, individuals with a severe milk allergy should not rely completely on kosher certification when selecting foods:

> The trace nuts and dairy disclaimer that is now printed on many products is there to warn consumers that although there are no nuts or dairy in the ingredients of the product itself, there is a possibility of parts per millions floating in the air and "contaminating" the product.
>
> The "contamination" would only affect consumers with extremely severe allergies who can detect even the most trace amounts of the substance that they are reacting to. A product that is labeled OU (and thereby certified kosher pareve) is halachically (by Jewish Law) pareve. The parts per million does not affect the status of a product, because parts per million are negligible and have no halachic significance.
>
> As an example, a factory might produce dairy and pareve products on two separate production lines. Nonetheless, airborne particles of milk or whey powder might float onto the pareve production line. Though a person might suffer an allergic reaction, the product is still halachically pareve.

Fortunately, for most individuals who choose to cut dairy from their diet for religious, personal, social, or medical reasons, kosher labeling can be a very useful tool.

If a product is kosher certified, then a kosher symbol will typically be found near the product name. That symbol may stand alone, or it may state "pareve," "parev," or "parve." In any of these cases, it indicates that the product was made without dairy ingredients (or meat ingredients, for that matter). In most (but not all) circumstances, this would also indicate that separate production lines or thorough cleaning processes have been utilized to minimize cross-contamination.

If the kosher symbol contains or is accompanied by a "D," "DE," or "Dairy," then the product either contains dairy within its ingredients or is simply manufactured on equipment that is shared with dairy-containing products and not thoroughly cleaned to pareve standards in between production runs. If your concerns do not lie with cross-contamination, then check the ingredients. It may still be a suitable product for you.

There are other notations, such as "M" and "Glatt," which denote a kosher product that contains meat. Under kosher certification requirements, any product containing meat should not contain dairy.

Kosher certification is issued by a number of different organizations throughout the world. For this reason, various organization-specific symbols are utilized to identify kosher products. Furthermore, each kosher-certifying organization may have varying standards. This is another reason why kosher labeling is not highly recommended as a decisive resource for strict diets. Nonetheless, it can be a quick and handy tool for most nondairy or vegan lifestyles, and for narrowing down potential food options.

DAIRY INGREDIENT LISTS

When all else fails, consult the following lists to verify whether the product you are considering is made without dairy ingredients. If any of the ingredients from the first list are within the product, then it most likely contains dairy in some form.

Definitely Dairy Ingredients

Acidophilus Milk

Ammonium Caseinate

Butter

Butter Oil

Butter Solids

Butterfat

Buttermilk

Buttermilk Powder

Calcium Caseinate

Casein

Caseinate (in general)

Cheese (all animal-based)

Condensed Milk

Cottage Cheese

Cream

Curds

Custard

Delactosed Whey

Demineralized Whey

Dry Milk Powder

Dry Milk Solids

Evaporated Milk

Ghee (see page 144)

Goat Cheese

Goat's Milk

Half-and-Half

Hydrolyzed Casein

Hydrolyzed Milk Protein

Iron Caseinate

Lactalbumin

Lactoferrin

Lactoglobulin

Lactose

Lactulose

Low-Fat Milk

Magnesium Caseinate

Malted Milk

Milk (all animal-based)

Milk Derivative

Milk Fat

Milk Powder

Milk Protein

Milk Solids

Nonfat Milk

Nougat

Paneer

Potassium Caseinate

Pudding

Recaldent

Rennet Casein

Sheep Cheese

Sheep's Milk

Skim Milk

Sodium Caseinate

Sour Cream

Sour Milk Solids

Sweet Whey

Sweetened Condensed Milk

Whey

Whey Powder

Whey Protein Concentrate

Whey Protein Hydrolysate

Whipped Cream

Whipped Topping

Whole Milk

Yogurt

Zinc Caseinate

Potentially Dairy Ingredients

ARTIFICIAL OR NATURAL FLAVORS/FLAVORING: These are vaguely named ingredients, which may be derived from a dairy source. A few of particular concern are butter, coconut cream, and egg flavors, though there are even dairy-free versions of these.

FAT REPLACERS: Brands such as Dairy-Lo and Simplesse are made with milk protein.

GALACTOSE: This is often a lactose by-product, but it can be derived from sugar beets or gums.

HIGH PROTEIN OR PROTEIN: Ingredients noted with no further details may be derived from milk proteins (casein or whey). This is particularly true in "high-energy" foods.

HYDROLYZED VEGETABLE PROTEIN: The processing phase may use casein, but only trace amounts would likely remain.

LACTIC ACID STARTER CULTURE: These may be prepared by using milk as an initial growth medium.

LACTOBACILLUS: This term is noted often as a probiotic. It is, in fact, bacteria, not a food by-product, and is named as such for its ability to convert lactose and other simple sugars into lactic acid. Though it is often utilized in milk products to create lactic acid, this ingredient on its own is not always a concern. However, in some cases it may have been cultured or produced on dairy, and thus have the potential to contain trace amounts.

MARGARINE: Milk proteins and lactose are used in several brands, but not all.

PREBIOTICS: These are indigestible carbohydrates gaining popularity in health foods. They are quite different from probiotics, which are living microorganisms. Prebiotics, such as galacto-oligosaccharides, lactosucrose, lactulose, and lactitol, may be derived from milk-based foods.

Rarely Dairy Ingredients

CALCIUM OR SODIUM STEAROYL LACTYLATE: Stearoyl lactylates are derived from the combination of lactic acid and stearic acid. They are generally considered nondairy and safe for the lactose intolerant and milk allergic. However, stearic acid may be animal derived, which could be a concern for vegans.

CALCIUM, SODIUM, OR POTASSIUM LACTATE: Lactates are salts derived from the neutralization of lactic acid, and are rarely a dairy concern. See the note below on Lactic Acid.

CARAMEL COLOR: Anything with caramel in its title may sound like a dairy red flag, but caramel color is typically derived from corn syrup (and occasionally from potatoes, wheat, or other carbohydrate sources). While lactose is a permitted carbohydrate in the production of caramel color, it is rarely if ever used.

LACTIC ACID: Lactic acid is created via the fermentation of sugars, and can be found in many dairy-free and/or vegan foods. Most commercially used lactic acid is fermented from carbohydrates, such as cornstarch, potatoes, or molasses, and thus dairy free. Though lactic acid can be fermented from lactose, its use is usually restricted to dairy products, such as ice cream and cream cheese.

Surprisingly Dairy-Free Ingredients/Food

Calcium Carbonate

Calcium Citrate

Calcium Phosphate

Calcium Propionate

Cocoa Butter

Cocoa Powder

Coconut Butter

Coconut Cream

Cream of Coconut

Cream of Tartar

Creamed Honey

Crème Liqueurs

Fruit Butters (Apple, Pumpkin, etc.)

Glucono Delta-Lactone

Lecithin Oleoresin

Malted Barley or other Grain-Based Malts

Malt Liquor

Malt Vinegar

Milk Thistle

Nut Butters (Peanut, Almond, etc.)

Shea Butter

WHERE THE DAIRY HIDES

So, where might one find dairy ingredients? There are the obvious foods, such as cow's milk (chocolate, whole, skim, malted, evaporated, etc.), buttermilk, half-and-half, cream, butter, cheese, ice cream, milkshakes, milk chocolate, and yogurt. However, did you know that the majority of processed foods also contain dairy? Some are fairly easy to spot, such as macaroni and cheese or creamy ranch salad dressing, while others may be more elusive. Below is a *partial* list of manufactured foods and non-food items where dairy ingredients may be hiding. A few just might surprise you . . .

BABY FORMULA AND BABY FOOD: If you are seeking a nondairy baby formula due to milk allergies, check with a physician. Babies can have much more sensitive and serious allergic reactions than adults.

BAKERY GOODS: It can be difficult to verify the ingredients of freshly baked goods. In general, muffins and quick breads frequently contain milk or buttermilk; scones are almost always rich with cream, buttermilk, or butter; and cookies typically contain butter and may contain milk chocolate. Though yeast breads appear safe, one of the most common dough conditioners utilized in bread is whey, a milk protein. In addition, some loaves and rolls may contain milk, dry milk powder, cheese, or buttermilk.

BAKING MIXES (pancakes, cakes, biscuits, etc.): Dry milk powder, buttermilk powder, and other milk solids are common in these products.

BATH PRODUCTS: Though your cleansers, hair products, and lotions are not food products, those who tend to have skin reactions to milk products (such as eczema) may want to avoid topical application (see page 77).

BEER: "Milk" beer has been around for some time, and may linger in breweries under the code name of "sweet stout." Quite often it makes itself known with a more obvious title, such as "milk stout" or "cream stout." These beers contain lactose, which adds sweetness, body, and calories to the finished beer. However, cream ales are usually dairy free. For tips on finding dairy-free beer, head to **GoDairyFree.org/dairy-free-alcohol**.

BREATH MINTS: A few contain casein-related ingredients.

CANDY: Much of the candy world (of the non-chocolate variety) is free game from a dairy-free point of view, but a surprise milk ingredient does pop up on occasion.

CANNED TUNA FISH: A few brands contain hydrolyzed caseinate.

CARAMEL: This is a suspicious food and ingredient, as it may be made simply from sugar and water, or it may contain milk, cream, or butter for body.

CEREAL: Dry and instant cereals vary significantly in ingredients, even among similar products. For example, one type of cereal may contain milk ingredients in the brand name, but not in the corresponding generic.

CHEESE ALTERNATIVES: Some brands of cheese alternatives (whether soy, rice, or almond based) are lactose free but still contain milk protein (casein) to create a more cheese-like consistency and texture.

CHEWING GUM: Some brands contain milk protein.

CHICKEN BROTH: Several brands use milk protein or solids, particularly in broth concentrates and bouillon cubes.

CHOCOLATE: Milk chocolate is a given, but some semi-sweet and dark chocolate brands also contain milk ingredients (even though they shouldn't in my opinion!).

CHOCOLATE DRINKS: Even the non-milk varieties may contain a bit of dairy to make them more substantial.

CLOTHING: It is not yet in the mainstream, but a few textile producers have come out with eco-fabrics that use milk fiber. Some clothing manufacturers are in the testing phases with using these weaves.

COCONUT MILK POWDER: A couple of dairy-free brands have emerged recently, but most brands available to consumers contain a small amount of milk protein. Manufacturers do have better access to dairy-free options of this ingredient.

COFFEE WHITENERS/CREAMERS: Milk is certainly white and creamy, and it has many uses in these foods.

COOKIES AND CRACKERS: It's common to find milk ingredients or by-products in processed foods such as these.

CREAM LIQUEURS: These may contain solid milk ingredients or caseinates, and shouldn't be confused with crème liqueurs, which are more of a syrup and typically made without dairy.

CUSTARD/PUDDING: Most prepared puddings, and a few dry mixes, contain milk ingredients.

DRUGS/MEDICATIONS: Lactose is sometimes used as a filler/base for prescription drugs and OTC medications (including antihistamines and birth control pills). Be sure to ask the pharmacist to review the ingredients of any prescription medications you will be taking before filling it.

EGG SUBSTITUTE: Some brands of egg substitute contain or are made from whey.

EGGNOG: This is typically richer in milk and cream than eggs. Visit **GoDairyFree.org/holiday-beverages** for an annually updated list of dairy-free and vegan "nogs."

FLAVORED SYRUPS: These may appear like pure colored sugar, but some harbor small amounts of milk.

FONDUE: Although there are some fondues made with stock, many are cheese-based and most chocolate fondues do contain dairy.

FRIED FOODS: The breading on fried foods may contain cheese, milk, buttermilk, or other milk-based ingredients.

GRANOLA & NUTRITION BARS: As with cookies, various milk additives may show up in bars.

GRAVIES: Some contain milk, milk powder, or milk solids for flavor and texture.

HOT COCOA MIX: The best varieties are pure cocoa and sugar, but some may contain milk ingredients for a creamier drink.

HOT DOGS: Convenience meats often contain fillers, and hot dogs are no exception. They can contain cheese, lactose, or other milk derivatives.

IMITATION CRAB MEAT: Most brands contain a milk ingredient or two, in addition to other surprise top allergens.

IMITATION MAPLE AND OTHER SYRUPS: Pure maple syrup is typically a safe selection. In the past, dairy was used in the production of maple syrup, but today, those production processes are very rarely used. However, imitation syrups can contain lactose, butter, or other ingredients derived from dairy.

INSTANT POTATOES: Many varieties contain milk products, most notably the "au gratin" or sour cream styles.

KOSHER PAREVE DESSERTS: Most pareve foods are okay, but it is said that those with highly sensitive milk allergies may have a problem with the desserts in particular.

LACTOSE-FREE MILK, CHEESE, AND OTHER DAIRY PRODUCTS: Lactose free does not mean dairy free. While these products have the milk sugar (lactose) removed, they are still most likely loaded with milk fat and milk proteins.

LATEX GLOVES: Some disposable latex gloves have milk protein (casein) in them. Interestingly enough, the use of such gloves by medical professionals during skin prick testing can potentially cause false-positive reactions and hives for their patients who are allergic.

MARGARINE: There are dairy-free options, but many contain milk ingredients.

MEAL REPLACEMENT/PROTEIN POWDERS AND BEVERAGES: Whey and dried milk powder are the two most common dairy ingredients in these drinks.

MILK BEVERAGES: Occasionally, a product pops up that actually has "almondmilk" or another dairy-free milk beverage in the title, but the product contains dairy, too.

POTATO CHIPS: Be extra cautious with flavored varieties, which may harbor buttermilk, whey, or cheese powder.

PROCESSED MEATS & SAUSAGES: Some "meat allergies" are actually dairy allergies in disguise. Lactose and milk protein (caseinates) are fairly common in processed meats, and milk powder is sometimes used as filler. Even less-processed meats are not a guarantee—turkey, chicken, and other meat may have been prepared with brines or marinades containing dairy. Because kosher dietary laws do not permit milk and meat in the same meal, seeking out kosher meat may be a good option. They should be stamped with a kosher symbol, but they will not be labeled as pareve, because pareve foods cannot contain meat.

SALAD DRESSINGS: Milk components or cheese may be added for flavor or thickening power to any dressing or vinaigrette.

SAUCES: Creamy options are obvious, but milk ingredients can linger in red sauces, too. And most pesto sauces contain cheese.

SEASONING BLENDS: Premixed spice packets, like taco seasoning, sometimes contain lactose or a powdered milk ingredient.

SHERBET: This is different from sorbet, which is typically dairy free. Sherbet almost always contains some amount of milk and/or cream.

SOUP: Obviously, the creamy varieties are of concern, but even some tomato- and chicken-based soups are not dairy free.

SOY "MEAT" PRODUCTS: Veggie hot dogs, sausages, and patties may harbor milk proteins, lactose, or even cheese for flavor and texture.

SPICE MIXES: Even some simple spice mixes contain whey powder or lactose.

SUGAR SUBSTITUTES: Some sweeteners, such as tagatose, are derived from dairy foods (lactose in this case). Also, certain forms of some sugar substitutes, such as Splenda Minis and certain brands of stevia, contain lactose (in very small quantities) as a filler ingredient.

TOOTHPASTE: Recaldent is a casein-containing ingredient that is sometimes added for cavity prevention.

WAX COATING ON FRUITS & VEGETABLES: Small amounts of soy or milk protein (casein) are often added to the wax in the production process. The FDA classifies the final fruits and vegetables as "safe," and they are still considered kosher pareve by most, if not all, certifiers.

WHIPPED TOPPING: Within FDA regulations, the term *nondairy* may be utilized on some foods, such as whipped toppings and creamers, which do in fact contain casein. See page 102 for more information.

WINE: Yes, I'm sorry, but milk protein is sometimes used in the fining process of wine, which could trigger an allergic response in highly sensitive individuals. Vegan and kosher wines are a good place to start when seeking milk-free wines. Kosher certification looks at the process in addition to the ingredients, so kosher-certified wines are typically produced without milk, but they may contain eggs. For more information and links to vegan wine resources, visit **GoDairyFree.org/dairy-free-alcohol**.

CHAPTER 9
SHOPPING LIST INSPIRATIONS

It never hurts to have a few ideas in your head before embarking on a supermarket trip, particularly when you have a special diet to consider. The following is a general list of suggestions to inspire your quest for dairy-less meals. Products do vary significantly by manufacturer, so always read the label on packaged foods to ensure that the ingredients are in fact dairy free, and contact the manufacturer whenever necessary to verify manufacturing processes.

DEPARTMENTS WITH UNLIMITED POTENTIAL

Produce

Go crazy in the produce department! I couldn't even begin to create a list for this category. Fresh fruits and vegetables should always be dairy free (well, almost always—read about waxed fruit and vegetables on page 111), and the choices are endless. As a dairy-free consumer, I am a big fan of avocados for luxurious dips, potatoes for creamy soups, and apples for a classic homemade crisp. Berries, salad greens, kiwis, squash, eggplant, peppers, whatever you fancy—try a new fruit or vegetable each week!

Meat

If you do not follow a vegan diet, this department also has a great deal to offer, but go for the real stuff: unadulterated chicken, turkey, beef, pork, buffalo, etc. Try to limit purchases of hot dogs, deli meats, and other processed options, as many brands contain dairy and/or nitrites. Pork and chicken are free of hormones by law (though they may have been treated with antibiotics). However, beef may have been treated with hormones and/or antibiotics. Whenever your budget permits, opt for organic selections or those labeled as free of antibiotics and added hormones. Always check the ingredients if you are considering a marinated cut.

Seafood

The whole seafood case is open for dairy-free business: wild salmon, halibut, tuna, real crab, prawns, oysters, and more. As with meats, read the label carefully when looking for marinated seafood or processed selections, such as imitation crab meat or seafood cakes. The purveyor should have the label if it came packaged, or should know the ingredients if they made it on-site.

COOK'S CORNER

Bottled Sauces

AMERICAN TRADITION: Mustard, mayo, relish, and ketchup are almost always dairy free, although egg-free consumers may want to seek out vegan mayonnaise. I highly recommend some of the natural mayonnaises, organic ketchups, and whole-grain mustards. The quality can take your burger, or veggie burger, to the next level.

ASIAN: Most Chinese, Japanese, Vietnamese, and Thai sauces are dairy free. Teriyaki, black bean, hoisin, soy, fish, chili garlic, sweet chili, sweet and sour, and oyster sauces can be found easily in most major grocers, and are all great for stir-fries. Thai curries, satays, and peanut sauces are other tasty considerations. Many Asian sauces do contain fish, so vegans should read labels carefully or look for vegan-specific brands.

MEXICAN: Hot sauce! Need I say more? Okay, I will anyway: I also like the wide variety of milk-free enchilada sauces and salsas of the green and red varieties. Mole and chimichurri are two of the richer sauce options that tend to be dairy free.

INDIAN: Many Indian sauces use yogurt, cream, or ghee. But some, like masala, jalfrezi, vindaloo, and rogan josh, are often dairy free.

ITALIAN: Most unadulterated tomato sauces are free of milk ingredients, unless cheese or cream is in their descriptive title. Marinara and arrabbiata, in particular, are usually dairy free. And don't shy away from the specialty section; rich sauces like caponata might be found, which is usually dairy free.

SALAD DRESSINGS: Anything highly processed is likely to contain milk ingredients, but if you choose from the better-quality options, you will likely find many variations of vinaigrette, sesame, French, Thousand Island, and honey mustard salad dressings that are a go.

CHUTNEYS: Mango is the most popular, but there are other chunky flavors on the shelves—and likely all are dairy free.

BRAND SPECIFIC: There are many brand-name condiments, from pesto to barbecue sauce and gravy to creamy dressing, that are free of milk ingredients. Read the ingredient statement to unearth your own healthy finds.

General Cooking

VINEGAR: Red wine, white wine, rice wine, white, apple cider, balsamic, raspberry, malt, rice (red, brown, white, seasoned)—did I get most of them?

OIL: All plant-based oils, including grapeseed, coconut, olive, avocado, peanut, flax, you name it, are dairy free. Plus, they are ideal for cooking and baking. Just be wary of butter oil (or ghee; page 144), which is made from dairy.

HERBS & SPICES: Experiment with plain herbs and spices; the flavors can yield restaurant-quality meals. Season with cinnamon, oregano, basil, rosemary, thyme, coriander, fennel . . . I could go on all day, but I think you get the picture.

"PASTES": Miso, curry, tamarind, and wasabi are very popular flavors throughout Asia. Other specialty pastes like Tunisian harissa and Moroccan tagine can spice up meals. And simple pastes like tomato, anchovy, or those made from herbs are usually dairy free. These selections are sometimes found in the refrigerated section and other times in shelf-stable packages in the international aisles.

BRAND SPECIFIC: Seasoning packets and spice mixes frequently contain dairy, but there are usually a few dairy-free options waiting to be discovered.

Basic Pantry Stocking

BEANS (DRIED OR CANNED): All varieties of plain beans (pinto, garbanzo, butter, black, etc.) are dairy free, and many are a good source of calcium and protein.

OLIVES: Sample the many varieties, which are perfect for adding bold flavor to cheese-free meals.

COCONUT MILK: The versatility of coconut milk extends far beyond curries (although I have nothing against curries). The canned milks and creams are almost always dairy free, but keep an eye on powdered coconut milk, which often contains casein.

LENTILS: These are easily found in the bulk department, or bagged with the grains. Go with plain brown, quick-cooking red, or French green lentils for a cheap, tasty, healthy, and very filling meal.

CHILI: Most (but not all) hearty canned chilies are dairy free and will soothe any savage beast.

CANNED VEGETABLES AND FRUIT: These are good in a pinch, and most kids (and husbands) enjoy canned fruit cocktails. Personally, I would be lost without some canned pumpkin on hand. And you may be surprised to learn that most brands of cream-style corn are dairy free.

BRAND SPECIFIC: Soups come in many varieties from various manufacturers, so assess them individually. Beyond broth-based options, there are several dairy-free creamy soups available.

BAKER'S DELIGHT

Baking at Home

FLOURS: All-purpose (white) is an easy option, but try wheat, brown rice, oat, amaranth, buckwheat, quinoa, and garbanzo flours to mix things up. These nutrient-dense flours will also add unique flavors to your sauces, coatings, and baked goods.

SWEETENERS: Natural sweeteners, such as coconut sugar, molasses, agave nectar, and pure maple syrup, can be excellent options. However, most sweeteners, including cane sugar, brown sugar, dark brown sugar, evaporated cane juice, and corn syrup, are free of milk ingredients. Be wary of sugar substitutes, which may be dairy derived or could contain milk as a filler ingredient.

COCONUT: Both the sweetened and unsweetened varieties are typically good dairy-free options.

CHOCOLATE: Cocoa powder, as well as semi-sweet, dark, baking, and bittersweet chocolate (chips, chunks, etc.), should in theory be dairy free. However, a few manufacturers may slip in milk products, usually in the form of milk solids or butterfat. In addition, most chocolate is at high risk for containing trace amounts of dairy, as it shares equipment with milk chocolate production. There are a few excellent "safe" brands, though. See page 154 for more details.

BAKING AGENTS: Thickeners, starches, yeast, baking soda, and baking powder should rarely cause a problem.

PURE FLAVOR: Real vanilla, almond, anise, cinnamon, rum, and other natural extracts are dairy free. Not surprisingly, you'll want to be wary of butter extract (though it can be dairy free).

MARSHMALLOWS: Not quite nutritious, but these fluffy white sugar pillows (vegan or regular) are handy for kids' treats or holiday baking.

BRAND SPECIFIC: Baking mixes, pancake/waffle mixes, and bread crumbs are great for quick meals and treats, though many do contain dry milk ingredients.

Bakery Fresh

There is an abundance of dairy-free baked goods on the market, but no single category stands out as mostly dairy free. You will probably have luck finding sourdough bread, bagels, and tortillas without dairy. And although many bakery items contain dairy, there are usually some nondairy sandwich loaves, English muffins, pitas, and even pastries. Don't hesitate to ask the baker if you don't see a label on any goods prepared in house.

SNACK TIME!

Fresh Dips

GUACAMOLE: Thick, creamy, indulgent, and yes, it is almost always dairy free. Beware of a few brands that may mix in sour cream.

HUMMUS: This spread made the garbanzo bean famous! Most flavors are made without dairy (including dessert varieties!), though a few add cheese or other milk-based ingredients. Other bean dips are sometimes dairy free, but check the ingredients to be sure.

SALSA: Okay, this one is a given, but it is still great stuff, with so many varieties to choose from.

BRAND SPECIFIC: Ingredients in dips vary widely, but you may discover some pâtés or spreads that are free from dairy ingredients.

Spreads

NUT BUTTERS: From natural peanut to almond, cashew, and sesame seed (tahini), nut and seed butters are all the rage. Many are now spiked with honey, fruit, and savory flavors. I have even spotted a few chocolate-blended nut butters and cookie butters that would be approved as nondairy. Use them for their oil and flavor in baking; incorporate them into dips, marinades, and sauces; or spread them on your favorite bread, rice cakes, or bagels.

OTHER "BUTTERS": Pumpkin butter is my favorite, but there are many varieties, such as apple, fig, and cherry.

JAMS & JELLIES: It may be out there, but I have yet to find a jam or jelly that isn't dairy free. Go traditional with strawberry, or jazz things up with international favorites like cloudberry preserves.

HONEY: Most grocers now carry a variety of flavored honeys plus "creamed" versions, which are typically spun without dairy. Honey may not be suitable for strict vegans.

Handy Snacks

DRIED FRUIT: Dried apples, cranberries, mango, cantaloupe, figs, and even kiwis have been spotted in the bulk food section and snack aisles (for a "convenience price"). Almost any fruit can be dehydrated, and manufacturers have certainly been taking advantage of this.

FREEZE-DRIED FRUIT & VEGETABLES: These crispy, natural bites have melt-in-your-mouth appeal and can also be used in snack recipes.

NUTS: All nuts are naturally dairy free, including almonds, walnuts, cashews, pecans, and macadamias. Choose raw, roasted, salted, or unsalted, and always check flavored varieties for added ingredients.

SEEDS: Flax, pumpkin, sesame, sunflower, etc.; follow the nut guidelines above for seeds.

GELATIN: Jell-O gelatin is in fact dairy free, but not suitable for vegans. Surprisingly, most flavors of their pudding are nondairy, too. See page 390 for some tricks on how to prepare them without dairy.

APPLESAUCE: Try the regular snack packs for kids, or pick a flavored variety.

FRUIT BARS AND LEATHERS: These aren't just for kids; they are a good way to address adult-size sugar cravings, too.

POPCORN: Very few microwave brands are dairy free. Try purchasing the far more economical bag of popcorn kernels and pop it up the old-fashioned way, in a pan with a touch of oil and salt (see page 275 for some stovetop recipes). You can also buy special microwave bags to pop those regular popcorn kernels in a jiffy.

RICE CAKES: The plain varieties are always dairy free, but not all the flavored ones are.

PICKLED VEGETABLES: From old-fashioned dill pickles to spicy cocktail vegetables, these can make a nice snack or addition to a party spread.

BRAND SPECIFIC: Granola bars, snack bars, cereal bars, and energy bars abound on store shelves. Though many contain dairy, a good selection do not. In addition, several brands of trail mix, crackers, puddings, prepared popcorn, and unflavored chips (baked or fried) are also suitable for a nondairy diet.

Just Desserts

GRAHAM CRACKERS: Though many brands contain honey, which may not be suitable for strict vegans, most brands of graham crackers (including gluten-free options) are dairy free.

SANDWICH COOKIES: You might be surprised to learn that most sandwich cookies, including many varieties of Oreos, are dairy-free and vegan. Traditional chocolate, vanilla, and even many of the seasonal flavors are made without milk.

SWEET POPCORN: Though some brands may use butter, kettle corn is a traditionally dairy-free treat. Also, Cracker Jack and some generic caramel popcorn brands are surprisingly free of milk ingredients.

RAW TREATS: Raw macaroons, tarts, and "cookies" are becoming more readily available in stores, and they are almost always dairy free. You can find some brands in the middle aisles, but many are sold refrigerated.

BRAND SPECIFIC: Of course most desserts are made with dairy, but there are brands of fig bars, crunchy cookies, and even brownies that are dairy free. Plus, there are many "top allergen-free" treats now popping up on the market, from cookies to chocolate bars.

GREAT GRAINS
For Sides and Meals

WHOLE GRAINS: From bulk foods to the international aisles, all grains (without seasoning, stuffing, or sauce) are dairy free. For gluten free, reach for quinoa, amaranth, buckwheat, millet, teff, brown rice, white rice, wild rice, or certified gluten-free oats. If gluten is okay, enjoy wheat, oats, barley, couscous, rye, kamut, triticale, and spelt.

PASTA: Choose from traditional dried semolina pasta shapes, or mix things up with one of the new blends, such as spelt, wheat, or kamut noodles. Lentil, quinoa, bean, and rice noodles are great gluten-free options. Other Asian noodles, like soba, udon, ramen, and lo mein, typically use wheat, but are also dairy free.

POLENTA: Seek out "chubs" of premade polenta that look like they should be refrigerated but are in fact shelf-stable. These are usually dairy free and packaged conveniently for "slice and heat" preparation.

BRAND SPECIFIC: Pre-seasoned, ready-to-cook pasta and rice dishes are a nice shortcut, and some options are made without dairy. Likewise, the potato-pasta hybrids known as gnocchi are delicious, and sometimes free of milk and cheese ingredients.

Cereal Aisle

HOT CEREALS: Those big tubs of oats are a healthy and very cheap breakfast option. The unflavored "cream of" (wheat, rice, whatever) hot cereals are also good choices. When you start looking at pre-flavored varieties, double-check the ingredients.

BRAND SPECIFIC: Cold cereal options are numerous; however, the ingredients do vary widely by brand.

KEEP IT COOL

Dairy Case

EGGS: Although they are located in the "dairy case," eggs come from chickens and are not related to milk. See page 6 for more information.

MILK BEVERAGES: Almond, coconut, soy, cashew, and rice milk beverages are often found in quart- or half-gallon-size containers in the refrigerated section. However, many brands can also be found in smaller shelf-stable packages in the middle aisles.

OTHER DAIRY ALTERNATIVES: Dairy-free options for replacing yogurt, butter, cheese, and creamer are becoming readily available and typically sit next to their dairy counterparts in the refrigerated section of grocers. Use caution, as dairy-based and lactose-free products may be intertwined with the dairy-free versions.

Vegan Options

TOFU: Soft, firm, extra firm, silken, pre-baked, lightly fried, dessert style . . . there are so many choices and an abundance of ways to use them in cooking, smoothies, and baking.

TEMPEH: This can be used like tofu in many savory recipes, but is fermented, firmer, and much more rustic in taste and texture. Many versions use grains or other nutritious add-ins.

BRAND SPECIFIC: There are many "meatless meats" and veggie burgers on the market, but several do contain casein, lactose, or straight-up cheese. Look for the options specifically labeled as "vegan."

Fresh Pasta

ASIAN STYLE: Won ton and gyoza wrappers, rice paper, and spring roll pastry are becoming more readily available. Some do contain eggs, but if you search around, a few vegan options will likely appear.

"UN-STUFFED": Fresh linguini or angel hair is always a deserved treat, but these do typically contain eggs.

GLUTEN-FREE ALTERNATIVES: Shirataki, kelp, and soy noodles are usually dairy free and vegan, and offer a nutritious way to experiment with new pasta flavors and textures.

BRAND SPECIFIC: Though many are cheese stuffed, dairy-free ravioli and pierogi can be found.

The Deep Freeze

DAIRY-FREE FROZEN DESSERTS: You may be shocked by the array of brands and flavors now available, from ice cream bars to an abundance of pints to full desserts. Coconut, almond, and cashew are the most popular bases for making dairy-free ice cream products, but soy, rice, fruit, or other bases may be used.

100 PERCENT JUICE BARS & SORBETS: These fruit-based desserts are naturally dairy free and oh so refreshing.

FROZEN FRUIT: A fantastic option for homemade smoothies, baking, or a cool snack.

FROZEN VEGETABLES: What a great invention, nicely chopped-up vegetables ready for cooking with or without defrosting. Be aware, there are some "creamed" varieties out there, which most likely contain dairy.

ASIAN MEALS: Check the labels, but thus far all of the frozen won tons, gyozas, and egg rolls (except for the Mexican-flavored ones) without sauce that I have spotted in the freezer section have been nondairy. For a healthy twist, try steaming gyozas and dumplings, boiling won tons in soup, or baking egg rolls with a brush of heart-healthy oil.

BRAND SPECIFIC: If you are a convenience lover, then you are still in luck. Numerous nondairy frozen entrées are available these days. Yes, there are even dairy-free pizzas!

THIRST QUENCHERS

JUICE: Juice is quick, hydrating, and often nutritious, especially the 100 percent pure and fresh-squeezed varieties. The selection is growing, so you might be able to choose from orange, pomegranate, pineapple, blueberry, carrot, cherry, and more.

BOTTLED WATER: Just a reminder in case your tap water is undesirable.

MILK BEVERAGES: In addition to the refrigerated varieties, smaller, shelf-stable packages are also available, with some brands and flavors sold in single-serve boxes.

TEA: Herbal teas are the most hydrating, and so many varieties are available, but white, green, and black teas are also pleasant dairy-free options.

COFFEE: Another naturally dairy-free beverage. Be cautious of coffee beverages: Though there are dairy-free varieties, many include milk-based ingredients.

BRAND SPECIFIC: When you are short on time and need a little extra energy, there are some packaged meal replacement beverages, energy drinks, and smoothies that are free of milk products.

PREPARED FOODS

Unless you are dealing with very sensitive food allergies, you need not write off the convenience deli. Look around; most grocers list the ingredients on the packaging or on a label near the foods. You might also seek out a natural food grocer that specializes in various diet requirements. Those with severe food allergies should note that deli departments are at high risk for cross-contamination due to the use of shared equipment (i.e., that multi-purpose cheese/meat/vegetable slicer).

SHOPPING RESOURCES

PRODUCT LISTINGS: I regularly update the review section of Go Dairy Free with product options of all types. To view, visit **GoDairyFree.org/product-reviews**.

QUICK LIST: For my everyday shopping list in a printable format, visit **GoDairyFree.org/news/dairy-free-shopping-list**.

BRANDS USED: For a listing of the brands used to test the recipes in this book, visit **GoDairyFree.org/gdf-brands**.

CHAPTER 10
GROCERY TIPS

Let's cut to the chase: I am frugal. I make it a point to buy the best quality possible, but I loathe paying too much for anything. Therefore, my collection of tips focuses on money-saving ideas and maximizing quality for a pocketbook-friendly yet delicious, dairy-free transition.

DON'T FORGET THE BASICS. My first instinct when I began to cook strictly dairy free was to find recipes created specifically for "free-from" diets. These are helpful, but I completely overlooked the simple dishes that I loved as a kid, and that are traditionally, without substitutions, dairy free. Meals such as Spanish rice, spaghetti, and chili are now weekly staples in our home, and each dish is so versatile that I can add whatever we have in the pantry.

DON'T THINK ABOUT WHAT IT IS, THINK ABOUT WHAT IT COULD BE. Dairy-free experimentation helped me unlock the potential of the produce department. When I see a good deal on cauliflower, I don't think about how my husband loathes this cruciferous vegetable. Instead, I imagine how much he will love the creamy soup I will make with it as the base (recipes on page 293 and page 349). Likewise, an abundance of in-season (and consequently cheap) zucchini prompts several loaves of his favorite zucchini bread (page 252).

VENTURE TO INTERNATIONAL MARKETS. Coconut milk and rice noodles are over $2 at my local grocery store, yet a quick trip the Asian market almost always yields these ingredients for half that, or even less. Likewise, tortillas at my neighborhood Mexican market and tahini from my local Middle Eastern food dealer are more affordable—and seem to be more authentic in taste. Moreover, most countries tend to rely less on dairy products than Western nations, resulting in specialty markets filled with interesting dairy-free options.

REACH FOR BOLD ACCENT FLAVORS. Cooking without the fatty tastes of cream, cheese, and butter means that I get to compensate in other areas, like flavor, to keep meals interesting. I splurge on spices, sun-dried tomatoes, miso, olives, Asian seasonings, and curry pastes. Luckily, a little goes a long way when it comes to these powerful additives, so even though they are more costly upfront, one package typically lasts for quite a while.

KEEP AN EYE ON ORGANIC. Yes, I am a penny-pincher, I swear, but I have a few great reasons (beyond the obvious) to consider organic foods. First, you may be surprised to learn that they are sometimes cheaper than their conventional counterparts, if not pretty close in price. Secondly, many organic packaged foods (but definitely not all) seem to be free of dairy. It is my theory that some organic manufacturers skip milk ingredients whenever possible as the organic versions tend to be very expensive. Be sure to check the label, though, as a few extravagant companies will undoubtedly splurge on organic dairy. Finally, "surprise" dairy ingredients are less likely to pop up, since organic food labels are usually easy to read and tend to contain mostly whole food ingredients.

DON'T RELY ON MAINSTREAM GROCERS FOR SPECIALTY PRODUCTS. Many of the "big guys" have added beautifully manicured natural food sections, and are consequently charging an arm and a leg for those "upscale" products. In most cases, it is actually cheaper to shop on the manufacturer's website or at a natural food store. However, I always do a quick cruise through those specialty aisles whenever we visit our local mega-grocer. Because their natural food sections are seldom popular, I occasionally strike gold with closeout items. I once scored 3 pounds of nutritional yeast (the most enormous bag you have ever seen) for less than $9.

LOOK FOR THE VEGAN LABEL. By definition, the vegan diet is free from all animal products, including dairy in all of its forms. While some products may be at risk for cross-contamination in manufacturing (always check!), the word *vegan* stamped on a food label gives you a good head start to finding some suitable dairy-free products.

CONSIDER HOMEMADE "MILK." Because of the rapid expansion in dairy-free options, milk beverages have become quite affordable in recent years. That said, making your own can be even less expensive. See chapters 12 and 16 for more information and recipes.

BUY TIMELY PRODUCE. When in season, produce is typically at its peak of quality and abundance, and harvested relatively nearby, rather than traveling thousands of miles before reaching your plate. Less transportation and greater availability equals a good price. Adjust your menu with the seasons and your grocery budget will thank you. For those items you must have year-round, find a reliable store with fair prices.

GO FOR WHOLE FOODS. As a rule of thumb, healthier processed food almost always costs more and contains less nutrients than fresh, whole foods.

SUPPORT LOCAL FARMERS. Great prices and fresh food abound at farmers' markets, where you can usually find everything from just-out-of-the-ground vegetables to free-range meats and local honey. Also, don't forget to visit local u-pick farms for a fun afternoon activity and bushels of inexpensive fruit.

CONSIDER MEAL HELPERS RATHER THAN COMPLETE MEALS. Obviously, making everything from scratch isn't feasible for everyone. I like to buy helpers that make cooking easier but don't break the budget, rather than buying the complete meal (i.e., frozen dinners). Soups and chili are wonderful for this. Pour them over rice or other grains and include your own add-ins (vegetables, last night's chicken, etc.) for a quick and nutritious meal.

GET THE MOST FOR YOUR MONEY. To save money and preserve quality, I rarely purchase lite canned coconut milk. It often contains additives, and is essentially regular coconut milk thinned with water. When I need 1 cup of a lite version, I simply use ¼ cup regular coconut milk plus ¾ cup water. For a slightly richer version, I increase the coconut milk to ⅓ cup and reduce the water to ⅔ cup. In essence, I get three to four cans of lite coconut milk for the price of one. How's that for a good deal?

FREEZE INGREDIENTS, NOT LEFTOVERS. Having all the necessary components ready to go in the freezer is a recipe for easy meals that are healthier than frozen entrées. Not to mention, you can stock up on frequently used foods when they go on sale. You may choose to purchase the ingredients frozen, or buy fresh and freeze them yourself. Some foods that freeze well include fruit (berries, mango, bananas, peaches, etc.), many vegetables (broccoli, spinach, green beans, corn, peas, etc.), ground flaxseed, ground nuts (in flour or "butter" form), won ton or gyoza wrappers, and filo pastry.

BULK UP. I scoop giant bags of organic rolled oats in the bulk foods section for a fraction of the cost I would pay for non-organic packaged oats. Spices and specialty grains are also excellent foods to purchase in bulk. If you do get hooked on bulk, make sure the bags are labeled to help tell those seeds and grains apart. But skip the bulk section if potential cross-contamination is a concern for you. And before you go wild filling your pantry with bags of bulk items, check the prices. There are many items, such as quinoa, that I often find for a cheaper price pre-packaged, even at Whole Foods! It is not uncommon for retailers to mark larger packages or bulk foods for a higher per-ounce price than smaller packages; deceptive, but true.

BROWSE ONLINE. Here's good news for those of you who can't find many dairy-free foods locally: There are numerous online retailers to order from! Purchasing online is often cheaper, too, but shop around as prices can vary widely. Also, keep shipping costs in mind. Many retailers will waive the shipping fee with a minimum purchase, so it's good to keep a running shopping list to make larger online orders all at once. For a list of online grocery retailers that carry dairy-free goods, see my online shopping guide at **GoDairyFree.org/ online-retailers.**

COUPONS! Yes, they do exist, even for specialty items. While you may occasionally spot soymilk discounts in your local paper, some of the best discounts are offered directly from the manufacturers themselves. I sign up for e-newsletters from all of my favorite manufacturers in order to receive coupons and other discount offers. Many natural food stores also provide coupon books at the store entrance, customized for their own offerings. For links to some great natural food coupon sites, visit **GoDairyFree.org/coupons.**

CHAPTER 11
THE WELL-EQUIPPED KITCHEN

Having a good supply of kitchen tools can be quite fun, but I think many of the small appliances out there are simply overkill. Here are the only small appliances and tools that I regularly use, plus a list of helpful gadgets that might fit your lifestyle. To see all of the kitchen tool brands that I'm currently recommending, visit **GoDairyFree.org/kitchen-tools**.

MY NECESSITIES

These are items that perhaps I could live without, but I really wouldn't want to. Each of these inexpensive appliances gets some use in my kitchen every week.

BLENDER: This handy gadget is the key to creating dairy-free creaminess. Although many bloggers will tell you that investing in a high-end, expensive blender is a must, I'm in the other camp. I do recommend getting a blender with both a full-size jar and personal-size cups, and corresponding blades. The smaller cups are great for making smoothies and can stand in as a mini food processor in a pinch. A high-speed blender can also be helpful, but it need not be a top-end model. I used a mid-range blender with attachments to create all of the recipes in this book, and it was less than $100 on sale during the holidays. If that is out of your budget, then a personal-size blender and spice grinder combo will also work great.

SPICE/COFFEE GRINDER: Since we are a household of two, I find that my spice grinder does just about everything I would need a food processor for, and with insanely quick cleanup. Of course, I use it to grind down cumin seeds and coffee beans. But it also works in a pinch to grind flax seeds for a nutritious recipe boost, to grind nuts (even into nut butter), and to make oat flour in an instant from my supply of whole oats. Some may dislike doing things in batches, but since I can make ⅓ cup oat flour in 30 seconds of whirling with a quick "wipe it out with a dry paper towel" cleanup, 1 cup is easily ready with my workspace clean in less than five minutes. A spice grinder with a personal-size blender attachment can be had for less than $30. But keep in mind that you will be rewarded with better grinding and blending power if you select a model that has 150 watts or more.

HAND MIXER: Want some nice toned arms? Skip the clunky stand mixer and go for a cheapo hand mixer. Don't think for a minute that these don't pack enough power; mine is in fact a little *too* turbocharged. Just make sure you pick out one that has a good range from low to high in power. I actually mix most things up by hand, but for whipping and creaming, a trusty little mixer is quite useful, and can be taken out and put away with ease.

ICE CREAM MAKER: If you really love ice cream, then do consider purchasing an ice cream maker. These gadgets allow you to whip up your own dairy-free frozen desserts from coconut milk, nuts, fruit, and other everyday ingredients. There are fancy models, but

I've purchased two ice cream makers on sale for $15 and both worked quite well. The first lasted for about five years before burning out and the new one is still going strong. The only caveat with cheap and mid-range ice cream makers is that you do have to plan ahead; the bowl requires overnight chilling before you can process the ice cream.

NUT MILK BAG: These washable nylon mesh bags create the dreamiest homemade milk beverages and can also be used for fine straining in other recipes. The cost for a good one is equivalent to buying about two packages of cheesecloth, but it will last for many more recipes and produce much cleaner results.

LITTLE LUXURIES

These aren't tools that I currently use, but I can admit to their usefulness depending on the size of your household and the types of foods that you regularly make.

FOOD PROCESSOR: I confess, food processors are quite useful, considering you can do anything from chopping to pureeing with the simple push of a button. Shopping for food processors can be overwhelming, though. Power, reliability, versatility, size, and ease of cleaning are all important factors to consider; higher-end models are often worth the splurge. Be sure to read reviews before investing in a food processor.

IMMERSION BLENDER: This handheld tool allows you to puree foods right in the pot or bowl and is a dream for making creamy soups. It skips the step of having to transfer the soup to a blender in batches, cutting out mess and the concern of handling and blending hot liquids.

YOGURT MAKER: If you are a true yogi, then this may be a good purchase. You can assemble your own yogurt-making setup at home, but yogurt makers are a nice, inexpensive, and clean way to get the job done.

BREAD MAKER: This once-trendy item can sit unused on the shelf, but dairy-free living may give you some extra motivation to dust it off. So many retail breads contain dairy that I find it easier (and tastier) to make my own at home. If you are a serious bread connoisseur (or your little ones devour two loaves a week), then this is definitely a nice piece of equipment to have.

SECTION 4

ALL YOU EVER WANTED TO KNOW ABOUT DAIRY SUBSTITUTES

CHAPTER 12
DISCOVERING THE MILKY WAY

Dairy-free milk alternatives have come a long way in the past decade. When I wrote the first edition of this book, the average grocery store carried a single variety of soymilk at best. But today, hundreds of dairy-free milk beverages are spilling over on store shelves, edging out dairy milk for prime retail space. In fact, the dairy industry has become so threatened that they've lobbied against these dairy-free beverages using the word *milk* in their names at all.

But it's important to note that not all "milks" are created equal. This chapter offers important information on nutrients, uses, taste profiles, and more.

MILK BEVERAGE KNOWLEDGE & TIPS

Over the years, I've gathered some wisdom about milk beverages that I think will be helpful for many of you.

Yes, They're Dairy Free

To the best of my knowledge, all of the nondairy milk beverages currently on the market are made without any milk ingredients (lactose or casein) whatsoever. In past years, a couple of brands attempted to add milk protein to some of their beverages. But they were met with such backlash for their odd ingredient choice that they did eventually remove the dairy from their products.

However, it isn't uncommon for dairy-free milk beverages to be processed or packaged on shared lines with dairy milk or in the same facility. Dairy-free milk beverages and dairy milk are both fluid products that require similar machinery and packaging. So in many cases, the same equipment or production center is used to save money or when other resources aren't available.

Nevertheless, strict allergen protocols are typically followed in the manufacture of dairy-free milk alternatives. And with fluid products, equipment is relatively efficient to clean between batches. Unlike powdered or sticky substances, milk isn't as likely to get "caught" in crevices. And there is also little risk of fluid milk making its way to dedicated dairy-free lines in other parts of the facility.

But of course, always read the ingredients to ensure that the product is made without dairy ingredients. And if a severe milk allergy is a concern for you, it's essential to always contact the manufacturer about their ingredients and processes, and decide if you feel they are "safe" for your needs.

In Fact, They Fit Many Dietary Needs

Dairy-free milk beverages also tend to be plant based and vegan, which means they are also cholesterol free. Most options are also gluten free, and many top food allergy–friendly milk beverages now exist.

In the past, soy caused a great deal of consumer concern in the dairy-free milk beverage category. But most varieties (aside from soymilk) now use ingredients like sunflower lecithin and rice bran oil to cut out every trace of soy. And it's rare to find a soymilk brand that isn't made with organic or non-GMO soy.

Beyond whole food concerns, the different brands hold an array of nutritional benefits. Some are close to homemade, with little to no additives and more of the natural nutrition from the base ingredients. Mainstream brands with a more refined consistency tend to contain less of the core ingredient but are often fortified with protein, calcium, vitamin D, vitamin B12, and other micronutrients to rival or even exceed the levels of cow's milk.

You're Naturally Drinking Less Sugar

Although plain and unsweetened varieties of dairy-free milk beverages typically taste a bit sweeter than cow's milk, most are amazingly lower in sugar. Low-fat or skim cow's milk has a whopping 12 to 16 grams of sugar per 1 cup serving! It's naturally high in lactose, the sugar that is known for upsetting stomachs worldwide.

Unsweetened varieties of dairy-free milk beverage usually have 0 grams of sugar per 1 cup serving. And even plain or "original" varieties usually have only 3 to 7 grams of sugar. However, some sweetened varieties can have a much higher level of added sugars, so be sure to keep an eye on the nutrition facts.

When Shopping, Look Around

Dairy-free milk beverages are sold in both refrigerated cartons and shelf-stable aseptic packages. The refrigerated versions must be kept chilled at all times, and can often be found in the dairy case or in their own dairy-free refrigerated section. The shelf-stable packages are usually clustered together in a middle aisle of the store, often near the cereals. They can be stored in your pantry, but once opened, they must be refrigerated.

Both the refrigerated and the aseptic packages tend to have a relatively generous shelf life, but once opened and refrigerated, they should be used up within a week or so.

Don't Forget to Shake Things Up

I mean this literally and figuratively.

Yes, it is true that ingredients in dairy-free milk beverages can settle. And there is nothing worse than dousing your cereal in chunky almond water, trust me. Give that package a quick shake (use caution, as the tops of some packages can leak when you shake them), pour, and enjoy the creamy consistency. This will also help disperse any fortified vitamins and minerals.

With store-bought varieties, you may need to shake the package only once or twice during the life of the carton. But with homemade milk beverages, you will need to shake or stir before each use.

And dairy-free milk beverages come in so many varieties that I recommend sampling as many options as possible. Each one has different flavor and consistency nuances, and brands can vary greatly in terms of ingredients and nutrition facts. Don't settle on one type immediately or banish dairy-free milk beverages just because the first ones didn't delight. Try new types and flavors as you see them on sale or by using the recipes in the Milking Plants chapter (starting on page 176).

Ultimately, It's Usually an Even Swap

Dairy-free milk beverage definitely isn't identical to cow's milk. But unsweetened varieties can be substituted 1:1 for low-fat or nonfat dairy milk in *most* recipes. For example, if a recipe simply calls for 1 cup of milk, you can substitute 1 cup of unsweetened almond milk beverage or other unsweetened dairy-free milk beverage. But it is important to consider the consistency and flavor profile of the milk beverage as it relates to your recipe.

I specified low-fat and nonfat milk above, because if your recipe goes so far as to name whole milk, then you may need a little more fat in the recipe. For whole milk, I have a few suggestions (this again is for a 1:1 ratio):

- If a mild coconut influence will work with the recipe, then try using lite coconut milk. It has just a touch more fat than your typical carton of whole milk.
- Try pureed soft silken tofu. It is just a bit higher in fat than soymilk, and it offers a thicker consistency.
- Whip up a quick batch of homemade milk beverage (recipes starting on page 177), but start with just 3 cups of water and add more, if needed, to get a whole milk consistency.
- Add a smidgen of oil to the recipe. Just a teaspoon or two whipped into the milk alternative should boost the richness of the dish to the level intended.

There are a few other situations where milk beverage isn't a perfect substitute. When making Jell-O pudding, for example, you must use one of my methods on page 390, or it most likely won't set up. Also, sweetened or naturally sweet milk beverages can make savory dishes taste "off," and milk beverages with a more pronounced taste, like hemp, can easily overpower in more delicate recipes. Protein-enriched milk beverages can also thicken oddly when heated.

THE ULTIMATE GUIDE TO DAIRY-FREE MILK BEVERAGES

I tested **twenty-five different types** of dairy-free milk beverages for you, and have summarized my top findings in this information-rich section.

The following information is based on pure plant-based milks that I made from scratch and experimented with at home. It does not reflect store-bought brands, which can contain varying levels of thickeners, emulsifiers, and fortification.

Most store-bought brands tend to have fewer natural phytonutrients and macronutrients, like fats, fiber, and protein, than homemade versions. This is because they use less of the primary ingredient and more additives to provide a very fluid "retail-friendly" consistency. However, many brands are fortified and may therefore contain more micronutrients, like calcium, vitamin D, and vitamin B12. Nonetheless, fresh blends from your kitchen, or very natural packaged brands, all contain their own array of micronutrients, depending on the base ingredients used.

I will discuss nutritional details and many other properties of pure dairy-free milk beverages in the pages that follow. They are listed in alphabetical order. For more tips and easy homemade recipes, see the Milking Plants chapter starting on page 176.

Almond Milk Beverage

TASTING NOTES: Mildly sweet, nutty, light but creamy mouthfeel, just a hint of astringency

COST PER QUART: $1.66 (based on $5.99/pound for almonds)

PREPARATION METHOD: Almonds are soaked, blended with water, and strained.

YIELD: 4½ to 5 cups milk beverage per 1 cup almonds

INGREDIENT USAGE: Expect 30 to 40 percent leftover fibrous pulp; none left over with INSTANT MYLK (page 178).

NUTRITION MERITS: Monounsaturated fats, protein, calcium, magnesium, manganese, copper, phosphorus, vitamin E, biotin, riboflavin

RECIPES: PURE NUT MYLK (page 177), INSTANT MYLK (page 178), NICE NUT CREAMER (page 188)

SUMMARY: Almond milk beverage is one of my top picks for homemade options. It has a very pleasing, versatile flavor and a reliable creaminess, and almonds are one of the most affordable nuts. It works beautifully in coffee or tea, is great over cereal or in smoothies, and can be used in most recipes. But its lightly nutty flavor profile should be kept in mind. Almonds with the skins on will produce a deeper, slightly more astringent, and less nutty flavor, but the skins are said to be high in flavonoids.

Brazil Nut Milk Beverage

TASTING NOTES: Full-bodied warm and earthy flavor, relatively creamy, light astringency, very slight powdery finish

COST PER QUART: $3.16 (based on $11.99/pound for Brazil nuts)

PREPARATION METHOD: Shelled Brazil nuts are soaked, blended with water, and strained.

YIELD: 5 cups milk beverage per 1 cup Brazil nuts

INGREDIENT USAGE: Expect 30 to 40 percent fibrous leftover pulp; none left over with INSTANT MYLK (page 178).

NUTRITION MERITS: Selenium (top source), copper, phosphorus, magnesium, manganese

RECIPES: PURE NUT MYLK (page 177), INSTANT MYLK (page 178)

SUMMARY: The thin skins on these nuts are very difficult to peel, but they are usually sparse, so they don't affect the flavor dramatically. It doesn't curdle or quickly separate, giving it potential in coffee or tea. But the flavor balance didn't wow, and it is a relatively expensive option.

Cashew Milk Beverage

TASTING NOTES: Rich, creamy, full-bodied mouthfeel and flavor, underlying light sweetness, surprisingly nutty and a touch earthy

COST PER QUART: $2.25 (based on $8.99/pound for cashews)

PREPARATION METHOD: Cashews are soaked, blended with water, and strained.

YIELD: 4½ to 5 cups milk beverage per 1 cup cashews

INGREDIENT USAGE: Expect 50 percent leftover fibrous pulp; none left over with INSTANT MYLK (page 178).

NUTRITION MERITS: Monounsaturated fats, protein, vitamin K, iron, magnesium, phosphorus, copper, zinc, manganese; cashews are also fairly high in magnesium

RECIPES: PURE NUT MYLK (page 177), INSTANT MYLK (page 178)

SUMMARY: One of the creamiest nut options, cashew milk beverage is quite versatile. Although I prefer the flavor profile of almonds in tea or coffee, it's pretty good in hot beverages and doesn't tend to curdle or separate. It also melds well in savory sauces, baked goods, and desserts. For better results with inexpensive but starchier milk beverages, like rice or oat, you can swap in part cashews.

Coconut Milk Beverage

TASTING NOTES: Very smooth and creamy, rich mouthfeel, lightly sweet flavor

COST PER QUART: $1.04 (based on $6.99/pound for unsweetened shredded coconut)

PREPARATION METHOD: Coconut shreds are blended with warm water and strained.

YIELD: 4¾ cups milk beverage per 1 cup unsweetened shredded coconut

INGREDIENT USAGE: Expect 50 percent very dry, fibrous leftover pulp.

NUTRITION MERITS: Manganese, medium-chain triglycerides (MCT) fatty acids, lauric acid

RECIPES: QUICK COCONUT MILK BEVERAGE (page 183)

SUMMARY: This was one of the smoothest and creamiest homemade milk beverages that I tested, with a lightly sweet flavor and relatively rich mouthfeel. It works well in tea and coffee, with a pleasant richness and creamy finish that doesn't quickly separate. It also offers great versatility for use in both sweet and savory applications, but for some people the coconut hints may shine through too much if not paired properly.

Hazelnut Milk Beverage

TASTING NOTES: Boldly flavored, nutty, rich, lightly creamy, only slightly astringent

COST PER QUART: $3.33 (based on $11.99/pound for hazelnuts)

PREPARATION METHOD: Hazelnuts are soaked, blended with water, and strained.

YIELD: 4½ cups milk beverage per 1 cup hazelnuts

INGREDIENT USAGE: Expect 50 percent fibrous leftover pulp; none left over with INSTANT MYLK (page 178).

NUTRITION MERITS: Vitamin E, monounsaturated fats, manganese, copper, magnesium, flavonoids (like quercetin)

RECIPES: PURE NUT MYLK (page 177), INSTANT MYLK (page 178)

SUMMARY: Hazelnut milk beverage begs for coffee. It provides a similar creaminess to many other nuts, but its pronounced flavor must be paired carefully. Use it in combination with chocolate, in smoothies, in baked goods, over cereal, or in desserts where its nutty notes will be welcome.

Hemp Milk Beverage

TASTING NOTES: Clean but grassy, relatively creamy, slight powdery finish, a touch astringent

COST PER QUART: $3.55 (based on $9.99/pound for shelled hemp seeds)

PREPARATION METHOD: Shelled hemp seeds are blended with water and strained.

YIELD: 4 cups milk beverage per 1 cup hemp seeds

INGREDIENT USAGE: Expect just 10 to 20 percent leftover fibrous pulp.

NUTRITION MERITS: Omega-3 fatty acids, gamma linolenic acid (GLA), magnesium, manganese, potassium, zinc, iron, thiamine, riboflavin, complete plant protein

RECIPES: HEALTHY HEMP MYLK (page 180), HAPPY HEMP CREAMER (page 188)

SUMMARY: Store-bought hemp milk failed to win me over, but something about the raw, natural taste and creamy finish of homemade hemp milk beverage intrigues my taste buds. Though pronounced in flavor, it's excellent in coffee or tea. It doesn't curdle and has a nice full-body finish. I also like it in other "earthy" applications, like smoothies, cereal, and bread.

Macadamia Milk Beverage

TASTING NOTES: Creamy but surprisingly light and fresh, mild flavor, gentle nutty notes

COST PER QUART: $3.75 (based on $14.99/pound for macadamia nuts)

PREPARATION METHOD: Macadamia nuts are soaked, blended with water, and strained.

YIELD: 4 cups milk beverage per 1 cup macadamia nuts

INGREDIENT USAGE: Expect 50 percent fibrous leftover pulp; none left over with INSTANT MYLK (page 178).

NUTRITION MERITS: Omega-9 fatty acids, manganese, copper, thiamine

RECIPES: PURE NUT MYLK (page 177), INSTANT MYLK (page 178)

SUMMARY: Precious macadamia nuts aren't the most economical base for homemade milk beverage. It is good in coffee or tea, with no curdling or separating, and has a relatively mellow flavor that offers good potential for sweet and savory applications. However, it wasn't as rich as expected, and I didn't think it offered quite enough "wow factor" to warrant the high price.

Oat Milk Beverage

TASTING NOTES: Light, rustic, powdery finish, watery (added oil helps create a milky consistency)

COST PER QUART: $0.40 (based on $1.99/pound for rolled oats)

PREPARATION METHOD: Rolled or quick oats are rinsed, toasted, and blended with water and a little oil.

YIELD: 4 cups milk beverage per 1 cup rolled oats

INGREDIENT USAGE: Expect just 20 percent leftover oat roughage.

NUTRITION MERITS: Lean protein, thiamine, manganese, magnesium, phosphorus, copper, biotin, zinc, unique antioxidants (avenanthramides), beta glucan fiber

RECIPES: UNASSUMING OAT MYLK (page 185)

SUMMARY: Oats are inexpensive, easy to find, and generally considered healthy, but they aren't the best base for milk beverage. I trialed many preparation methods, and the best way was also one of the simplest. But it's still impossible to override the very fibrous, starchy composition that makes oats special. I recommend making oat milk beverage in small batches and using it immediately, as it doesn't store well. It is pretty good in smoothies and cereal, but it does best in other applications where a little extra starch won't hurt. I don't recommend it in hot beverages, as it adds very little body and isn't a great flavor match.

Peanut Milk Beverage

TASTING NOTES: Earthy, mild but bright peanut taste, just lightly creamy, slightly astringent with a lightly powdery finish
COST PER QUART: $0.87 (based on $2.99/pound for shelled blanched peanuts)
PREPARATION METHOD: Shelled peanuts are soaked, blended with water, and strained.
YIELD: 4½ cups milk beverage per 1 cup shelled peanuts
INGREDIENT USAGE: Expect 30 to 50 percent fibrous leftover pulp; none left over with INSTANT MYLK (page 178).
NUTRITION MERITS: Vitamin E, thiamine, niacin, protein, folate, magnesium, phosphorus, copper, manganese, omega-9 fatty acids, flavonoids (like resveratrol)
RECIPES: PURE NUT MYLK (page 177), INSTANT MYLK (page 178)

SUMMARY: Rumor has it that peanut milk is on the retail horizon, and I can see why. Though not quite perfect on the creamy consistency front, it has a bright, beloved flavor that adores salt and sweetener. And did you see the cost? It's very inexpensive, relatively good in coffee or tea, and can add flair to smoothies and cereals. It should also work well in sweet and savory recipes, as long as the somewhat pronounced peanut taste is a good flavor match.

Pecan Milk Beverage

TASTING NOTES: Pleasant nutty undertones, quite astringent, only mildly creamy
COST PER QUART: $2.65 (based on $11.99/pound for shelled pecans)
PREPARATION METHOD: Shelled pecans are soaked, blended with water, and strained.
YIELD: 4 cups milk beverage per 1 cup shelled pecans
NUTRITION MERITS: Thiamine, copper, manganese, monounsaturated fats
INGREDIENT USAGE: Expect 50 percent fibrous leftover pulp.
RECIPES: PURE NUT MYLK (page 177)

SUMMARY: This milk beverage has a wonderful fragrance and a flavor that loves maple syrup. It doesn't curdle, but it also tends to separate and doesn't emulsify and cream as well as many other bases. For this reason, I preferred it with less water (about 3½ cups) to up the creaminess and make it more fulfilling in smoothies or cereals. I don't recommend it in coffee or tea due to the astringent flavor and lack of body.

Pine Nut Milk Beverage

TASTING NOTES: Creamy, rich, nutty, smooth finish, very slight astringency

COST PER QUART: $4.16 (based on $18.99/pound for pine nuts)

PREPARATION METHOD: Pine nuts are briefly soaked, blended with water, and strained.

YIELD: 5½ cups milk beverage per 1 cup pine nuts

INGREDIENT USAGE: Expect about 20 percent fibrous leftover pulp.

NUTRITION MERITS: Vitamin E, vitamin K, phosphorus, magnesium, zinc, copper, manganese

RECIPES: PURE NUT MYLK (page 177)

SUMMARY: These little nuggets of gold do offer a touch of luxury over most other milk beverage bases. Their high oil content creates a very creamy consistency that's fantastic for savory sauces and offers good body in coffee and tea. The addictively nutty flavor is relatively seamless in many applications, but the high price keeps this milk beverage from being an everyday staple.

Pistachio Milk Beverage

TASTING NOTES: A little sweet, very nutty, intense but not overpowering, creamy, light powdery and astringent finish

COST PER QUART: $4.15 (based on $16.99/pound for shelled pistachios)

PREPARATION METHOD: Shelled pistachio nuts are soaked, blended, and strained.

YIELD: 4½ cups milk beverage per 1 cup shelled pistachio nuts

INGREDIENT USAGE: Expect 40 to 50 percent fibrous leftover pulp; none left over with INSTANT MYLK (page 178).

NUTRITION MERITS: Thiamine, vitamin B6, phosphorus, copper, manganese, lutein, protein

RECIPES: PURE NUT MYLK (page 177), INSTANT MYLK (page 178)

SUMMARY: The fun and somewhat boisterous flavor of pistachio milk beverage has an undying love for honey. I think it is best in baked goods or sweet applications that aren't too delicate. It doesn't curdle in hot beverages, but the bold flavor didn't play very nicely with coffee or tea.

Potato Milk Beverage

TASTING NOTES: Starchy, slight gelatinous mouthfeel, pronounced potato flavor

COST PER QUART: $0.45 (based on $0.99/pound for potatoes)

PREPARATION METHOD: Peeled and cooked potatoes are mashed and blended with water and oil.

YIELD: 5 cups milk beverage per 1 cup plain mashed potato

INGREDIENT USAGE: All

NUTRITION MERITS: Vitamin B6, potassium, copper, vitamin C, kukoamines (potential blood pressure–lowering compounds)

RECIPES: TWO-POTATO MYLK (page 183)

SUMMARY: Potato milk beverage has been a top request over the years, but on its own, it isn't stellar. It's very watery and lacks body. To give it a milky consistency a little oil is a must, but this still doesn't override the very potato-y flavor. Nonetheless, potato milk beverage or even just mashed potatoes can be used in savory sauces and soups for a creamier edge that blends well.

Pumpkin Seed Milk Beverage

TASTING NOTES: Light but semi-rich mouthfeel, mild seedy flavor, slightly bitter
COST PER QUART: $2.15 (based on $6.99/pound for shelled pumpkin seeds)
PREPARATION METHOD: Shelled pumpkin seeds are soaked, blended, and strained.
YIELD: 4 cups milk beverage per 1 cup pumpkin seeds
INGREDIENT USAGE: Expect 40 to 60 percent fibrous leftover pulp.
NUTRITION MERITS: Manganese, copper, vitamin K, phosphorus, magnesium, zinc, iron, broad-spectrum vitamin E, protein
RECIPES: SIMPLY SEED MYLK (page 179), INSTANT MYLK (page 178, seed butter version)

SUMMARY: Pumpkin seeds give this milk beverage a pretty light-green hue. Although it isn't as seedy in taste as sunflower seed milk beverage, the slightly pronounced flavor didn't wow for straight sipping or hot beverages. Nonetheless, it doesn't curdle and could work in recipes where the bitterness isn't an issue. And it is pretty good in smoothies, cereal, and hearty baked goods when a touch of sweetener is added.

Rice Milk Beverage

TASTING NOTES: Clean, light, watery, a little flat, very powdery
COST PER QUART: $0.58 (based on $1.59/pound for rice)
PREPARATION METHOD: Rice is rinsed, toasted, soaked, blended with water and oil, and strained.
YIELD: 4½ cups milk beverage per 1 cup rice
INGREDIENT USAGE: Expect 50 to 60 percent leftover dry rice bits.
NUTRITION MERITS: Manganese, magnesium, selenium, thiamine, niacin, vitamin B6, phytonutrients (like lignan) in brown rice only
RECIPES: CLEAN RICE MYLK (page 184)

SUMMARY: Rice milk beverage is another "you get what you pay for" option. Although inexpensive, it readily separates in hot beverages and requires added fat to gain a milky consistency. I rinse and toast the grains to get rid of as many health concerns as possible without fully cooking the grains. When fully cooked, rice becomes very starchy and produces milk beverage with a pasty mouthfeel. White rice milk beverage has a very "plain" taste that can be integrated into almost any recipe where a creamy finish isn't needed. Brown rice milk beverage is much nuttier, has higher arsenic concerns, and is a little fussier to work with if homemade.

Soymilk Beverage

TASTING NOTES: Creamy, rich, very smooth, a bit beany, very bitter (see Summary)
COST PER QUART: $2.21 (based on $5.33/pound for organic soybeans)
PREPARATION METHOD: Soybeans are soaked, blended with water, strained, and boiled.

YIELD: 4 cups milk beverage per 1 cup organic soybeans

INGREDIENT USAGE: Expect 50 percent leftover okara, which feels a bit like playdough.

NUTRITION MERITS: Complete plant protein, vitamin K, thiamine, riboflavin, folate, iron, calcium, magnesium, potassium, phosphorus, copper, manganese

RECIPES: ORGANIC SOY MYLK (page 180)

SUMMARY: Pure soymilk takes some tricks to tame. It's very bitter and thus benefits from relatively long cooking times and adding sweetener. Once balanced, it's still a little beany, but it has a very smooth and creamy consistency. Soymilk producers use patented processes to remove the natural bitterness (from saponins), which is why they can produce unsweetened versions that are appealing. With homemade versions, it's best to stick with smoothies, cereals, or other sweet and hearty applications. Unsweetened store-bought versions do work well in savory dishes where the beany flavor complements and some light creaminess is desired. Homemade and store-bought soymilk beverages both tend to curdle, so I don't recommend them for hot beverages or where separation is a big concern. Please note that soybeans *must* be cooked before consumption.

Sunflower Seed Milk Beverage

TASTING NOTES: Very seedy and savory with a mild hint of bitter; not very rich, but has a creamy, non-powdery finish

COST PER QUART: $0.79 (based on $2.99/pound for sunflower seeds)

PREPARATION METHOD: Sunflower seed kernels are soaked, blended with water, and strained.

YIELD: 4½ cups milk beverage per 1 cup sunflower seed kernels

INGREDIENT USAGE: Expect 30 to 50 percent fibrous leftover pulp; none left over if using the Seed Butter option of INSTANT MYLK (page 178)

NUTRITION MERITS: Vitamin B6, folate, pantothenic acid, phosphorus, iron, zinc, copper, magnesium, manganese, niacin, thiamine, selenium, vitamin E

RECIPES: SIMPLY SEED MYLK (page 179), INSTANT MYLK (page 178, seed butter version)

SUMMARY: Sunflower seeds boast many nutritional benefits, but they fall short in their milking potential. For some reason, the resultant milk beverage separates significantly when added to just about anything. It also has a very pronounced flavor that won't easily meld in many dishes. But it is pleasant in smoothies and cereal when lightly sweetened and works in bolder savory sauces.

Tiger-Nut Milk Beverage

TASTING NOTES: Creamy, smooth, full-bodied but light, natural sweetness, fruity notes, no bitterness, distinctive finish

COST PER QUART: $3.98 (based on $12.00/pound for tiger nuts)

PREPARATION METHOD: Peeled tiger nuts are soaked, blended with water, and strained.

YIELD: 4⅓ cups milk beverage per 1 cup peeled tiger nuts

INGREDIENT USAGE: Expect 60 to 70 percent leftover pulp with a coconut-like texture.

NUTRITION MERITS: Prebiotics, vitamin E, iron

RECIPES: EYE OF THE TIGER-NUT MYLK (page 182)

SUMMARY: Tiger nuts are actually tubers, not tree nuts. But they're higher in fat than their potato cousins, yielding a much creamier milk beverage. They're also quite high in resistant starch (prebiotics that feed probiotics), resulting in a relatively thick consistency that must be stirred to emulsify into hot beverages. Tiger-nut milk beverage is naturally sweet and works well in smoothies, homemade ice cream, and baked goods.

Walnut Milk Beverage

TASTING NOTES: Lightly sweet, nutty, astringent and lightly powdery finish, creamy but lacks body
COST PER QUART: $2.09 (based on $8.99/pound for shelled walnuts)
PREPARATION METHOD: Shelled walnuts are soaked, blended with water, and strained.
YIELD: 4½ cups milk beverage per 1 cup shelled walnuts
NUTRITION MERITS: Vitamin B6, folate, pantothenic acid, phosphorus, iron, zinc, copper, magnesium, manganese, niacin, thiamine, selenium, vitamin E
INGREDIENT USAGE: Expect 30 percent fibrous leftover pulp.
RECIPES: PURE NUT MYLK (page 177)

SUMMARY: I shunned the idea of walnut milk at first due to the nut's high astringency. But it melds quite well in coffee and tea, and has potential in savory sauces. It also takes well to a touch of sweetener for use in smoothies and cereals.

Milk Beverages Tested but Not Listed

BEAN MILK BEVERAGES: Though less bitter than soybeans, other beans like navy, black, and cannellini beans are much lower in fat but high in protein and fiber. The result is far from milky and creamy and definitely not worth the labor in my opinion.

FLAX MILK BEVERAGE: Flax seeds don't blend into creamy milk like some other seeds can. Store-bought versions use an emulsification with flaxseed oil to get the right consistency. At home, without using too many additives, I had to use a high ratio of oil to mimic the proper creaminess. I recommend sticking with store-bought if flax milk beverage is your favorite.

MILLET MILK BEVERAGE: Millet is slightly less bitter than quinoa, but it has the same downfalls when made at home. There aren't many store-bought brands available for this type, either.

PEA MILK BEVERAGE: This is a more recent allergy-friendly milk beverage on the market, but it isn't made by milking peas. It's a blend of pea protein and various other ingredients to make a milky beverage. It's not easily replicated at home and varies by brand. Store-bought brands tend to have a fairly versatile flavor profile, but can have a slight powdery finish.

QUINOA MILK BEVERAGE: Both store-bought and homemade versions tend to be bitter and watery, and aren't nearly as versatile as other types of milk beverages. At home, it is best to fully cook quinoa, which results in more of a starchy sludge than a creamy milk beverage.

SWEET POTATO MILK: I've included sweet potatoes in my TWO-POTATO M
183), but on their own, the flavor is oddly sweet and unctuous. I think it
tial in soups or even baked goods where the flavor melds, but it isn't con
versatile than potato milk.

THE ESSENTIAL GUIDE TO COCONUT MILK

Coconut milk seems like such a straightforward ingredient. But confusion about the type of coconut milk to use is a top reason for failed dairy-free recipes. I highly recommend reading all of the information in this section. Then you can buy the different types, find your favorite brands, and get ready to enjoy hundreds of dairy-free recipes.

The Four Key Types of Coconut Milk (Must Read!)

There are four versions of "coconut milk" currently on the market, and it's **essential** to understand the differences. I keep each one on hand, as they work miracles in dairy-free recipes, but aren't always interchangeable. If you use coconut milk beverage in a homemade whip, it likely won't set up. And traditional coconut milk is a bit too rich for that morning bowl of granola. So here's my easy-to-follow reference guide to ensure that you get every recipe right.

Coconut Milk Beverage

This is the thinnest type of coconut milk, and it was discussed in the previous section. But here are some more key points to remember:

- It contains around 5 grams of fat per cup.
- It has a consistency similar to 2 percent dairy milk.
- It is sold in shelf-stable and refrigerated packages, in large quart or half-gallon sizes.
- It is good for everyday multipurpose uses for drinking, smoothies, and cereal.
- It is available unsweetened, sweetened, and flavored.
- Unsweetened plain versions can be used in place of low-fat dairy milk in most recipes, including baking and sauces.
- It adds minimal coconut flavor to recipes.
- It is easy to make your own with my QUICK COCONUT MILK BEVERAGE recipe (page 183).
- On its own, it will not help to thicken pies, fudge, whip, etc.
- It does not thicken or create coconut cream when chilled.
- Do *not* use it when a recipe specifically calls for just "coconut milk." (You might see some recipe creators label coconut milk beverage as simply "coconut milk." Please politely ask them to stop doing this, so we can all avoid confusion!)

Lite Coconut Milk

Notably creamier, but still pourable, this version of coconut milk has many qualities and specific uses of its own:

contains around 15 grams of fat per cup.

- It is a thinner, lower-fat version of traditional coconut milk.
- It is thicker and creamier than coconut milk beverage.
- It is sold in shelf-stable cans or small aseptic packages that contain just 11 to 15 ounces, often in the Asian section of grocers.
- It is not available sweetened or in flavors.
- It is traditionally used in Asian and tropical cuisines for sweet and savory dishes.
- It can be used in place of light cream or half-and-half in most recipes.
- It may add a hint of coconut flavor, depending on the recipe.
- It will thicken only a little when chilled and does not produce thick coconut cream.
- You can quickly make 1 cup of lite coconut milk by blending ⅓ cup regular coconut milk (see below) with ⅔ cup water.

Coconut Milk

Steeped in tradition, this is classic coconut milk. I refer to it as "full-fat coconut milk" in this book, to help avoid confusion. Some may call it "regular coconut milk" or just "coconut milk." However it's identified, these are the facts:

- It contains around 45 grams of fat per cup.
- It is pure coconut milk made from the grated meat of a mature coconut.
- It is sold in shelf-stable cans or small aseptic packages that contain just 11 to 15 ounces, often in the Asian section of grocers.
- It is not available sweetened or flavored.
- It has a thick, creamy consistency that doesn't pour easily unless warm.
- It can be used in place of heavy cream in most recipes.
- Shake before opening if using in a recipe calling for heavy cream; chill and don't shake if using in a recipe calling for heavy whipping cream (see Coconut Cream, below).
- It is traditionally used in Asian and tropical cuisines for sweet and savory dishes.
- It may add some notable coconut flavor, depending on the recipe.
- When chilled, it should thicken significantly and separate into coconut water on the bottom and coconut cream on the top.
- If it doesn't form a thick cream layer when chilled, then it is either a poor-quality batch or the brand contains too many additives—it may still work as a substitute for heavy cream, but shouldn't be used in place of heavy whipping cream or in recipes that need to "set up."

Coconut Cream

Though coconut cream can be purchased, I recommend reading these notes to avoid suffering the failed recipe consequences of a dud brand:

- It contains around 72 grams of fat per cup.

- It is very thick coconut milk with most of the water removed.

- It is sold in shelf-stable cans or small aseptic packages that contain just 11 to 15 ounces, often in the Asian section of grocers, but you can also make it from coconut milk.

- To make coconut cream, place regular, full-fat coconut milk or store-bought coconut cream in the refrigerator for several hours or overnight, and scoop the thick cream that forms from the top.

- Good-quality coconut milk (see Coconut Milk) should always separate and thicken when chilled to create ½ to 1 cup of coconut cream per package or can.

- Some brands of coconut cream are just glorified coconut milk, so you may get more coconut cream from a trusted, rich coconut milk.

- Leftover coconut water from coconut cream separation can be used in smoothies or baking.

- It does get fluffy but does not thicken further or become voluminous like dairy cream when whipped—what you see is what you get, so make sure it's a thick cream to start with.

- It can be used in place of heavy whipping cream in most recipes.

- It works very well in chilled desserts that need to set up.

- It will most likely add some coconut flavor, but this still depends on the recipe.

- It should not be confused with cream of coconut, which is discussed on page 162.

Since coconut milk quality can vary greatly among brands, I have included the ones I used to create the recipes in this book at **GoDairyFree.org/gdf-ingredients**.

Making Your Own Coconut Milk

To make full-fat coconut milk, finely grated coconut meat is steeped in hot water until it is cool enough to handle. It is then squeezed until dry; the white fluid is strained to remove all of the pulp. Canned coconut milk, as we find it in stores, usually has a stabilizer added, such as guar gum. Some brands may have other additives, which can reflect a poorer-quality product.

I usually purchase coconut milk since it is so inexpensive and easy to find. But to control quality, many people do prefer to make their own. If you would like to give it a whirl, try one of the following methods:

- Put equal parts chopped fresh coconut meat and boiling water in a bowl, and allow it to sit for 1 hour. Strain the rich coconut water through a double layer of cheesecloth or a tea towel. Squeeze the coconut pulp in the cheesecloth to extract as much of the "milk" as possible. Discard the coconut pulp or use it for another food or skincare application.

- Put 1 cup dried unsweetened coconut and 1 cup water in a pan and bring to a boil. Remove the pan from the heat and allow it to cool for few minutes. Mix the coconut water in a blender at high speed, and then strain it through cheesecloth as directed on the previous page.

- For a shortcut to lite coconut milk, whisk ½ cup hot water into 1 cup coconut milk powder. Use caution when purchasing coconut milk powder. Several brands use milk-based ingredients (such as sodium caseinate) to "improve" the product. See my current dairy-free recommendations at **GoDairyFree.org/gdf-ingredients**.

- For "raw" coconut milk, blend 1 cup raw coconut meat with 3 cups coconut water (from the inside of the coconut) in a blender or food processor until smooth. Young Thai coconuts work particularly well for this, but feel free to experiment with your favorite variety.

CHAPTER 13

HOW TO MOO-VE BEYOND BUTTER

"But you can eat butter, right?" If you haven't heard this question yet, you will. While it might seem logical to many that butter is in fact a dairy product, to some people it stands alone in its very own food group. Be vigilant when someone tells you that a particular dish doesn't contain dairy. When I inquire further with the more specific question, "Does it contain butter or was butter used in the preparation?" at least 50 percent of the time the answer is yes.

IS DAIRY BUTTER OKAY FOR YOU?

You may be wondering if butter is really a concern for your particular situation. If you are dairy free for political, religious, social, allergy, or general health reasons, then odds are you will avoid all dairy products, including butter. But when it comes to lactose intolerance or other dietary concerns, butter often meets controversy.

Butter is created by churning fresh or fermented cream or milk. It is mostly butterfat (80 to 85 percent) surrounded by tiny droplets, which consist mostly of water and milk proteins (like casein and whey). Be warned: I have actually seen some websites that incorrectly state that butter does not contain casein or whey. It is true that butter contains less milk protein than milk or cheese, but it still contains some milk protein.

If your allergy or intolerance is not hypersensitive, then you may be very lucky. Butter is unknowingly slathered on sandwich buns, stirred into fresh pasta, and even used to prepare the grill in many restaurants. The staff may not even realize when butter is used. If you can tolerate the small amounts of milk protein or lactose that might make their way into your food from these unintentional additions, then your life could be much simpler. However, even these small amounts can elicit reactions in many milk-allergic individuals. You and your physician must decide what level of dairy, if any, is safe for you or your loved one before risking consumption of any butter.

Contrary to popular belief, butter is not lactose free, but it is very, very low in lactose. It may contain as little as 0.1 percent lactose, unless milk solids are added back to the butter, which would pump that level up a bit. Since butter is considered a very low lactose food, it can be consumed by many lactose-intolerant individuals without fear of symptoms. Of course, this varies from person to person, and with the severity of the intolerance.

THE EXTENDED BUTTER FAMILY

Clarified butter and ghee have been around for hundreds of years, but they've recently regained popularity in many countries. They are still versions of dairy butter, but they are "purified" for higher quality and may be referred to as "butter oil."

Clarified butter is produced by melting butter and allowing the milk solids, water, and butterfat to separate by density. The water evaporates, while the whey proteins float on top (and are skimmed off) and the casein proteins sink to the bottom (where they are left behind when the butterfat is poured). In essence, clarified butter is almost pure butterfat. Many cooks like clarified butter because it has a much longer shelf life than butter and a higher smoke point for better use in sautéing.

Ghee is basically clarified butter that is brought to higher temperatures. Once the water has evaporated, the milk solids brown and are then removed, leaving behind the butterfat. This process gives ghee a unique flavor that is popular in the Middle East and South Asia, and produces antioxidants that lengthen its shelf life to up to eight months.

In theory, clarified butter and ghee should be safe for milk allergies. However, those with milk allergies must be warned that these two types of butter may still have a lingering milk protein or two. There is no guarantee that traces of casein or whey won't be left behind, which is why these products are still on my dairy ingredient list (page 106).

Lactose-intolerant individuals may be a little better off with these buttery ingredients. While it is possible that trace amounts of lactose may remain, the lactose levels in ghee and clarified butter are typically so low that only in rare instances would it create a lactose intolerance reaction.

But clarified butter and ghee are still off-limits for vegans, and usually for those who shun dairy for political or social reasons. These butter oils are questionable for people with religious or general health concerns. Some versions of the paleo diet, for example, permit the use of ghee.

WHEN BUTTER ISN'T BUTTER

One of the most common dairy concern questions I receive is about chocolate, but it isn't what you might think. Milk chocolate or milk added to dark and semi-sweet chocolate is a definite concern, and cross-contamination of milk ingredients in chocolate manufacturing is a big risk. But some dairy-free consumers are unsure if they can enjoy chocolate at all. They fear one of the core ingredients: cocoa butter.

To ease your minds, many foods with the word *butter* in their title are in fact okay for dairy-free consumers. In pure form, they're safe for milk allergies and intolerances, too. When we speak of butter in relation to dairy-free living, we are only speaking of dairy butter (from the milk of a cow, goat, sheep, or other mammal). Luckily, the following buttery foods are plant-based and thus free from dairy.

- Cocoa/cacao butter (chocolate lovers rejoice!)
- Coconut butter
- Peanut butter
- Tree nut butter (almond, cashew, macadamia nut, etc.)
- Seed butter (hemp seed, sesame seed [tahini], sunflower seed, pumpkin seed, etc.)

- Fruit butter (pumpkin, apple, pear, etc.)
- Shea butter*
- Mango butter*

* Used exclusively in skincare and beauty products.

Keep in mind that fancy new versions of foods are constantly coming on the market, so you should always check ingredients on these "butters," as they may have some milk ingredients added for a unique flavor.

BUTTERY SUBSTITUTES

Margarine has been around for generations and has offered an inexpensive, direct 1:1 substitute for dairy butter for millions of families. But not all margarine is created equal.

At its core, margarine is an oil and water emulsification that is heavier on the oil. It's whipped and salted to create spreads and sticks that mimic the flavor and solid form of butter. It received a bad rap when manufacturers started using partially hydrogenated oils (trans fats) for consistency and stability. And many margarine brands contain milk in some form.

Fortunately, several brands have emerged in recent years with dairy-free and non-hydrogenated options. They are often called "buttery spread" or "buttery sticks" to differentiate themselves from old-school margarines. Buttery sticks usually have a slightly different formula than buttery spread that makes them better for baking.

Some people note an "off" flavor when cooking or baking with certain brands of buttery spread or sticks. This may be due to flaxseed oil or other low-heat oils used in the formula, which can taste burnt or rancid if heated too much. If you find yourself with this problem, look for a brand that doesn't use flaxseed oil and contains just medium- to high-heat oils (page 147).

In this book, any recipes that list margarine or buttery spread as an option were tested with dairy-free, non-hydrogenated buttery spread and/or my BAKEABLE BUTTER recipe (page 192). You can see which brands I used at GoDairyFree.org/gdf-ingredients.

Like margarine, shortening is a potential butter substitute that also suffers from a bad reputation. It's usually dairy free, but partially hydrogenated oils are often used to create the perfect emulsification. Some natural food companies have begun using palm oil (see page 149) and/or coconut oil to create non-hydrogenated shortenings. These shortenings are usually dairy free, soy free, and allergy friendly.

Non-hydrogenated shortening can be used as a 1:1 swap for butter in several applications, like pie crusts and frosting. It makes frosting easier to work with but does create a different mouthfeel than butter. In other general baking applications, you should typically test with just ¾ cup for every 1 cup of butter that the recipe calls for, and add more shortening or liquid as needed. I don't recommend shortening for general cooking.

ALL ABOUT OIL

When I discovered the possibilities of oil, I was hooked! Though it might take a bit of experimentation at times, oil can be utilized as an excellent substitute for butter in most applications, even in baking. Obviously, oil will work very well as a substitute for butter in sautéing or roasting. But in baking, much less oil is sometimes required, as it can yield a greasy product if used as a 1:1 substitution.

As a fat equivalent, they say that ⅞ cup (¾ cup + 2 tablespoons) of vegetable oil (or other good baking oil) equals 1 cup of butter. I agree that ¾ to 1 cup of oil substitutes well for butter in recipes such as cake. However, for cookies and bars, this is a bit generous. I modified a cookie recipe to use just ½ cup of oil in place of the 1 cup of butter called for, and those little chocolate chip morsels are always gobbled up with huge smiles (recipe on page 359). Any more oil and the cookies turn out quite greasy.

Each recipe varies, but in general, I use half to three-quarters the amount called for when substituting oil for solid or softened butter in baked goods. I then add a little milk beverage, usually 1 to 3 tablespoons, to get the right moisture level.

If a recipe specifically calls for a certain amount of melted butter or for clarified butter or ghee, then you should be able to replace it with the equivalent amount of oil.

I have included some charts on the following pages that list the smoke points of various oils to help you select the best oil(s) for use in your recipes. The smoke point is the temperature at which cooking oil begins to break down, and literally smokes. When this happens, the oil is essentially burning, losing its nutritional benefits and creating carcinogens. As you might expect, burnt oil does not leave the best taste on your food, either.

Keep in mind that this is just a general guide, as smoke points can vary depending upon the refining process and the source of the oil. As you will notice, the more refined the oil, the higher the heat it can take. However, unrefined oils are typically considered much more nutritive.

I've also included a "neutral taste" column. Neutral oils can be used in most recipes without notably affecting the overall taste. For non-neutral oils, keep the mild flavor profile in mind when pairing with recipes. For example, avocado oil shines in Mexican dishes and can be used in rich chocolate desserts, but may be too deep for a delicate white cake.

No-Heat Oils

Best for Dressings, Marinades, and Dipping

The following oils have a low smoke point and should not be heated. Luckily, these unrefined oils tend to have a rich flavor that complements food nicely when drizzled on as a finishing touch.

TYPE OF OIL	SMOKE POINT °F	SMOKE POINT °C	NEUTRAL TASTE
Olive Oil, Extra-Virgin	200–250	93–121	No
Borage Oil, Unrefined	225	107	No
Canola Oil, Unrefined	225	107	Yes

TYPE OF OIL	SMOKE POINT °F	SMOKE POINT °C	NEUTRAL TASTE
Flaxseed Oil, Unrefined	225	107	No
Safflower Oil, Unrefined	225	107	Yes
Sunflower Oil, Unrefined	225	107	Yes

Low-Heat Oils

Best for Light Sautéing and Sauces

These oils are suitable for lightly sautéing vegetables, simmering a sauce over low heat, or low-heat baking. Of course, they will also suit no-heat applications nicely, acting as a base for salad dressings or drizzled atop your meal.

TYPE OF OIL	SMOKE POINT °F	SMOKE POINT °C	NEUTRAL TASTE
Red Palm Oil	300	149	No
Corn Oil, Unrefined	320	160	Yes
Olive Oil, Unrefined	320	160	No
Peanut Oil, Unrefined	320	160	No
Safflower Oil, Semi-Refined	320	160	Yes
Soybean Oil, Unrefined	320	160	Yes
Walnut Oil, Unrefined	320	160	No
Hemp Seed Oil, Unrefined	330	165	No
Canola Oil, Semi-Refined	350	177	Yes
Coconut Oil, Unrefined	350	177	No
Sesame Oil, Unrefined	350	177	No
Soybean Oil, Semi-Refined	350	177	Yes

Medium-Heat Oils

Best for Baking and Sautéing

These oils tend to have a nice neutral or light flavor, making them good all-purpose oils for baking and normal sautéing, or in cold or hot applications acting as the carrier for salad dressings and sauces.

TYPE OF OIL	SMOKE POINT °F	SMOKE POINT °C	NEUTRAL TASTE
Macadamia Nut Oil	390	199	No
Coconut Oil, Refined	400	204	Yes

continued on next page . . .

TYPE OF OIL	SMOKE POINT °F	SMOKE POINT °C	NEUTRAL TASTE
Walnut Oil, Semi-Refined	400	204	No
Canola Oil, Refined	400–475	204–246	Yes
Almond Oil, Refined	420	216	Yes
Cottonseed Oil	420	216	Yes
Grapeseed Oil	420	216	Yes
Virgin Olive Oil	420	216	No

High-Heat Oils

Best for Frying and All-Purpose Cooking

These oils sit at the top of the oil pyramid, but as you will notice, most are quite refined. This means that they have undergone a chemical process in most cases to make them more resilient to high temperatures. For this reason, some of them may not possess the same nutritive properties or full-bodied flavor of lower-heat oils.

TYPE OF OIL	SMOKE POINT °F	SMOKE POINT °C	NEUTRAL TASTE
Sunflower Oil, Refined	440	227	Yes
Corn Oil, Refined	450	232	Yes
Palm Fruit Oil, Refined	450	232	Yes
Peanut Oil, Refined	450	232	Yes
Safflower Oil, Refined	450	232	Yes
Sesame Oil, Semi-Refined	450	232	No
Soybean Oil, Refined	450	232	Yes
Olive Oil, Extra-Light	468	242	Yes
Tea Seed Oil	485	252	Yes
Rice Bran Oil	490	254	Yes
Avocado Oil	520	271	No

A Few Extra Oil Notes

- *Canola Oil:* This is also known as rapeseed oil, and is a major crop of Canada. It is often genetically modified, but you can purchase certified non-GMO or organic canola oil.
- *Extra-Virgin Olive Oil:* This oil is sometimes recommended for sautéing and stir-frying. Some say that the smoke point is actually closer to 375°F or even as high as 400°F.

This could be true, but the evidence is controversial. To preserve the most nutritional benefit and flavor, I have chosen to err on the cooler side of the recommendations.

- *Soybean Oil:* Soy oil often hides under the guise of vegetable oil. Like canola, it is a major GMO crop. You can purchase non-GMO or organic soy and vegetable oils.

GOING COCONUTS

Coconuts are rich in saturated fat, the type of fat that makes butter solid. It's what makes coconut milk set up into a luxurious cream. And that benefit carries over into coconut oil, the fat extracted from coconuts.

Coconut oil can be melted and used as a pourable liquid, but it sets up into a solid at temperatures below 76ºF. When solid, it can be cut into biscuits or help fudge set up. It also has a more buttery mouthfeel than most other oils.

But coconut oil does have a few limitations. I don't recommend using it to grease pans, because it can "glue" the food to the pan once cool. Melted coconut oil also solidifies very quickly when it hits cold liquid or batter and will "bead up," creating little coconut oil bits throughout. If you want coconut oil to remain liquid as you add it, bring your other ingredients to room temperature first. Also, coconut oil doesn't soften or cream very well. Butter has sugars and proteins that help it maintain a "soft" state at certain temperatures. Coconut oil is pure fat, so it only maintains the states of solid and liquid well. This is where coconut butter steps in.

Coconut butter is ground coconut—fat, sugar, protein, and all. Although it does melt into a liquid and can set up into a firm solid, it can also maintain a softened state. The two main drawbacks of coconut butter are that it isn't quite as creamy as dairy butter and it tastes profoundly like coconut. It isn't a neutral-tasting ingredient, so applications for it are a bit more limited.

And coconut butter can be quite expensive. Fortunately, it's easy to make at home. Start with grated or flaked coconut, toast it if desired, and then puree it in your blender or food processor until it takes on the consistency of a smooth paste. If a little more moisture is needed, simply blend in a little melted coconut oil.

For a more versatile homemade butter that does soften, I emulsify coconut oil with a neutral-tasting oil (see page 146) and some liquid. See my favorite BAKEABLE BUTTER recipe on page 192.

PALM OIL PRESERVATION

If you aren't a fan of coconut oil, or if you are allergic to it, then palm oil could be a good solution. It also solidifies and is a key ingredient in natural, non-hydrogenated brands of shortening. There are three general types of palm oil to know about:

- *Red palm oil* is unrefined oil from palm fruit. It's very rich in color due to its high beta-carotene content. It's also about 50 percent saturated fat, so it does get solid at lower temperatures but remains somewhat soft at room temperature.

- *Palm oil or palm fruit oil* is also the oil from palm fruit, but it's refined for a more neutral flavor. It's white because the beta-carotene is lost in refinement.
- *Palm kernel oil* is oil derived from the nut-like core of the palm fruit. It's also white and contains about 80 percent saturated fat, giving it properties more similar to coconut oil.

Unfortunately, palm oil has met with bad press in recent years due to deforestation issues and destruction of orangutan habitats related to its production. But there are a few important facts to keep in mind:

- *Consumption doesn't quit, it just shifts.* The problem with palm oil is that it's so darn useful. Various industries demand this oil, causing the need to plant more and more trees. But overall demand doesn't stop. If you force a move away from palm oil, then more resources will be used for replanting, and the new oil darling may be less productive. Palm trees produce four to ten times more oil than most other vegetable oil crops based on land usage. And other vegetable oils, including coconut oil, face their own environmental and social challenges.
- *Some palm oil sources are highly sustainable.* Many natural food brands are sourcing sustainable palm oil that is produced on existing farmlands and not threatening habitats. These are vegan and sometimes organic farms that enable brands to certify their products with the Roundtable on Sustainable Palm Oil (RSPO). You can see the big list of companies that are certified by the RSPO at **RSPO.org**.

LOW-FAT FRUIT SUBSTITUTES

If you don't think your baked good recipe will falter with less fat, then you can try a fruit-based alternative. Pureed apples, prunes, bananas, pineapple, and pears can provide body and give a little jolt of health and flavor to sweets and quick breads. Here are a few tips to help maximize your results:

- Because the fruit will add more sweetness than butter, reduce the sugar in your recipe.
- Think of the flavor of your recipe to judge which fruit will work best. For example, prune puree blends nicely with chocolate desserts, such as brownies, while pineapple adds a tropical flair to quick breads.
- Use just ½ cup of fresh fruit puree for 1 cup of butter. I also recommend adding 1 to 4 tablespoons of oil, depending on the moisture of the recipe. Baked goods without any fat tend to be a bit gummy.
- If you don't have fresh fruit on hand, drained applesauce, strained baby food fruit, or a puree of water with any dried fruit (prunes, apples, apricots, peaches, etc.) will work in a pinch. To make a dried fruit puree, blend 1 cup pitted prunes or other dried fruit with ½ cup hot water until smooth. Use this puree plus 2 to 4 tablespoons of oil in place of 1 cup of butter in baked goods.

CHAPTER 14

CHEESE, CHOCOLATE & CREAMER TIPS

This chapter is about the addictive "three Cs," as I like to call them. The top three concerns I hear from people going dairy free are: How can I live without cheese? Does this mean no chocolate? And what will I put in my coffee? The information that follows, plus countless recipes in this book, will help alleviate all of your fears.

CUTTING THE CHEESE

My primary advice to new dairy-free dieters is to **take a cheese break**. Many dairy-free cheese brands and recipes taste good, they really do. But most don't taste like cheese. If you haven't broken the cheese addiction cycle (page 68) and you jump right into dairy-free cheese, disappointment could derail your efforts. Give the cheese cravings time to subside, which usually happens if you are truly following a strict dairy-free diet. Then introduce some cheesy dairy-free foods. This will allow your taste buds to simply decide "good" or "bad" without comparing.

And once you're ready to venture into the cheesy dairy-free world, you'll find no shortage of options.

Store-Bought Dairy-Free Cheese Alternatives

In the past twenty years, the world of dairy-free cheese has not only risen, it has flourished. A wide variety of cheese alternatives are now available both in stores and online. Does this mean that finding the perfect cheese substitute is no longer a problem? Well, no. Unfortunately, mimicking cheese without the use of casein, the all-powerful, super-binding milk protein, is a great challenge. Nonetheless, manufacturers are getting closer with every attempt, and most people are able to find a cheese alternative or two that they enjoy.

But when you do shop, be sure to carefully check the ingredients. Cheese alternatives that contain casein and don lactose-free labels sit right alongside dairy-free cheese alternatives. Lactose isn't really required to give cheese its signature texture, so if you do come across a cheese alternative that melts and tastes exactly like real cheese, do a double-check on the label. There is a good chance some casein (milk protein) is hidden within.

For information on many dairy-free cheese alternative brands, visit **GoDairyFree.org/cheese-reviews**.

Simple Swaps

Cheese is essentially salt and fat with a little umami thrown into the mix. This means that some dishes that aren't cheese heavy may just need a little boost when the cheese is omitted:

- Add more salt! I often see complaints of a "flavorless" meal when cheese is removed from a recipe because the cook failed to add some flavor back in. Sprinkle in extra salt, to taste, and add a drizzle of good-quality oil.

- Dust your dish with a little nutritional yeast. Trust me—it isn't as weird as it sounds. This flaky ingredient is like cheese seasoning, and it can be sprinkled on top of or stirred into almost any dish that would benefit from the underlying flavor of cheese. Start with just 1 teaspoon per serving and add more as desired.

- Finely dice kalamata or green olives and sprinkle them over your entrée as you would Parmesan. Though very different in taste, olives offer just the right amount of bold flavor that can often seem lacking without a sprinkling of cheese. Use the ones stuffed with garlic or jalapeño for an even bigger flavor boost.

- Toast bread crumbs in a pan with some olive oil and minced garlic, and season to taste with salt. It's not cheese, but is a delicious way to replace Parmesan sprinkles atop vegetables, pasta, or casseroles.

- Thinly slice smoked or baked tofu for a mozzarella- or provolone-like experience in sandwiches or with crackers.

UNIQUE INGREDIENTS FOR HOMEMADE CHEESE ALTERNATIVES

Beginning on page 195, I have over a dozen recipes for making your own dairy-free cheese alternatives. Most are quite easy, but they may require a "new to you" ingredient or two. Here is a rundown of the ingredients you are likely to see in various cheesy dairy-free recipes.

Agar-Agar

Also known simply as agar, this is a vegetable gelatin made from algae or seaweed. It's useful as a gelatin substitute in vegan recipes and it helps homemade dairy-free "cheese" set up. It replaces some of the binding power that milk protein provides to dairy cheese.

Agar-agar is sold in Asian stores and in many natural food stores, but it can also be found online. It comes in powder or flake form. The powder is more concentrated and more commonly used, but if you can only find flakes, then you can substitute 1 tablespoon of the flakes for every 1 teaspoon of the powder called for. The flakes will also take longer to dissolve in water.

Miso

This rich, salty, fermented condiment is very popular in Japanese cooking. It comes in many colors, ranging from creamy white to red and dark brown, and it may be made from soybeans, rice, chickpeas, or barley. Some varieties of miso are soy free and some are gluten free, so shop around if you have additional free-from needs.

Miso adds a unique umami taste to recipes, and when combined with other ingredients, can provide a cheesy flavor vibe. I typically use white miso in cheesy recipes, but don't be afraid to experiment with some of the darker, more intense varieties.

Look for tubs of miso in the refrigerated section of Asian markets and natural foods stores. Though perishable, it will keep in the refrigerator for many months once opened.

Nutritional Yeast

I hate the name but love the versatility. Cheesy in taste and usually loaded with B vitamins, nutritional yeast has become a staple ingredient for nondairy and vegan recipes.

Nutritional yeast can be found in flake or powder form in bulk food departments or pre-packaged in natural food stores and supplement shops. If you can't find it in your area, nutritional yeast is readily available online. And because it's so lightweight, and usually used in small amounts, a 1-pound package will last for many recipes.

Don't confuse nutritional yeast with baker's or brewer's yeasts, which shouldn't be used as substitutes. Baker's yeast is active yeast used for rising bread, while nutritional yeast is inactive yeast with a more pleasant flavor. Because it's inactive, nutritional yeast is often considered safe for anti-candida diets. Brewer's yeast is quite bitter, and lacks the nutty, cheesy flavor of nutritional yeast.

Tahini

Otherwise known as sesame seed paste or butter, tahini has a very sharp, bold, and often bitter taste that makes it a poor option for slathering on bread. However, when just a bit is added to recipes, it can be a special ingredient that makes the flavor pop. Such is the case with hummus, and often with dairy-free cheese alternatives.

Luckily, a little goes a long way with tahini. A single jar can last for quite a while. You can find tahini at most grocery stores, in Middle Eastern markets, or online.

Tofu

Tofu is very versatile in dairy-free recipes, and it comes in two primary types, silken and regular (all the tofu varieties that aren't designated as silken).

Silken tofu ranges from soft to extra firm and will produce the smoothest product when processed. This is great for any creamy applications, from sauces to pies. The most popular brand of silken tofu is sold in shelf-stable aseptic packages, but many stores still stock it in the refrigerated section.

Regular tofu (which is usually labeled simply as "tofu") also ranges from soft to extra firm and is best when a chunkier finish is preferred, as in dairy-free feta (recipe on page 196). It's usually sold in the refrigerated section.

Both varieties can be purchased organic, and most brands on the market are certified non-GMO. Tofu tends to be a domestic product, and you may even be able to find a small local tofu maker in your area. But if you are having trouble finding a specific variety in your area, seek out an Asian food market or shop online.

For most recipes, you will want to ensure the tofu is well drained and pressed to remove any excess water prior to use. If you're a regular tofu user, you may opt to purchase an inexpensive tofu press. But for the rest of us, firmly pressing tofu between paper towels or a clean kitchen towel is enough.

CHOCOHOLICS REJOICE!

I'm about to make some of you very happy: Pure chocolate is actually a dairy-free food. To make it, cacao beans are roasted, ground, and melted into chocolate liquor. Sometimes the liquor is further processed to make cocoa solids and cocoa butter, both of which are naturally dairy free.

It's what manufacturers often add to chocolate for better marketability (i.e., milk solids, butter oil, cream) that can pose a problem for dairy-free consumers. Of course, dairy-based milk and white chocolates are off-limits. But milk-based ingredients can linger in many brands and varieties of semi-sweet and dark chocolate, too.

Fortunately, there are numerous brands of semi-sweet and dark chocolate that are made without dairy ingredients. There are even some dairy-free "milk" and white chocolate varieties, too! But it's important to note that some of these milkless chocolates may be made on shared lines with milk-containing chocolate. With some companies, strict allergen protocols are followed, but not with others. It's essential to assess whether the trace amounts of potential milk cross-contamination could be an issue for you. If so, always contact the manufacturer (regardless of what their label does or doesn't say) to determine if the product is safe for your needs.

The good news is that a number of allergy-friendly chocolate manufacturers have dedicated dairy-free lines, or even a dairy-free facility. Go to **GoDairyFree.org/gdf-ingredients** to see the brands that I used to test the recipes in this book.

You can also visit **GoDairyFree.org/chocolate-reviews** to see all of the chocolates we have reviewed to date. The reviews include a variety of chocolate brands that are made without dairy ingredients—some are allergen-safe, while some are better for those who do not have severe allergy concerns.

You can also make your own dairy-free and even allergy-friendly chocolate! I have included recipes in this book for WHITE CHOCOLATE (page 428), MYLK CHOCOLATE (page 427), QUICK CHOCOLATE CHUNKS (page 426), and PEANUT BUTTER CHIPS (page 429).

THERE IS DAIRY-FREE CREAMER

Creamer has been one of those gray areas for dairy-free consumers over the years. As explained on page 102, foods labeled as nondairy can contain a small amount of milk protein. This is a notorious concern with nondairy creamers. They may be lactose free, but many aren't truly dairy free.

Luckily, many truly dairy-free creamers have emerged over the years. Most are sold in the refrigerated section of grocers, near the milk beverages. However, there are also a few shelf-stable options that you can find in natural food stores or online. For a big list of the dairy-free and vegan creamer options, see **GoDairyFree.org/creamers**.

Some people opt to simply use dairy-free milk beverage for their coffee or tea creamer, but a lot of packaged brands lack body or separate when added to hot beverages. On the contrary, many homemade milk beverages, without any additives, work beautifully in coffee and tea. See chapter 12 to learn which milk beverages work best in hot caffeinated drinks.

I've also taken some of my favorite milk beverage bases and made a range of easy homemade dairy-free creamers. The recipes include NICE NUT CREAMER (page 188), HAPPY HEMP CREAMER (page 188), LITE COCONUT CREAMER (page 187), and SARAH'S NO-FUSS COCONUT CREAMER (page 187).

CHAPTER 15

ESSENTIAL DAIRY SUBS

Do you have a few dairy-rich recipes that you or your family just can't live without? In this chapter I'll share easy swaps for commonly used dairy products to make your old recipes new again.

The first edition of this book included a special section on substituting eggs, since eggs are the most common co-concern among dairy-free consumers. In this edition, every recipe is either egg free or has a fully tested egg-free option, so I've removed that section. But I have expanded it and posted it online for your use at **GoDairyFree.org/egg-subs**.

POWDERED MILK

Dairy-free milk powders can be difficult to locate in stores, but several brands are readily available online. They're shelf-stable, so they ship easily and can be stored in the cupboard for convenience. Like dairy milk powders, dairy-free milk powders can be reconstituted, for milk beverage on demand. They can also be used in homemade mixes or other recipes, like bread.

The most common types of dairy-free milk powders available are soymilk powder, rice milk powder, potato milk powder, and coconut milk powder. Many brands of coconut milk powder do have a little bit of caseinate (milk protein) mixed in. But in recent years, a few purely dairy-free brands have emerged. Be sure to read the ingredient label carefully, and visit **GoDairyFree.org/gdf-ingredients** to see the dairy-free brand I used to test recipes for this book.

Milk powders tend to be creamier than protein powders, but in some recipes, dairy-free protein powders may work as a substitute. I recommend very fine protein powders, like pea protein, for the best results. Brown rice protein powders in particular tend to be very grainy.

In some recipes, you may be able to bypass the milk powder altogether. In bread machine recipes, for example, the ingredient list may include dry milk powder *and* water. In this case, you can substitute a dairy-free milk beverage or lite coconut milk for the water, and omit the milk powder.

BUTTERMILK

Just as regular cow's milk can be soured to create a quick buttermilk stand-in, dairy-free milk beverage can easily be "soured" to create a faux version. But beyond the basic formula, I have a few extra tips to ensure easy, foolproof results.

Basic Buttermylk

To make 1 cup of dairy-free buttermilk alternative for recipes, put 1 tablespoon lemon juice, apple cider vinegar, or white vinegar in a glass measuring cup and add enough unsweetened plain dairy-free milk beverage to make 1 cup.

You can simply adjust the ratios of this formula up or down, depending on how much buttermilk your recipe calls for.

Why Dairy-Free Buttermylk Works

The acid in buttermilk provides tenderness, full-bodied flavor, and lift when used with baking soda in baked good recipes. As it reacts with the baking soda, it also neutralizes the unpleasant flavor that baking soda can leave behind. The vinegar or lemon juice in the dairy-free buttermylk formula above provides an equivalent level of acid to ensure that your recipe still performs in all of these areas.

The Dairy-Free Buttermylk Myth

In traditional homemade buttermilk substitute recipes, milk is allowed some time to curdle with the added acid. Most dairy-free alternative recipes follow the same instructions. But this can cause frustration because some types of milk beverage won't do a darn thing when an acid is added, while others can turn into a lumpy mess. In reality, the curdling isn't a necessary step for most recipes. You're using the milk beverage for creaminess while the acid is doing all the heavy lifting—literally. It doesn't usually matter if the two curdle together before adding, as they will function properly as individuals in the recipe.

How to Resolve Curdling Chaos

As mentioned, some milk beverages will look exactly the same after an acid is added while others may separate almost instantly. If it becomes too gloppy or clumpy, just whisk to smooth it out, or, if needed, give it a quick blend to emulsify. Problem solved and recipe saved!

Choosing the Milk Beverage

It's important to consider the flavor profile of your recipe when picking the best milk beverage for your dairy-free buttermilk. Most types will work, so it is really about your preference in taste. I prefer to use unsweetened plain milk beverage since buttermilk is sour, not sweet. But if sweetened, vanilla, or even chocolate milk beverage suits your recipe, you can use it as the base for your dairy-free buttermylk.

Choosing the Acid

White vinegar has the most neutral taste and is the most versatile for making dairy-free buttermylk. Apple cider vinegar also works well in most recipes, since it just adds a light sweetness and a little body but has the same underlying neutral flavor profile as white vinegar.

Citrus is a little more finicky. Lemon juice, or even lime juice, adds the right amount of acid, but it will impart more flavor to your recipe. In some baked goods, lemon juice can make the results taste a little "off." I use citrus only if the flavor pairs very well with the recipe.

HALF-AND-HALF

Moving down the fat scale, we have finally arrived at the lightest of the three standard creams, half-and-half. Because half-and-half isn't used much for thickening, the following substitution ideas can be used somewhat interchangeably in recipes. Just be sure to consider the flavor profile of the recipe when selecting the best option.

Dairy-Free Creamer

In most cases, dairy-free creamer can be used as a 1:1 substitute for half-and-half, and you may even find an option in the creamer section labeled as dairy-free half-and-half. If purchasing, be sure to pick up a dairy-free variety (page 154) that isn't sweetened. For homemade, my NICE NUT CREAMER (page 188) or HAPPY HEMP CREAMER (page 188) will work well in place of half-and-half in many recipes, but omit the sweetener and extract.

Coconut Milk

Combine ½ cup plus 1 tablespoon full-fat coconut milk (shaken) with 7 tablespoons unsweetened dairy-free milk beverage to get 1 cup of half-and-half substitute. If you want to tame the coconut flavor, use a milk beverage like cashew or almond.

Pureed Tofu

Blend one part soft silken tofu puree with one part unsweetened dairy-free milk beverage to obtain a low-fat alternative to half-and-half. One 12-ounce package of silken tofu produces about 1½ cups of pureed tofu.

Thickened Dairy-Free Milk Beverage

Blend ⅞ cup plain, unsweetened dairy-free milk beverage with 2 tablespoons melted dairy-free buttery spread or your favorite oil. This will make a scant 1 cup of dairy-free half-and-half for use in most recipes.

Nutty Half-and-Half

Put ½ cup raw cashews or almonds (preferably blanched) in your spice grinder or food processor and process into a powder, about 30 seconds. Put the ground nuts and 1¼ cups water in your blender. Blend until smooth and creamy, about 1 to 2 minutes.

This makes about 1½ cups of dairy-free half-and-half that I enjoy most in neutral or sweet recipes.

For more of a savory finish, blend ½ cup of pine nuts with 1¼ cups of water until smooth and creamy, about 1 to 2 minutes. Pine nuts do not need to be pre-ground, but I recommend pouring the cream through a fine-mesh strainer or a double layer of cheese-cloth for the smoothest consistency.

LIGHT CREAM

Light cream contains about half the fat of heavy cream, and consequently has a much thinner consistency. As you might expect, leaner versions of the cream substitutes above will work quite well in place of light cream.

Coconut Milk

Shake a can or package of full-fat coconut milk and use it as a 1:1 substitution for light cream in recipes. When emulsified, full-fat coconut milk has a rich consistency that is nearly identical to light cream. It works surprisingly well in lighter white sauces, creamy soups, and desserts. I do not recommend using lite coconut milk in this case, because it is much lower in fat and lacks some of the richness and body that light cream provides.

Pureed Tofu

Blend soft silken tofu until smooth. One 12-ounce package of soft silken tofu will make about 1½ cups of pureed tofu "light cream." Use it as a 1:1 substitution for light cream when the recipe needs some body but a lower fat substitute is suitable. This is a good option for thickening power in sauces and soups, and it usually works quite well in baking applications.

Thickened Dairy-Free Milk Beverage

Blend ⅞ cup plain, unsweetened dairy-free milk beverage with 3 tablespoons melted dairy-free buttery spread or your favorite oil. This will make about 1 cup of light cream for use in sweet or savory recipes. It works fairly well in sauces, soups, and desserts that need a more neutral flavor profile.

Nutty Light Cream

Put ½ cup raw cashews or almonds (preferably blanched) in your spice grinder or food processor and process into a powder, about 1 minute. Put the ground nuts and ¾ cup water in your blender. Blend until smooth and creamy, about 1 to 2 minutes. This makes about 1 cup of light dairy-free cream that works well in sweet and most savory recipes, but it does have a slight underlying sweetness.

For more of a savory finish, blend ½ cup of pine nuts with ¾ cup of water until smooth and creamy, about 1 to 2 minutes. Pine nuts do not need to be pre-ground, but I recommend pouring the cream through a fine-mesh strainer or a double layer of cheesecloth for the smoothest consistency.

HEAVY CREAM

For years I completely avoided cream sauce recipes, assuming that a dairy-free equivalent would be impossible. After I finally gave in to some experimentation, I discovered a whole world of foods that could provide the feeling of comfort I had been missing. No, they aren't identical, but they are rich, creamy, satiating, and, according to my palate, delicious.

Store-Bought Dairy-Free Cream

Over the years, a few dairy-free heavy creams have come and gone from the market. At last check, there were still a few options in Europe. In North America, there are a few options for sweet dairy-free whipped cream, but unsweetened is much harder to locate. Fortunately, there are many easy alternatives made from everyday ingredients.

Coconut Milk or Cream

Allow an 11- to 15-ounce can or package of full-fat coconut milk or coconut cream (not cream of coconut) to chill in the refrigerator for 2 hours or longer. Coconut cream will rise to the top and can easily be skimmed for use. A good-quality coconut milk or cream should yield ½ to 1 cup of coconut cream per package. Substitute equal parts coconut cream for the dairy cream in recipes. This works particularly well in sauces for seafood and poultry, and can also be used in place of the cream in desserts.

Good-quality, cold coconut cream will whip, but it doesn't get thicker or more voluminous like heavy whipping cream does. It fluffs up a bit, but what you see is pretty much what you will get with coconut cream.

In recipes where a very rich cream isn't completely necessary, you may be able to directly substitute full-fat coconut milk (shaken), rather than just the separated cream, for the heavy cream.

Pureed Tofu

Blend firm silken tofu until smooth or blend together one part extra firm silken tofu with one part unsweetened rice or soymilk. One 12-ounce package of silken tofu will make about 1½ cups of pureed tofu "cream." This works as an excellent substitute for milk and cream when a thickener is needed in sauces and soups, but higher fat content isn't necessary. It also provides nice structure in chocolate or other richly flavored desserts where the "beaniness" of tofu isn't as noticeable. Pureed tofu can be substituted 1:1 for heavy cream.

Pureed Vegetables

White vegetables, such as cauliflower and potatoes, can add a healthy dose of creamy texture to sauces and soups without the added fat. Simply boil the vegetables in some water (a ratio of ½ pound of cauliflower florets or chopped potatoes to 1½ to 2 cups of water works well). Once tender, puree the vegetables and cooking water together in your blender or food processor until creamy. Add more liquid as needed to reach your desired consistency. For a richer finish, blend in 2 tablespoons of your favorite oil or dairy-free buttery spread.

Thickened Dairy-Free Milk Beverage

Blend ⅔ cup plain, unsweetened dairy-free milk beverage with 5 to 6 tablespoons melted dairy-free buttery spread or your favorite oil. This will make a scant 1 cup of heavy cream for use in sweet or savory recipes. I like this option in sauces, soups, and desserts that need a more neutral flavor profile. But it will set up only a bit when chilled (if using coconut oil or buttery spread) and will not whip.

Nut Cream

Put ½ cup raw cashews or almonds (preferably blanched) in your spice grinder or food processor and process into a powder, about 1 minute. Put the ground nuts and ½ cup water in your blender. Blend until smooth and creamy, about 1 to 2 minutes. This makes about ¾ cup of heavy dairy-free cream that works well in sweet and most savory recipes, but it does have a slight underlying sweetness. Also, it will thicken as it sits or when cooked, but it won't whip.

For cream that is well suited to dishes like lasagna and moussaka, blend ½ cup of pine nuts with ½ cup of water until smooth and creamy, about 1 to 2 minutes. Pine nuts do not need to be pre-ground, but I recommend pouring the cream through a fine-mesh strainer or a double layer of cheesecloth for the smoothest consistency.

EVAPORATED MILK

Mimicking evaporated milk is relatively easy since it is simply a lower-moisture version of milk. It's used in sweet and savory recipes where a little extra richness is needed, and should not be confused with sweetened condensed milk (page 162).

Dairy-Free Creamer

In most cases, dairy-free creamer can be used as a 1:1 substitute for evaporated milk. If purchasing, be sure to pick up a dairy-free creamer (page 154) that isn't sweetened. For homemade, my NICE NUT CREAMER (page 188) will work well in place of evaporated milk in many recipes, but omit the sweetener and extract.

Lite Coconut Milk

Depending on the recipe, you may find lite coconut milk to be a suitable substitute for evaporated milk. Although lower in protein, lite coconut milk tends to have a similar fat level to evaporated milk, and it can provide just the right body and thickness for many recipes, including baked goods.

Simple Evaporated Mylk

Evaporated milk is merely milk with a little more than half of the water cooked off. You can use this methodology to make a dairy-free version of evaporated milk at home. Simply pour 3¾ cups unsweetened dairy-free milk beverage into a medium saucepan over medium-low heat. Cook, stirring frequently, until the volume has reduced to 1½ cups, about 30 minutes. This makes the equivalent of one 12-ounce can of evaporated milk for using in recipes. This technique does work best with richer milk beverages, like coconut, cashew, or soy. Also, I do not recommend using a milk beverage with added protein, as they tend to separate more when cooked.

Instant Evaporated Mylk

A quick substitute for evaporated milk can be whipped up from that handy stash of dairy-free milk powder (page 156) in your cupboard. Put ½ cup plus 1 tablespoon plain dairy-free milk powder in a blender or bowl. Pour in 1½ cups boiling water. Blend or whisk until the powder has dissolved completely. This makes 1½ cups or the equivalent of one 12-ounce can of evaporated milk for using in recipes.

SWEETENED CONDENSED MILK

Sweetened condensed milk is essentially sweetened evaporated milk, but it takes an extra step or two and additional ingredients. For that reason, I've included my EVERYDAY SWEETENED CONDENSED COCONUT MILK (page 191), RICH SWEETENED CONDENSED COCONUT MILK (page 190), and INSTANT SWEETENED CONDENSED MYLK (page 192) in the recipe section. However, there are some store-bought options that I want to briefly discuss.

Store-Bought Alternatives

In recent years, a few brands of soymilk-based and coconut milk–based sweetened condensed milk alternatives have emerged. They are easiest to find in natural food stores or online. They are usually quite expensive, and some brands contain less than a full 14-ounce can equivalent. For those reasons, I make my own at home using one of the recipes mentioned above.

Cream of Coconut

Canned cream of coconut is typically sold in or near the liquor department of grocery stores. It is the "special" ingredient used to make tropical drinks such as piña coladas. Do not confuse it with coconut cream. Cream of coconut is very sweet and can be substituted 1:1 for sweetened condensed milk in many recipes.

SOUR CREAM

Sour cream is a beloved food throughout North America for both recipes and as a cool, creamy garnish. I have several homemade versions of dairy-free sour cream, including my recipes for Silken Sour Cream (page 189), Sour Cashew Cream (page 189), and Sour Coconut Cream (page 190). I even have a less tangy Coconut Crème Fraîche recipe (page 191). But there are a few store-bought shortcuts that you might want to know about.

Dairy-Free Sour Cream

There are a few of brands of dairy-free sour cream alternatives on the market, and they can be quite convincing. Most are soy based, but there are emerging brands made with nuts or other allergy-friendly ingredients. Look for them on the refrigerated shelves next to dairy sour cream or in a special dairy-free section.

Dairy-Free Yogurt

Unsweetened plain dairy-free yogurt can be used as a 1:1 substitute for sour cream in dips and salad dressings. From a consistency perspective, dairy-free yogurt will also work in place of sour cream in baked goods, but with a slightly different flavor flair. See the pages that follow for a bigger discussion on dairy-free yogurt.

Mayonnaise

In dips or salad dressings, natural mayonnaise or vegan mayonnaise is a great substitute for sour cream. Although it looks rich, creamy, and dairy full, mayonnaise is made from an emulsion of oil and eggs. And unless it has some strange milk additives, it should not contain dairy in any form. Nonetheless, there are many vegan mayonnaises on the market, which are both dairy free and egg free.

YOGURT

When I wrote the first edition of this book, dairy-free yogurt was a scarce commodity. Now we have a plethora of choices at the store and in our own kitchens. For homemade, enjoy the Cultured Coconut Yogurt recipe (page 223). For other yogurt substitution options, read on.

Dairy-Free Yogurt

As mentioned above, you can make your own dairy-free yogurt, but the refrigerated section at many natural food grocers overflows with options. No two brands are alike in ingredients, taste, or consistency, so if you don't find one that pleases, move on to the next. The most popular dairy-free yogurts are coconut, almond, or cashew based. However, there are other types, including top food allergen–free ones.

Coconut Cream

Chill a can or package of full-fat coconut milk for a few hours or overnight. Skim the cream from the top and use it in cold recipes as a 1:1 substitute for yogurt. Be aware that coconut cream is much higher in fat than most brands of yogurt, and it won't provide the characteristic tang of yogurt. For some added tang, squeeze in a little bit of lemon juice.

Pureed Tofu

Puree firm silken tofu to create a 1:1 substitute for yogurt in most recipes. One 12-ounce package of firm silken tofu will make about 1½ cups of puree. Pureed tofu will hold its shape whether chilled or heated, so it provides more versatility than coconut cream. However, it does have a beany flavor, making it best for heartier or more flavorful recipes. It also lacks the tang of yogurt, so you may want to squeeze a little lemon juice into your dish.

Buttermylk

It is thinner than average yogurt, but dairy-free buttermylk (options beginning on page 157) makes a relatively good substitute for yogurt in marinades and general cooking. I also recommend it in baked goods, dressings, and sauces when a lot of thickness isn't needed. For a slightly thick consistency, use lite coconut milk to make your dairy-free buttermylk alternative. It can be used as a 1:1 substitution for yogurt.

When You Just Need Probiotics

Yogurt is far from the only option for enjoying dairy-free probiotics. Of course, there are some good supplements (see **GoDairyFree.org/probiotics** for dairy-free options). But you can also get a good bacteria boost from dairy-free kefir or drinkable yogurt; kimchi, sauerkraut, or other fermented vegetables; and fermented soy products like natto, tempeh, and miso. Heat-stable probiotics are also being added to countless packaged foods, from chocolate to cereal to baking mixes.

SECTION 5

THE RECIPES

QUICK RECIPE NOTES

The following chapters include **OVER 250 RECIPES** to ensure that you have all of the bases covered in your dairy-free transition and beyond. Here are just a few things that I want to tell you about them:

NO SUBSTITUTES ARE REQUIRED. It is not necessary to purchase any specialty dairy alternatives to make the recipes in this book. Although I do list "dairy-free milk beverage" and "dairy-free buttery spread" as ingredients in several of the recipes, I've included from-scratch recipes for each of these in the early chapters. Other substitutes, like dairy-free yogurt, are listed only as options, and are not crucial to any of the recipes.

YOU CAN SEE WHAT I USED. I have included links to the foods, specific products, and brands that I used for creating these recipes at **GoDairyFree.org/gdf-ingredients** for your reference. I also have a list of my favorite helpful kitchen tools at **GoDairyFree.org/kitchen-tools**.

I COVERED THE BASES. This is an essential mix of recipes you will need for spontaneous special occasions (like cake), weeknight dinners (like pastas and sides), lunchboxes (like pinwheels), and adapting your own recipes (like condensed "cream of" soups).

I KEPT IT REAL. Going dairy free isn't about living without. I've included both nutritious and indulgent options, because we all need a cookie or ice cream cone now and then. And since inhaling bowls of raw kale isn't likely to happen in most households, I've interspersed ways to enjoy healthy-bone foods and other nutritious ingredients in your everyday diet.

I'M ALL ABOUT OPTIONS. I've spent over a decade creating recipes for publications and brands that cover various special diet needs, beyond dairy free. So although the recipes that follow are intended for "just dairy free," I have included tested gluten-free and allergy-friendly options wherever possible.

I DO HAVE PREFERENCES. For some ingredients in my recipes, I list options equivalently. For example, the ingredient might say "peanut butter, almond butter, or sunflower seed butter." This means that each option produced optimal results. But for other ingredients, I put options in parentheses like this: "(can substitute . . .)." In those cases, the main ingredients are preferred for *best* results, but you "can substitute" an ingredient in the parentheses in a pinch or if your diet requires it. The ingredient will still work, and the result will still taste delicious.

I APPRECIATE THE PLANT-BASED COMMUNITY. There are already hundreds of vegan books on the market, so this one needed to cover the broader topic of dairy-free living. But because I am very grateful to the vegan community, every recipe in this book is either naturally vegan or has a fully tested vegan option. The options were created by me and by the talented vegan author Hannah Kaminsky.

DON'T MISS THE INDEX. I have a complete recipe list beginning on page 167 for easy scanning. It includes the page number for each recipe and columns for quickly identifying gluten-free, tree nut–free, peanut-free, and soy-free recipes. I do include columns for vegan and egg free, too, but *all* of the recipes can be made egg-free and vegan.

RECIPE & FOOD ALLERGY INDEX

V = Vegan; **EF** = Egg Free; **GF** = Gluten Free;
NF = Tree Nut Free; **PF** = Peanut Free; **SF** = Soy Free

O = Option; **C** = Contains Coconut

RECIPES	PAGE	V	EF	GF	NF	PF	SF
Milking Plants							
Pure Nut Mylk	177	✓	✓	✓	O	✓	✓
Instant Mylk	178	✓	✓	✓	✓	✓	✓
Mighty Mylk	178	✓	✓	✓		✓	✓
Simply Seed Mylk	179	✓	✓	✓	✓	✓	✓
Healthy Hemp Mylk	180	✓	✓	✓	✓	✓	✓
Organic Soy Mylk	180	✓	✓	✓	✓	✓	
TOFU MYLK	181	✓	✓	✓	✓	✓	
Eye of the Tiger-Nut Mylk	182	✓	✓	✓	✓	✓	✓
Two-Potato Mylk	183	✓	✓	✓	✓	✓	✓
Quick Coconut Milk Beverage	183	✓	✓	✓	C	✓	✓
Clean Rice Mylk	184	✓	✓	✓	✓	✓	✓
CREAM OF RICE CEREAL	184	✓	✓	✓	✓	✓	✓
Unassuming Oat Mylk	185	✓	✓	✓	✓	✓	✓
Cream of the Crop							
Sarah's No-Fuss Coconut Creamer	187	✓	✓	✓	C	✓	✓
Lite Coconut Creamer	187	✓	✓	✓	C	✓	✓
Nice Nut Creamer	188	✓	✓	✓		✓	✓
Happy Hemp Creamer	188	✓	✓	✓	✓	✓	✓
Silken Sour Cream	189	✓	✓	✓	✓	✓	
Sour Cashew Cream	189	✓	✓	✓		✓	✓
Sour Coconut Cream	190	✓	✓	✓	C	✓	✓
Rich Sweetened Condensed Coconut Milk	190	✓	✓	✓	C	✓	✓
Everyday Sweetened Condensed Coconut Milk	191	✓	✓	✓	C	✓	✓
Coconut Crème Fraîche	191	✓	✓	✓	C	✓	✓
Instant Sweetened Condensed Mylk	192	✓	✓	✓	✓	✓	✓
Bakeable Butter	192	✓	✓	✓	C	✓	✓

RECIPES	PAGE	V	EF	GF	NF	PF	SF
Light Buttery Spread	193	✓	✓	✓	C	✓	✓
Instant Whipped Butter	194	✓	✓	✓	C	✓	✓
Cheesy Alternatives							
Dairy-Free Feta-ish	196	✓	✓	✓	✓	✓	
Almond Ricotta or Baked Feta	196	✓	✓	✓		✓	✓
Tofu Ricotta	197	✓	✓	✓	✓	✓	
Rich & Nutty Ricotta	198	✓	✓	✓		✓	✓
Cashew Cheeze Wheel	198	✓	✓	✓		✓	✓
Cashew Cream Cheeze	199	✓	✓	✓		✓	✓
Seedy Cheeze	200	✓	✓	✓	✓	✓	✓
Cottage-Style Cheeze	201	✓	✓	✓	✓	✓	
Pine Nut Parma Sprinkles	202	✓	✓	✓		✓	✓
Sunflower Grated Parma	202	✓	✓	✓	✓	✓	✓
Sneaky Cheesy Sauce	203	✓	✓	✓		✓	✓
STOVETOP MAC & CHEEZE	203	✓	✓	O		✓	✓
BAKED MAC & CHEEZE	203	✓	✓	O		✓	✓
Easy Orange Cheesy Sauce	204	✓	✓	✓	✓	✓	✓
STOVETOP MAC & CHEEZE	204	✓	✓	O	✓	✓	✓
Melty Mozza Cheeze	205	✓	✓	✓		✓	✓
Sliceable Sandwich Cheeze	206	✓	✓	✓		✓	✓
Powdered Cheeze Mix	207	✓	✓	✓	O	✓	✓
INSTANT CHEEZE SAUCE	207	✓	✓	✓	O	✓	✓
Blends to Brews							
Wild Blue Smoothie	209	✓	✓	✓	✓	✓	✓
The Big Squeeze Smoothie	210	✓	✓	✓	✓	✓	✓
Gingersnap Super Smoothie	210	✓	✓	✓	C	✓	✓
Just Peachy Power Smoothie	211	✓	✓	✓	✓	✓	✓
Pumpkin Pie Protein Shake	212	✓	✓	✓	✓	✓	✓
PUMPKIN PIE SPICE	212	✓	✓	✓	✓	✓	✓
Chocolate Frostee	213	✓	✓	✓	C	✓	✓
Mocha Frappé-ccino	213	✓	✓	✓	✓	✓	✓
Vanilla Mylkshake	214	✓	✓	✓	C	✓	✓
Strawberry Mylk	214	✓	✓	✓	✓	✓	✓
Chocolate Mylk	215	✓	✓	✓	✓	✓	✓

RECIPES	PAGE	V	EF	GF	NF	PF	SF
Instant Vanilla Chai Latte	216	✓	✓	✓	✓	✓	✓
CINNAMON-SPICE CHAI MIX	216	✓	✓	✓	✓	✓	✓
SPICY CHAI MIX	216	✓	✓	✓	✓	✓	✓
Hot Drinking Chocolate	217	✓	✓	✓	✓	✓	✓
Classic Hot Cocoa	218	✓	✓	✓	✓	✓	✓
Toasty Carob Mylk	218	✓	✓	✓	✓	✓	✓
Warming Up to Molasses Mylk	219	✓	✓	✓	O	✓	✓
Rise & Dine!							
Easy Everyday Blender Waffles	221	✓	✓	✓	✓	✓	✓
Essential Cinnamon-Raisin Granola	222	✓	✓	✓	O	✓	✓
Cultured Coconut Yogurt	223	✓	✓	✓	C	✓	✓
Instant Berry-Banana Yogurt	224	✓	✓	✓	✓	✓	✓
Baked French Toast Sticks	224	O	O	✓	C	✓	✓
NUTTY MAPLE-CINNAMON DIP	225	✓	✓	✓	O	✓	✓
Back to School Breakfast Cookies	226	✓	✓	✓	✓	✓	✓
Dukkah Avocado Toast	227	✓	✓	✓	✓	✓	✓
Pillowy Wholesome Pancakes	228	✓	✓		✓	✓	✓
Eggs Benedict with Blender Hollandaise Sauce	229	O	O	✓	C	✓	✓
In an Instant Oatmeal Packets	230	✓	✓	✓	✓	✓	✓
Best Darn Biscuits & Gravy	231	✓	✓	✓	C	✓	✓
EASY HOMEMADE BREAKFAST SAUSAGE	231	O	✓	✓	✓	✓	✓
Crustless Confetti Mini Quiche	232	✓	✓	✓	✓	✓	✓
Bakeshop Bites							
Cinn-full Overnight Cinnamon Rolls	234	✓	✓		✓	✓	✓
Bakery-Style Blueberry Muffins	235	O	O		✓	✓	✓
The Most Versatile Muffins	236	✓	✓		✓	✓	✓
Chunky Monkey Muffins	237	✓	✓	✓	✓	✓	✓
Any Day Pumpkin Muffins	238	O	O		✓	✓	✓
Pear-fectly Good Vanilla Muffins	239	✓	✓		✓	✓	✓
My Favorite Maple Bran Muffins	240	✓	✓		✓	✓	✓
Baked Cake Donuts with Maple Icing	240	O	O		C	✓	✓
Raised Glazed Donuts	242	✓	✓		✓	✓	✓
Double Chocolate Scones with Vanilla Glaze	244	✓	✓		C	✓	✓

RECIPES	PAGE	V	EF	GF	NF	PF	SF
Strawberry Danish Scones	246	✓	✓		C	✓	✓
Flaky French Croissants	248	O	O		✓	✓	✓
Fresh Bread							
Iced Lemon Loaf	251	O	O		✓	✓	✓
Glazed Zucchini-Pineapple Bread	252	✓	✓		✓	✓	✓
Breakfast-Worthy Banana Bread	254	✓	✓		✓	✓	✓
Sarah's Cinnamon Raisin Bread	255	✓	✓		✓	✓	✓
Whole-Grain Sandwich Bread	256	✓	✓		✓	✓	✓
Four-Ingredient Baking Powder Biscuits	258	✓	✓	O	C	✓	✓
Heavenly Honey Wheat Pull-Apart Rolls	260	✓	✓		✓	✓	✓
Speedy Wheat Buns	261	O	O	✓	✓	✓	✓
Simply Slider Buns	262	✓	✓	✓	✓	✓	✓
Snack on This							
Jammin' Grain Bars	264	✓	✓		C	✓	✓
Chewy No-Bake Granola Bars	266	✓	✓	✓	O	✓	✓
Chocolate, Nuts & Sea Salt Nice Bars	267	✓	✓	✓		✓	✓
Chocolate Peanut Butter Oat Cups	268	✓	✓	✓	✓	✓	✓
Pineapple-Coconut Protein Bites	269	✓	✓	✓	C	✓	✓
Power Fudgies	270	✓	✓	✓	O	✓	✓
Apple a Day "Donuts"	270	✓	✓	✓	C	✓	✓
Chocolate Pistachio Figs	271	✓	✓	✓	O	✓	✓
Pinwheels	272	✓	✓	✓	✓	✓	✓
Un-Sushi Snackers	273	✓	✓	✓	✓	✓	✓
Five-Minute Nachos	274	✓	✓	✓		✓	✓
Please Pass the Cheeze Popcorn	275	✓	✓	✓	✓	✓	✓
PERFECT STOVETOP POPCORN	275	✓	✓	✓	✓	✓	✓
Easy Cheesy Crackers	276	✓	✓	✓	✓	✓	✓
Garlic & Herb Baby Cheezes	277	✓	✓	✓		✓	✓
Lay It on Thick							
Pizza Dip	279	✓	✓	✓	O	✓	✓
Baba Ghanoush	280	✓	✓	✓	✓	✓	✓
Rawesome Nut Dip	281	✓	✓	✓		✓	✓
Super Spinach & Artichoke Dip	282	✓	✓	✓		✓	✓

RECIPES	PAGE	V	EF	GF	NF	PF	SF
Company's Coming Nacho Dip	283	✓	✓	✓	o	✓	✓
Buttery Carrot Spread	283	✓	✓	✓	c	✓	✓
Fresh Strawberry Chia Jam	284	✓	✓	✓	✓	✓	✓
Rockin' Raspberry Chia Jam	284	✓	✓	✓	✓	✓	✓
Five-Star Ranch Dressing or Dip	285	✓	✓	✓	✓	✓	✓
Japanese Restaurant–Style Dressing	286	✓	✓	✓	✓	✓	✓
Dreamy Honey Dijon Dressing	286	✓	✓	✓		✓	✓
All-in Asian Dressing or Dip	287	✓	✓	✓	✓	✓	
Kickin' Chipotle Dressing	288	✓	✓	✓	✓	✓	✓
Balsamic Tahini Dressing	288	✓	✓	✓	✓	✓	✓
Soup for the Soul							
Classic Condensed Cream of Mushroom Soup	290	✓	✓	✓	✓	✓	✓
Healthy Condensed Cream of Chicken Soup	291	✓	✓	✓		✓	✓
Roasted Eggplant & Tomato Soup	292	✓	✓	✓	✓	✓	✓
Curried Cauliflower Bisque	293	✓	✓	✓	✓	✓	✓
GARAM MASALA	293	✓	✓	✓	✓	✓	✓
Light Vichyssoise	294	✓	✓	✓	✓	✓	✓
Comforting Corn Chowder	295	✓	✓	✓	c	✓	✓
Cream of Asparagus Soup	296	✓	✓	✓	✓	✓	✓
African Peanut Stew	297	✓	✓	✓	✓	✓	✓
Mexican Bean Soup	298	✓	✓	✓	✓	✓	✓
Warming Winter Squash Soup	299	✓	✓	✓	✓	✓	✓
Hearty Mushroom Barley Stew	300	✓	✓	o	✓	✓	✓
Creamy Potato Miso Soup	301	✓	✓	✓	✓	✓	✓
Cheesy Broccoli Soup	302	✓	✓	✓		✓	✓
Pizza Night							
White Cheeseless Pizza	304	✓	✓	o		✓	✓
Roasted Ratatouille Pizza	304	✓	✓	o	✓	✓	✓
Cheesy Pepperoni Pizza	306	✓	✓	o	✓	✓	✓
Thai Chick-Un Pizza	307	✓	✓	o	✓	o	✓
Pesto Polenta Pie	308	✓	✓	✓	c	✓	✓
Personal Portobello Pizzas	309	✓	✓	✓	✓	✓	
No-Rise Pizza Crust	310	✓	✓		✓	✓	✓

RECIPES	PAGE	V	EF	GF	NF	PF	SF
Ancient Grain Pizza Crust	311	✓	✓		✓	✓	✓
Gluten-Free Classic Pizza Crust	312	✓	✓	✓	✓	✓	✓
Roasted Tomato Pizza Sauce	313	✓	✓	✓	✓	✓	✓
Creamy Garlic Pizza Sauce	314	✓	✓	✓		✓	✓
Avocado Pesto Pizza Sauce	314	✓	✓	✓	c	✓	✓
Thai Peanut Pizza Sauce	315	✓	✓	✓	✓	o	✓
So Many Pasta-bilities							
Greek Pasta Salad	318	✓	✓	✓	✓	✓	
Portobello-Ricotta Ravioli	318	✓	✓		✓	✓	o
Almost Too Easy Alfredo	320	✓	✓	✓		✓	✓
Pasta Primavera	321	✓	✓	✓	✓	✓	✓
Creamed Spinach Pasta	322	✓	✓	✓			✓
Homemade Cheeze Tortellini	323	✓	✓		✓	✓	✓
Spaghetti X's & O's	324	✓	✓	✓	✓	✓	✓
Shells 'n' Butternut Bake	324	✓	✓	✓		✓	✓
Brazilian-Style Stroganoff	326	✓	✓	✓		✓	✓
Sesame Soba Noodles with Kale	327	✓	✓	✓	✓	✓	✓
Chinese Five-Spice Noodles	328	✓	✓	✓	✓	✓	✓
Lasagna Béchamel	329	✓	✓	✓	✓	✓	✓
Very Veggie Lasagna	330	✓	✓	✓	o	✓	o
More Marvelous Mains							
Paleo Eggplant Cannelloni with Fresh Tomato-Basil Sauce	333	✓	✓	✓		✓	✓
Guacamole Enchiladas in Red Sauce	334	✓	✓	✓	✓	✓	✓
Mushroom & Sage Stuffed Bell Peppers	335	✓	✓	✓	✓	✓	✓
Rustic Roasted Eggplant Puttanesca	336	✓	✓	✓	✓	✓	✓
Deconstructed Falafel Bowls with Tahini Sauce	337	✓	✓	✓	✓	✓	✓
Lentil Curry in a Hurry	338	✓	✓	✓	c	✓	✓
Tofu Saag Paneer	339	✓	✓	✓	c	✓	
Power Stir-Fry	340	✓	✓	✓	o	✓	
Hawaiian Teriyaki Bowls	341	✓	✓	✓	✓	✓	✓
Grilled Cheeze Sandwiches	342	✓	✓	✓	o	✓	✓
Build Your Own Taco Bar	342	✓	✓	✓	✓	✓	✓
EASY GUACAMOLE	343	✓	✓	✓	✓	✓	✓

RECIPES	PAGE	V	EF	GF	NF	PF	SF
Sweet Potato & Black Bean Taquitos	344	✓	✓	✓	✓	✓	✓
Veggie Tostadas with Avocado Crema	345	✓	✓	✓	c	✓	✓
Warm Sides							
Bring on the Bok Choy	347	✓	✓	✓	✓	✓	✓
Kale & Sweet Onion Sauté	348	✓	✓	✓	✓	✓	✓
Broccoli Dijon	348	✓	✓	✓	✓	✓	✓
Creamy Cauliflower Gratin	349	✓	✓	✓	✓	✓	✓
Mashed Potatoes & Miso-Mushroom Gravy	350	✓	✓	✓	✓	✓	✓
Anytime Oven-Roasted Potatoes	352	✓	✓	✓	✓	✓	✓
Seasoned Oven Fries	353	✓	✓	✓	✓	✓	✓
Roasted Sweet Potato & Greens Salad	354	✓	✓	✓	✓	✓	✓
Blackstrap Barbecue Beans	355	✓	✓	✓	✓	✓	✓
Spanish-Style Barley	356	✓	✓		✓	✓	✓
Creamy Poblano Baked Risotto	356	✓	✓	✓	c	✓	✓
Multi-Grain Pilaf	357	✓	✓	✓	✓	✓	✓
The Cookie Jar							
Never Enough Chocolate Chip Cookies	359	✓	✓		✓	✓	✓
Coffeehouse Cookies	360	✓	✓		✓	✓	✓
Soft and Chewy Oatmeal Cookies	361	✓	✓		✓	✓	✓
Maple Pumpkin Spice Cookies	362	✓	✓		✓	✓	✓
Fudge Brownie Cookies	363	✓	✓	o	✓	✓	✓
Girl Scout Caramel Delight Cookies	364	✓	✓		c	✓	✓
Raw Cookie Dough Bites	365	✓	✓	✓		✓	✓
Enchanted Bars	366	✓	✓	✓	c	✓	✓
Chia Berry Crumb Bars	367	✓	✓	✓	✓	✓	✓
O'Henry Bars	368	✓	✓	✓	✓	✓	✓
Fabulous Fudge Brownies	368	o	o	✓	✓	✓	✓
Lemon Streusel Squares	370	✓	✓		c	✓	✓
Take the Cake							
Banana Crumb Coffee Cake	373	✓	✓		✓	✓	✓
Sweet Apple Snackin' Cake	374	✓	✓		✓	✓	✓
Yellow Birthday Cake	374	o	o		✓	✓	✓

RECIPES	PAGE	V	EF	GF	NF	PF	SF
Pineapple Upside-Down Cake	376	O	O		✓	✓	✓
Simply Wonderful White Cake	377	✓	✓		✓	✓	✓
Chocolate Wacky Cake	378	✓	✓		✓	✓	✓
Carrot Spice Cupcakes	378	O	O	O	✓	✓	✓
Orange Chocolate Chunk Cupcakes	380	✓	✓		✓	✓	✓
Chocolate Mug Cake	381	✓	✓		✓	✓	✓
Vanilla Mug Cake	382	✓	✓		✓	✓	✓
Mini Berry Cheezecakes	383	✓	✓	✓		✓	✓
Whipped Vanilla Icing	384	✓	✓	✓	✓	✓	✓
Cream Cheeze Frosting	384	✓	✓	✓	C	✓	✓
Buttercream Frosting	385	✓	✓	✓	✓	✓	✓
Peanut Butter Fudge Frosting	386	✓	✓	✓	✓	O	✓
Fudgy Chocolate Frosting	386	✓	✓	✓	✓	✓	✓
Dark Chocolate Ganache Frosting	387	✓	✓	✓	✓	✓	✓
Butterless Spice Frosting	388	✓	✓	✓		✓	✓
Pudding, Mousse & Pie, Oh My!							
Double Chocolate Pudding	391	✓	✓	✓	✓	✓	✓
Buttahscotch Pudding	392	✓	✓	✓	✓	✓	✓
Versatile Vanilla Pudding	393	✓	✓	✓	✓	✓	✓
Creamsicle Chia Pudding	394	✓	✓	✓	C	✓	✓
Chocolate-Covered Banana Mousse	395	✓	✓	✓	✓	✓	
Death by Chocolate Mousse	396	✓	✓	✓	C	✓	✓
Key Lime Mousse Pie	397	✓	✓	✓	C	✓	✓
Crazy for Coconut Cream Pie	398	✓	✓	✓	C	✓	✓
Maple & Brown Sugar Apple Crisp	399	✓	✓	✓	✓	✓	✓
Easy Peasy Pie Crust	400	✓	✓		✓	✓	✓
Cookie Crumb Crust	401	✓	✓	✓	✓	✓	✓
Ice Cream Social							
Purely Vanilla Ice Cream	403	✓	✓	✓	✓	✓	✓
Chocolate Puddin' Pop Ice Cream	404	✓	✓	✓	C	✓	✓
Fresh Strawberry Ice Cream	405	✓	✓	✓	C	✓	✓

RECIPES	PAGE	V	EF	GF	NF	PF	SF
Very Cherry Nice Cream	405	✓	✓	✓	O	✓	✓
Peanut Butter Parad-Ice Cream	406	✓	✓	✓	C	O	✓
Snickerdoodle Cashew Ice Cream	407	✓	✓	✓		✓	✓
Tropical Coconut Ice Dream	408	✓	✓	✓	C	✓	✓
Mint Stracciatella	409	✓	✓	✓	C	✓	✓
Decadent Dark Chocolate Sorbet	410	✓	✓	✓	✓	✓	✓
Oatmeal Cookie Ice Cream Sandwiches	410	✓	✓	✓	✓	✓	✓
Mango-Orange Sherbet Bars	412	✓	✓	✓	C	✓	✓
Piña Colada Pops	412	✓	✓	✓	C	✓	✓
Fruit 'n' Cream Pops	413	✓	✓	✓	C	✓	✓
Chocolate Magical Shell	414	✓	✓	✓	C	✓	✓
Peanut Butter Magical Shell	414	✓	✓	✓	C	O	✓
Hot Fudge Sauce	415	✓	✓	✓	C	✓	✓
Sweet & Silky Butterscotch Sauce	415	✓	✓	✓	C	✓	✓
Sweet Everythings							
Chocolate-Dipped Coconut Crispy Cups	419	✓	✓	✓	C	✓	✓
Irresistibly Easy Buckeyes	420	✓	✓	✓	✓	✓	✓
Anytime Truffles	420	✓	✓	✓	C	✓	✓
Fabulous Fudge Bites	421	✓	✓	✓	C	✓	✓
Dulce de Coco	422	✓	✓	✓	C	✓	✓
Goes-with-Everything Chocolate Ganache	423	✓	✓	✓	C	✓	✓
Cool Whipped Coconut Cream	424	✓	✓	✓	C	✓	✓
Fruit Whip	425	✓	✓	✓	C	✓	✓
Cocoa Whip	425	✓	✓	✓	C	✓	✓
Quick Chocolate Chunks	426	✓	✓	✓	✓	✓	✓
Mylk Chocolate	427	✓	✓	✓	C	✓	✓
White Chocolate	428	✓	✓	✓	C	✓	✓
Peanut Butter Chips	429	✓	✓	✓	✓		✓
No-Bake Crumble Topping	430	✓	✓	✓		✓	✓

CHAPTER 16

MILKING PLANTS

Homemade Milk Beverage Recipes

GOOD TO KNOW FOR THIS CHAPTER

A NUT MILK BAG IS WORTH IT. They cost just $5 to $15 (depending on the size and brand), are reusable for hundreds of batches (saving you money in cheesecloth), make cleanup a breeze, and help make the smoothest homemade milk beverages.

YOU CAN FORTIFY HOMEMADE MILK BEVERAGE. Just like store-bought brands, you can pump up the micronutrients, and it's even cost-effective. Calcium citrate and magnesium citrate are sold in affordable powder form for easily blending in. They will add a slight powdery finish, depending on how much you use. Vitamin D can be purchased in liquid form with a dropper and usually contains hundreds of servings per bottle.

GO THICK OR THIN. The water amounts are based on my preferred consistency from testing, but you can make the milk beverages lighter or richer by increasing or decreasing the water amount, respectively.

IT WILL USUALLY SETTLE. Most homemade milk beverages will separate in the refrigerator and need to be shaken, blended, or stirred before every use. It's a minor inconvenience for the freshest option.

SWEETENER IS UP TO YOU. If desired, most types of sweeteners will work well in homemade milk beverage, including cane sugar, agave nectar, honey, maple syrup, stevia, and even one or two pitted dates. It just comes down to your flavor and ingredient preference.

MORE DETAILS ARE PROVIDED. See The Ultimate Guide to Dairy-Free Milk Beverages section, starting on page 130, for a full breakdown of the different types of milk beverages.

PURE NUT MYLK

MAKES 4½ CUPS

Tree nuts and peanuts have a wonderful balance of nutrients for making dairy-free milk beverages. The fat provides a creamy consistency, the protein helps create structure and body, and the carbohydrates lend pleasant flavors to each sip. This recipe is a great option if you like to soak nuts before consuming them. Some argue that soaking helps to increase nutrient absorption and improve digestion.

> 1 cup tree nuts or peanuts (see Nut Variations below)
> 4 cups water, plus additional for soaking
> Pinch salt
> Sweetener, to taste (optional)

1. Put the nuts in a container and cover with a few inches of water. Cover and place in the refrigerator to soak for several hours (see Soaking Times Note below). Drain and rinse the nuts.
2. Put the soaked nuts in your blender and add 2 cups of the water. Blend until smooth and creamy, about 2 minutes. Add the remaining 2 cups water and salt. Blend until smooth, about 1 minute.
3. Pour the milky mixture through a nut milk bag or a few layers of cheesecloth lining a sieve to strain. Squeeze the pulp to extract as much milky goodness as possible.
4. If desired, return the milk beverage to your blender and blend in some sweetener.
5. Store in an airtight container in the refrigerator for up to 1 week. Stir before each use; it will separate as it sits.

SOAKING TIMES NOTE: *Soak pine nuts for just 2 hours or less. Most of the other nuts will be ready after 4 to 6 hours, but they can soak for up to 24 hours.*

NUT PULP USES: *Nut pulp is very fibrous and quite flavorless. However, you can add it to hot cereal or stir it into homemade granola before baking to avoid waste.*

....

NUT VARIATIONS

See chapter 12 for full details on all the nut options that I tested with this recipe. If using almonds (one of my favorites), I recommend purchasing blanched almonds or peeling the almonds after they've soaked. They are easy to peel, but there are a lot of them! If needed, I usually peel them while watching TV, to justify some downtime. Whichever type you choose, use a raw variety.

....

INSTANT MYLK

MAKES 3 TO 4 CUPS

This super-speedy milk beverage recipe results in almost no leftover pulp. Consequently, it makes roughly double the quantity of the soaking method. My go-to nut for this recipe is cashews, but the other nuts listed grind and blend well, too.

> ½ cup raw cashews, blanched almonds, macadamia nuts, pistachios, peanuts, hazelnuts, or Brazil nuts *or* ¼ cup nut butter or seed butter
> 3 to 4 cups water
> Sweetener, to taste (optional)
> ½ teaspoon pure vanilla flavoring or extract (optional)
> Pinch salt (omit if using salted nut butter)

1. If using nuts, put them in your spice grinder or small food processor. Process until powdered or beginning to take on a thick butter consistency, about 1 minute.

2. Put the ground nuts *or* nut butter or seed butter in your blender and add 2 cups of the water. Blend until smooth and creamy, about 1 minute. Add the remaining 1 to 2 cups water (as desired for richness), sweetener (if using), vanilla (if using), and salt. Blend until smooth, about 1 minute.

3. If desired, pour the milky mixture through a nut milk bag or a few layers of cheesecloth lining a sieve to strain. There won't be a notable amount of pulp, but this will help remove any leftover nut bits.

4. Store in an airtight container in the refrigerator for up to 1 week. It will thicken as it sits, but you can blend in more water, if needed. Stir before each use; it will also separate as it sits.

MIGHTY MYLK

MAKES 3 TO 4 CUPS

This lightly sweet milk beverage has a slightly creamy, low-fat milk consistency. It's naturally rich in micronutrients, with about 88 milligrams of calcium and 68 milligrams of magnesium per cup. It also boasts a healthy dose of plant-based iron, some protein, and vitamin E.

> ½ cup raw almonds (preferably blanched)
> 2 tablespoons raw sesame seeds
> 3 to 4 cups water
> 2 tablespoons maple syrup
> 1 teaspoon pure vanilla flavoring or extract

1. Put the almonds and seeds in your spice grinder or food processor and process until powdered, about 1 minute.

2. Put the nut-seed powder in your blender and add 1 cup of the water. Blend until smooth and creamy, about 1 minute. Add the remaining 2 to 3 cups water (as desired for richness). Blend until smooth, about 1 minute.

3. Pour the milky mixture through a nut milk bag or a few layers of cheesecloth lining a sieve to strain. There won't be a notable amount of pulp, but this will help remove any leftover nut and seed bits.

4. Return the milk beverage to your blender and blend in the maple syrup and vanilla.

5. Store in an airtight container in the refrigerator for up to 1 week. It will thicken as it sits, but you can blend in more water, if needed. Stir before each use; it will also separate as it sits.

SIMPLY SEED MYLK

MAKES 3 TO 4 CUPS

Seeds tend to be a little more bitter than nuts, so I don't consider the sweetener and vanilla optional in this recipe. But feel free to customize the recipe to your taste.

¾ cup raw pumpkin seeds or sunflower seeds
3 to 3½ cups water, plus additional for soaking
1 to 2 tablespoons sweetener of choice, or to taste
¾ teaspoon pure vanilla flavoring or extract
Pinch salt

1. Put the seeds in a container and cover with a few inches of water. Cover and place in the refrigerator to soak for 12 to 24 hours.

2. If using pumpkin seeds, simply drain and rinse the seeds. If using sunflower seeds, rub the seeds between your fingers to release most of the skins. They will tend to float to the top. Drain off the water slowly, along with most of the skins. You can repeat this process, if desired, but the remaining skins won't negatively affect the flavor.

3. Put the seeds in your blender and add 2 cups of the water. Blend until smooth and creamy, about 2 minutes. Add the remaining 1 to 1½ cups water (as desired for richness) and blend until smooth, about 1 minute.

4. Pour the milky mixture through a nut milk bag or a few layers of cheesecloth lining a sieve to strain. Squeeze the pulp to extract as much milky goodness as possible.

5. Return the milk beverage to your blender and blend in the sweetener, vanilla, and salt.

6. Store in an airtight container in the refrigerator for up to 1 week. Stir before each use; it will separate as it sits.

SEED PULP USES: Seed pulp is very fibrous and quite flavorless. However, you can add it to hummus, BABA GHANOUSH (page 280), or hot cereal or stir it into homemade granola before baking to avoid waste.

HEALTHY HEMP MYLK

MAKES 4 CUPS

Homemade hemp milk beverage tastes so much better than packaged varieties. I add a touch of vanilla to temper the grassiness, and maple syrup for a perfectly sweet flavor complement. I recommend enjoying hemp mylk raw or just lightly heated to preserve the abundant omega-3 fatty acids. It is delicious in smoothies, over cereal, or gently warmed with spices.

> 1 cup shelled hemp seeds
> 4 cups water
> 1½ to 2 tablespoons maple syrup (can substitute favorite sweetener)
> 1 teaspoon pure vanilla flavoring or extract
> Pinch salt

1. Put the hemp seeds and 2 cups of the water in your blender. Blend until smooth and creamy, about 2 minutes. Add the remaining water, 1 cup at a time, and blend until it reaches your desired consistency.
2. Pour the milky mixture through a nut milk bag or a few layers of cheesecloth lining a sieve to strain. Squeeze the pulp to extract as much milky goodness as possible.
3. Return the milk beverage to your blender and blend in the maple syrup, vanilla, and salt.
4. Store in an airtight container in the refrigerator for up to 1 week. Stir before each use; it will separate as it sits.

HEMP SEED PULP USES: There won't be much pulp remaining, but you can stir that small amount of fibrous leftovers into hot cereal, a smoothie, or cooked grains to avoid any waste.

ORGANIC SOY MYLK

MAKES 4 CUPS

There's a good reason why most people don't make their own soymilk. Manufacturers have patented processes for extracting the bitterness that naturally occurs in soybeans. Unfortunately, we don't have that luxury at home. But after testing nearly every method, I found that cooking the beans for a little longer than usual helps quite a bit. Then a final touch of sweetener negates most of the remaining bitterness. For unsweetened soymilk beverage, I would stick with pre-packaged versions.

> 1 cup organic dry soybeans
> 8 cups hot water, as needed, plus additional for soaking and topping off
> 2 tablespoons cane sugar (can substitute your favorite sweetener), or to taste
> Pinch salt

1. Put the soybeans in a container and cover with a few inches of water. Cover and place in the refrigerator to soak for 24 hours.
2. Drain and rinse the soaked soybeans. Remove any remaining hard soybeans (those can be cooked and tossed into a meal for extra protein).

3. Put 2 cups of the slightly softened soybeans in your blender and add 2 cups of the hot water. Blend until relatively smooth and creamy, about 2 minutes.

4. Pour the milky mixture into a medium saucepan, through a nut milk bag or a few layers of cheesecloth lining a sieve to strain. Squeeze the pulp to extract as much milky goodness as possible.

5. Return the remaining soybean pulp to your blender. Add 2 cups hot water and blend until creamy, about 1 minute. Pour the milky mixture through the nut milk bag or cheesecloth into the saucepan again, and squeeze to extract more of the milky goodness. Repeat this step 2 more times, using up the remaining 4 cups of water and fully extracting as much richness from the beans as possible.

6. Place the pan over medium heat and bring the soymilk beverage to a boil. Reduce the heat to medium-low and simmer for about 35 minutes, whisking often. If a skin develops (this can happen several times), simply whisk it in or remove it, if preferred.

7. Whisk in the sugar and salt and cook, whisking often, for another 5 minutes.

8. Pour the thickened soybean milk beverage into a 4-cup glass measuring cup and add enough fresh water to make 4 cups. Whisk to combine.

9. Store in an airtight container in the refrigerator for up to 1 week. Stir before each use; it might separate a little as it sits.

SOYMILK MAKING NOTES:

- *I don't waste time removing the skins from the soybeans, as it's very tedious and has little, if any, effect on the resultant taste.*

- *If you don't like the beaniness of soymilk, add 1 pandan leaf or a slice of fresh ginger to the soymilk before boiling. Remove it once cooked. Or add ½ teaspoon vanilla or almond extract after cooking to help influence the flavor.*

TOFU MYLK RECIPE

Tofu tastes much beanier and isn't as smooth, rich, and creamy as traditionally made soymilk, but in a pinch, you can use it. Blend a 12-ounce package of soft silken tofu with 3 to 4 cups of water for quick, protein-rich soymilk. This can be a speedy option for recipes when you run out of milk beverage, since some brands of silken tofu are shelf stable. It also works well in smoothies.

EYE OF THE TIGER-NUT MYLK

MAKES 4¼ CUPS

Although it may be new to you, tiger-nut milk beverage has been around for quite some time, but it was traditionally known as Spanish-style horchata. No matter what you call it, this prebiotic-packed milk beverage is rich, creamy, naturally sweet, and nut free. Despite the confusing name, tiger nuts (or chufas) are actually tubers, not tree nuts. I have tested this recipe with unpeeled tiger nuts and sliced tiger nuts, but the whole peeled ones yielded superior results.

> 1 cup whole peeled tiger nuts
> 4 cups water, plus additional for soaking

1. Put the tiger nuts in a container and cover with a few inches of water. Cover and place in the refrigerator to soak for 12 to 24 hours. Drain and rinse the tiger nuts.
2. Put the soaked tiger nuts in your blender and add 2 cups of the water. Blend until smooth and creamy, about 2 minutes. Add the remaining 2 cups water. Blend until smooth, about 1 minute.
3. Pour the milky mixture through a nut milk bag or a few layers of cheesecloth lining a sieve to strain. Squeeze the pulp to extract as much milky goodness as possible.
4. Store in an airtight container in the refrigerator for up to 1 week. Stir before each use; it will separate as it sits.

....

FLAVOR VARIATIONS

Tiger nuts are lightly sweet and bold in flavor on their own, which is why I don't suggest any sweetener in the main recipe. But this milk beverage does take well to flavors. After straining, you can blend in any of the following:

- 1 or 2 soft pitted Medjool dates
- 1 to 2 tablespoons maple syrup
- ½ teaspoon ground cinnamon plus a pinch salt
- ½ teaspoon vanilla, almond, or hazelnut extract

....

TWO-POTATO MYLK

MAKES 3 CUPS

Potato milk has been a top allergy-friendly milk beverage request over the years. It's tricky to make because potatoes are high in starch but low in fat. Adding oil helps create a milky emulsification, and using a combination of sweet and white potatoes creates more balanced flavors. Even so, it's a unique-tasting milk beverage with a mild natural sweetness. If you aren't a fan of the flavor for sipping, try it in smoothies, baked goods, or soups.

> ¼ cup mashed cooked sweet potatoes (white flesh)
> ¼ cup mashed cooked white or yellow potatoes
> 1 tablespoon grapeseed, rice bran, or other neutral-tasting oil (see page 146)
> 2½ cups water
> Pinch salt

1. Put the potatoes, oil, water, and salt in your blender. Blend until smooth and creamy, about 2 minutes.
2. Store in an airtight container in the refrigerator for up to 2 days. Whisk before each use; it might separate a little as it sits.

COOKING TIP: *To cook the potatoes, slice the unpeeled white or yellow potatoes in half and the unpeeled sweet potatoes into large sections and place them in a steamer. Steam for 20 to 30 minutes, or until quite tender. Once cool, the skins peel right off.*

QUICK COCONUT MILK BEVERAGE

MAKES 4¾ CUPS

This milk beverage recipe has become one of my favorites for ease, creaminess, pleasant flavor, and cost. I use warm water in this recipe to extract as much richness as possible. The coconut shreds are rich in coconut oil, which solidifies rather than emulsifying when cold water is added. Once fully blended, you can then chill the milk beverage.

> 5 cups warm water
> 1 cup unsweetened shredded coconut
> Pinch salt
> Sweetener, to taste (optional)
> ½ teaspoon pure vanilla flavoring or extract (optional)

1. Put 2 cups of the warm water in your blender and add the coconut and salt. Blend until relatively smooth and creamy, about 2 minutes. Add the remaining 3 cups warm water and blend until smooth, about 1 minute.
2. Pour the milky mixture through a nut milk bag or a few layers of cheesecloth lining a sieve to strain. Squeeze the pulp to extract as much milky goodness as possible.
3. If desired, return the milk beverage to your blender and blend in some sweetener and/or the vanilla.
4. Store in an airtight container in the refrigerator for up to 1 week. Stir before each use; it will separate as it sits.

CLEAN RICE MYLK

MAKES 4½ CUPS

Like other grains, rice is low in fat but high in starch—a combination that results in a watery but starchy milk beverage when cooked. To avoid the hazards of raw rice, and to forgo the poor texture of cooked rice, I toast the grains, soak them, and then blend with a little oil to emulsify. This method results in a simple "clean" milk beverage. I prefer to use white rice rather than brown rice to minimize the arsenic load, and because the toasted brown rice can taste a bit overpowering.

> 1 cup white rice
> 3 to 4 cups water, plus additional for soaking
> 1 tablespoon rice bran oil or other neutral-tasting oil (see page 146)
> Pinch salt
> Sweetener, to taste
> 1 teaspoon pure vanilla flavoring or extract (optional)

1. Rinse the rice in a fine-mesh sieve under cold water and let it air-dry for a few minutes.
2. Put the rice in a skillet over medium heat. It should finish drying out as the pan heats up, but stir to prevent sticking. Continue stirring until the grains no longer look opaque and are lightly toasted, about 3 to 5 minutes.
3. Put the toasted rice in a container and cover with a few inches of water. Cover and place in the refrigerator to soak for 12 to 24 hours. Drain and rinse the rice.
4. Put the soaked rice in your blender and add 1 cup of the water. Blend until the rice is finely ground and has released some milkiness, about 2 minutes. Add the remaining 2 to 3 cups water (as desired for richness). Blend until relatively smooth, about 1 minute.
5. Pour the milky mixture through a nut milk bag or a few layers of cheesecloth lining a sieve to strain. Squeeze the pulp to extract as much milky goodness as possible.
6. Return the milk beverage to your blender and add the oil and salt. Blend until emulsified and relatively creamy, about 1 minute.
7. Blend in your favorite sweetener and the vanilla (if using).
8. Store in an airtight container in the refrigerator for up to 1 week. Whisk before each use; it might separate a little as it sits.

CREAM OF RICE CEREAL RECIPE

The leftover sediment from homemade rice milk beverage makes great hot cereal. For every ¼ cup of sediment, use ½ to ¾ cup of water, depending on how thick you like it. Boil the water with a generous pinch salt and thoroughly whisk in the rice sediment to prevent lumps. Cook the rice, while whisking, until thick and creamy, about 3 minutes. Add buttery spread or your favorite sweetener, to taste.

UNASSUMING OAT MYLK

MAKES 1 CUP

Oats release a starch that makes them a bit slimy when wet or cooked. This "slime" can make homemade oat milk beverage a bit unpleasant. I've tried several recipes, including the ones that suggest rinsing the oats again and again to wash away the starchiness. But the only thing that method accomplished was wasting excessive amounts of water. After much experimentation, I finally settled on this much easier recipe. Adding a touch of oil helps banish wateriness, and the almost instant small batch lets you use it immediately, since it is best when fresh.

¼ cup rolled oats (certified gluten free, if needed)
⅞ cup cold water
1 teaspoon grapeseed, rice bran, or other neutral-tasting oil (see page 146)
Pinch salt
Sweetener, to taste (optional)

1. Rinse the oats in a fine-mesh strainer under cold water.
2. Put the wet oats in your blender and add the cold water. Blend until relatively smooth, about 1 minute.
3. Pour the milky mixture through a nut milk bag or a few layers of cheesecloth lining a sieve to strain. Do not squeeze to extract more oat milk.
4. Return the milk beverage to your blender and add the oil and salt. Blend until emulsified and relatively creamy, about 1 minute.
5. Blend in your favorite sweetener, if desired.
6. Oat milk beverage is best used immediately. If stored in the refrigerator, it will usually release more starches. If needed, store leftovers in an airtight container in the refrigerator for up to 2 days. Blend briefly before using; it might separate a little as it sits.

CHAPTER 17

CREAM OF THE CROP
Dreamy Dairy Substitute Recipes

GOOD TO KNOW FOR THIS CHAPTER

FRESH IS BEST. Store-bought creamers can contain so many thickeners and emulsifiers that some actually perform poorly in coffee and tea. Homemade versions, without additives, tend to submerge and enrich beautifully on their own.

VINEGAR AND SALT PREVENT BACTERIA GROWTH. Like many of you, I'm not a big fan of culturing at home. But the recipes in this chapter that sit at room temperature aren't fermenting. They develop flavor better at room temperature, but the ingredients naturally inhibit bacteria rather than creating it.

NOT ALL CANS OF FULL-FAT COCONUT MILK ARE CREATED EQUAL. Some brands tend to be more fluid due to additives and/or water, and sometimes you can just get a "bad" batch in terms of richness. If in doubt, always chill the product before using to see if it forms a thick, spoonable creamy layer.

BUT DON'T LEAVE IT IN THE PACKAGE. I empty the coconut milk contents of the can or package into an airtight container before chilling. Once set, it's much easier to use from the container as needed.

THERE'S ANOTHER NATURAL COLOR. Many recipes use turmeric to give buttery spread a yellow hue, but it also influences the taste. Sustainable red palm oil is saturated with beta-carotene, and just a little bit of it colors an entire batch without notably altering the recipe.

SARAH'S NO-FUSS COCONUT CREAMER

MAKES 1¾ CUPS

This recipe was created by my coffee-loving associate editor, Sarah Hatfield. She tested various nut bases but kept coming back to coconut milk. "I really enjoy full-fat coconut milk in my coffee. I keep it in a jar in my refrigerator and use it just like half-and-half. When I want something a little fancier, I add a bit of sweetener and extract. Almond extract is my favorite."

> 1 (14-ounce) can full-fat coconut milk
> ¼ cup agave nectar or sweetener of choice
> ½ to 1 tablespoon vanilla, almond, peppermint, maple, or hazelnut extract, to taste
> Pinch salt

1. Put the coconut milk, sweetener, extract, and salt in your blender. Blend until smooth and creamy, about 1 minute.
2. Store in an airtight container in the refrigerator for up to 1 week. Stir before each use; it will thicken and separate as it chills.

LITE COCONUT CREAMER

MAKES 1⅓ CUPS

After making countless batches of EVERYDAY SWEETENED CONDENSED COCONUT MILK (page 191), I realized that the rich, sweet syrup could be a perfect coffee creamer. I reduced the sweetener, added extract, and *voilà*—a luxurious coffee creamer.

> 1 (14-ounce) can lite coconut milk
> ¼ cup cane sugar or agave nectar
> Pinch salt
> ½ to 1 tablespoon vanilla, almond, peppermint, maple, or hazelnut extract, to taste

1. Put the coconut milk, sweetener, and salt in a small saucepan and whisk to combine.
2. Place the saucepan over medium heat and bring the liquid to a gentle boil. Reduce the heat to low and simmer, whisking occasionally, for 5 to 10 minutes. It should thicken just a bit, to a rich milk beverage consistency.
3. Remove the pan from the heat and whisk in the extract. Let cool completely.
4. Store in an airtight container in the refrigerator for up to 1 week. It will thicken as it chills.

NICE NUT CREAMER

MAKES 2¾ CUPS

My favorite nut to use for this creamer is blanched or peeled almonds, but cashews and hazelnuts also work well. If you want a slightly creamier base and don't mind a nuttier flavor, you can reduce the water to 2 cups.

> 1 cup almonds (preferably blanched)
> 2½ cups water, plus additional for soaking
> 1 to 3 tablespoons sweetener, to taste (optional)
> ½ to 1 teaspoon vanilla, almond, or hazelnut extract, to taste (optional)
> Pinch salt

1. Put the almonds in a container and cover with a few inches of water. Cover and place in the refrigerator to soak for 12 to 24 hours.
2. Drain and rinse the almonds. If the almonds aren't blanched, I recommend peeling them for optimum flavor and creaminess. It's easy to peel a soaked almond, but there are a lot of them! I do this while watching TV or listening to music. If you don't have time to peel them, the flavor will be a little deeper and more rustic.
3. Put the soaked almonds in your blender and add the 2½ cups water. Blend until relatively smooth and creamy, about 2 minutes.
4. Return the nut creamer to your blender and blend in the sweetener (if using), extract (if using), and salt.
5. Store in an airtight container in the refrigerator for up to 1 week. Stir before each use; it will thicken and separate as it chills.

HAPPY HEMP CREAMER

MAKES 2 CUPS

Something about this creamer just puts a smile on my face. It's full-bodied, sweet, and a bit grassy. But somehow that very natural taste works with coffee and tea for a comforting brew.

> ¾ cup shelled hemp seeds
> 1½ cups water
> 1½ to 2 tablespoons maple syrup, to taste
> ¾ teaspoon vanilla extract
> Pinch salt

1. Put the hemp seeds and water in your blender. Blend until relatively smooth and creamy, about 2 minutes.
2. Pour the milky mixture through a nut milk bag or a few layers of cheesecloth lining a sieve to strain. Squeeze the pulp to extract as much milky goodness as possible.
3. Return the hemp creamer to your blender and blend in the maple syrup, vanilla, and salt.
4. Store in an airtight container in the refrigerator for up to 1 week. Stir before each use; it will thicken and separate as it chills.

SILKEN SOUR CREAM

MAKES 1⅓ CUPS

This is a cost-effective, make-ahead recipe with excellent versatility. Refrigerating it for a few hours (or even overnight) before use gives the flavors some time to marry.

1 (12-ounce) package firm silken tofu
1 tablespoon grapeseed, rice bran, or other neutral-tasting oil (see page 146)
2 to 4 teaspoons lemon juice, to taste
2 teaspoons apple cider vinegar
1 teaspoon agave nectar or sweetener of choice
½ teaspoon salt

1. Put the tofu, oil, lemon juice, vinegar, sweetener, and salt in your food processor or blender. Process until the mixture is smooth and creamy, about 1 minute.
2. Store in an airtight container in the refrigerator for up to 1 week.

SOUR CASHEW CREAM

MAKES 8 OUNCES OR ¾ CUP

This sour cream alternative is a bit different when tasted straight, but even my husband admitted that the flavor was spot-on when used in recipes. I swirl a large dollop of this into my MEXICAN BEAN SOUP (page 298) and everyone loves it.

1 cup raw cashews
¼ cup water, plus additional as needed (see Instant Variation below)
2 to 3 tablespoons lemon juice, to taste
1 tablespoon grapeseed, rice bran, or other neutral-tasting oil (see page 146)
1 to 2 teaspoons apple cider vinegar, to taste
Generous ¼ teaspoon salt, or to taste

1. Put the cashews in your spice grinder (in batches, if needed) or food processor. Process until they pass the powdered stage and begin to clump a bit, about 1 minute.
2. Put the ground cashews in your blender and add the water, lemon juice, oil, vinegar, and salt. Blend until very smooth, about 3 minutes.
3. Transfer the sour cashew cream to an airtight container and chill in the refrigerator for at least 1 hour. It will thicken as it chills. If it thickens too much, add more water, 1 tablespoon at a time, until it reaches your desired consistency.
4. Store in an airtight container in the refrigerator for up to 1 week.

....

INSTANT VARIATION

If using immediately with no time for refrigeration, reduce the water to 2 tablespoons. Add more water, as needed, to reach your desired consistency.

....

SOUR COCONUT CREAM

MAKES A SCANT 1¼ CUP

This recipe was inspired by the recipe creators at So Delicious Dairy Free. Their full-fat coconut milk is so rich that I was able to use the entire 11-ounce package in this recipe. But if you are using a brand of coconut milk that is somewhat thin or tends to have a moderate amount of coconut water, chill it and use just the thicker coconut cream that sets up when making this sour cream alternative.

> 1 cup + 2 tablespoons full-fat coconut milk or coconut cream
> 1 tablespoon apple cider vinegar
> ⅜ teaspoon salt

1. In a small bowl, whisk together the thick coconut milk or cream, vinegar, and salt until smooth.
2. Cover the bowl with cheesecloth or a paper towel and secure it with a rubber band.
3. Let the mixture sit at room temperature, away from sunlight, for 48 hours. This allows the flavors to develop much better than if refrigerated. This isn't fermenting; the vinegar and salt naturally inhibit bacteria growth.
4. After the 2 days, store in an airtight container in the refrigerator for up to 1 week.

RICH SWEETENED CONDENSED COCONUT MILK

MAKES 1¾ CUPS (EQUIVALENT BY VOLUME TO JUST UNDER 1½ [14-OUNCE] CANS)

I use this special recipe when making a dessert that calls for more than a can of sweetened condensed coconut milk and will benefit from extra richness, like my LEMON STREUSEL SQUARES (page 370). It also works very well in recipes that need to "set up" when chilled, like my KEY LIME MOUSSE PIE (page 397).

> 2 (14-ounce) cans full-fat coconut milk
> ½ cup cane sugar (see Sweetener Note on page 191)
> 1 teaspoon vanilla extract
> Generous pinch salt

1. Pour the coconut milk into a medium saucepan over medium heat. Whisk in the sugar, and bring the mixture to a boil. Reduce the heat to low and simmer, whisking occasionally, for 45 to 55 minutes, or until the mixture reduces to 1¾ cups.
2. Remove the pan from the heat and whisk in the vanilla and salt. Let cool completely.
3. Store in an airtight container in your refrigerator for up to 1 week. It will thicken a bit as it chills.

EVERYDAY SWEETENED CONDENSED COCONUT MILK

MAKES 1¼ CUPS (EQUIVALENT BY VOLUME TO 1 [14-OUNCE] CAN)

This is my new go-to for substituting sweetened condensed milk in most recipes. It's relatively inexpensive and has a thick but pourable consistency that's spot-on for the original. It is far lower in sugar than traditional sweetened condensed milk, but it's actually a touch sweeter!

1 (14-ounce) can lite coconut milk
½ cup cane sugar (see Sweetener Note below)
½ teaspoon vanilla extract
Generous pinch salt
½ cup unsweetened plain dairy-free milk beverage (preferably cashew or coconut)

1. Pour the coconut milk into a small saucepan over medium heat. Whisk in the sugar, and bring the mixture to a boil. Reduce the heat to low and simmer, whisking occasionally, for about 25 minutes, or until the mixture reduces to ¾ cup. It will be very thick and a bit "gloppy."
2. Remove the pan from the heat and whisk in the vanilla and salt. Let cool for 10 minutes.
3. Vigorously whisk in the milk beverage until very smooth.
4. Store in an airtight container in your refrigerator for up to 1 week. It will thicken a bit as it chills.

SWEETENER NOTE: Plain white cane sugar (or beet sugar) produces the most neutral, versatile flavor in this recipe. Other sweeteners like brown sugar, coconut sugar, agave nectar, honey, and maple syrup can be substituted, but since you are concentrating the liquid, the sweetener will heavily influence the resultant flavor. Make sure the bolder flavor profile suits your recipe.

COCONUT CRÈME FRAÎCHE

MAKES 1¼ CUPS

This lightly tangy, perfectly creamy recipe was a lucky by-product of my SOUR COCONUT CREAM (page 190) recipe tests. It's the perfect finish for sweet and savory recipes.

1¼ cups full-fat coconut milk or coconut cream
1 tablespoon apple cider vinegar
¼ teaspoon salt

1. In a small bowl, whisk together the coconut milk or cream, vinegar, and salt until smooth.
2. Cover the bowl with cheesecloth or a paper towel and secure it with a rubber band.
3. Let the mixture sit at room temperature, away from sunlight, for 48 hours. This allows the flavors to develop much better than if refrigerated. This isn't fermenting; the vinegar and salt naturally inhibit bacteria growth.
4. After the 2 days, store in an airtight container in the refrigerator for up to 1 week.

INSTANT SWEETENED CONDENSED MYLK

MAKES 1¼ CUPS (EQUIVALENT BY VOLUME TO 1 [14-OUNCE] CAN)

This is a wonderful recipe when you're in a hurry, or if you need a non-coconut option. It uses the handy dairy-free milk powder (page 156) in your cupboard, and, in a pinch, plain or vanilla dairy-free protein powder may be substituted.

1 cup + 2 tablespoons unsweetened plain dairy-free rice milk powder
¾ cup cane sugar
½ cup hot water
2 tablespoons coconut, grapeseed, rice bran, or neutral-tasting oil (see page 146)
¼ teaspoon vanilla extract
Generous pinch salt

1. Put the milk powder and sugar in your blender. Blend for 30 seconds, or until powdered.
2. Add the hot water, oil, vanilla, and salt. Blend until thickened and creamy, about 2 minutes. Let cool completely.
3. Store in an airtight container in your refrigerator for up to 1 week. If it separates as it chills, whisk or blend the mylk before using.

COCONUT MILK POWDER VARIATION

Substitute 1½ cups dairy-free coconut milk powder for the rice milk powder, optionally use coconut oil for the oil, and increase the vanilla extract to ½ teaspoon. This version will thicken if refrigerated for 1 hour or longer, especially if you opt to use coconut oil.

BAKEABLE BUTTER

MAKES 2 CUPS (1 POUND)

This very versatile recipe uses a couple of well-tested new tricks. First, lecithin isn't simply stirred into the recipe; it's properly emulsified. Second, xanthan gum is added to help bind that emulsification so it doesn't break when baking. I put this recipe to the ultimate tests—including batches of vegan (egg-free) Toll House–style cookies at high altitude. There was no greasy separation, just perfect chewy cookies. Use this recipe as a 1:1 substitute for dairy butter, margarine, or dairy-free buttery spread in recipes or simply enjoy it slathered on toast or a baked potato!

½ cup unsweetened plain dairy-free milk beverage
2 teaspoons liquid soy lecithin or sunflower lecithin (for soy free)
¾ cup grapeseed, rice bran, or other neutral-tasting oil (see page 146)
1 cup coconut oil, melted
1 teaspoon sustainable red palm oil, for color (optional)
½ teaspoon xanthan gum (can substitute guar gum)
½ teaspoon salt, or to taste

1. Put the milk beverage in a blender, food processor, or medium mixing bowl. With the motor or a hand mixer running, slowly drizzle in the lecithin. Continue mixing until it is completely incorporated, about 1 minute (this may take a little longer with a hand mixer).
2. With the motor or mixer still running, add just a few drops of the neutral oil. Once it has emulsified, very slowly drizzle in the remaining neutral oil, followed by the coconut oil.
3. Add the red palm oil (if using), xanthan gum, and salt. Process or mix to combine.
4. If it isn't already in a bowl, pour the emulsified liquid into a medium mixing bowl. Place the bowl in an ice water bath within a larger bowl or pot. Immediately begin mixing with your hand mixer on low speed until softly whipped. It will thicken before your eyes in just a couple of minutes!
5. Store in an airtight container in the refrigerator for up to 1 week.

LIGHT BUTTERY SPREAD

MAKES 1¼ CUPS

This uniquely rich and flavorful butter alternative contains less than 4 grams of fat per tablespoon. It's good for spreading on baked goods, melting atop rice or potatoes, roasting, and using as a dredge for breading. But for sautéing and baking, I would stick with my BAKEABLE BUTTER (page 192) and INSTANT WHIPPED BUTTER (page 194).

> ¼ cup non-GMO yellow cornmeal or dry polenta
> 1¼ cups water, plus additional as needed
> ½ teaspoon + ¼ to ½ teaspoon salt, divided
> ⅓ cup coconut oil
> ⅜ teaspoon lemon juice
> Pinch sugar (optional)

1. Put the cornmeal or polenta in your spice grinder and whiz until powdered, about 30 seconds.
2. Put the ground cornmeal, water, and ½ teaspoon salt in a small saucepan over medium heat. Bring the mixture to a boil while whisking. Reduce the heat to medium-low and cook, whisking often, until a thick polenta consistency forms, about 15 minutes.
3. Remove the pan from the heat and whisk in the coconut oil. Let cool for 5 minutes.
4. Scrape the cooked and cooled cornmeal mixture into your blender. Add the lemon juice, ¼ teaspoon salt, and sugar (if using). Blend until emulsified and smooth, about 2 minutes. Taste test and blend in up to ¼ teaspoon additional salt, if desired.
5. Pour the mixture into a container, cover, and refrigerate for 1 to 2 hours.
6. Whip the spread with a whisk, adding water as needed if it is too firm or not creamy enough for your needs.
7. Store in an airtight container in the refrigerator for up to 3 days.

INSTANT WHIPPED BUTTER

MAKES 1⅛ CUPS

This easy buttery spread takes just 5 minutes to make, from measuring cups to perfectly whipped pillows. It is great as a spread or topper, and we even enjoy it melted and drizzled on popcorn. It also works for sautéing, and can be used in some baked good recipes where oil is a suitable swap for butter, like bread or cake.

> ½ cup coconut oil, melted
> ½ cup grapeseed, rice bran, or other neutral-tasting oil (see page 146)
> 1 teaspoon sustainable red palm oil, melted, for color (optional)
> ⅛ teaspoon salt, or to taste
> Optional add-ins (see below)

1. Put the coconut oil, neutral oil, and red palm oil (if using) in a medium mixing bowl. Place the bowl in an ice water bath within a larger bowl or pot.
2. Immediately begin mixing with your hand mixer on low speed until softly whipped. It will thicken before your eyes in just a couple of minutes! Scrape the bowl to ensure that no coconut oil has solidified to the sides.
3. Add the salt and any optional add-ins desired. Mix with your hand mixer on medium speed to combine and lightly whip.
4. Store in an airtight container in the refrigerator for up to 1 week if you used optional add-ins or up to 1 month if you didn't. It will solidify a bit more as it chills, but you can re-whip it with a fork or whisk, if desired.

....

ADD-IN VARIATIONS

Some of these flavor additions also work in combination, like the herbs, umami, and garlic, or the sweet with the spice.

HERBS: Up to 2 tablespoons chopped fresh herbs, such as chives, rosemary, thyme, or sage

GARLIC: 2 to 4 minced raw or roasted garlic cloves or ¼ teaspoon garlic powder

UMAMI: 1 to 2 teaspoons nutritional yeast flakes or white miso

SWEET: Maple syrup, agave nectar, honey, or cane sugar, to taste

SPICE: 1 teaspoon ground cinnamon, paprika, or smoked paprika

CITRUS: 1 tablespoon fresh-squeezed lemon juice

....

CHAPTER 18

CHEESY ALTERNATIVES

Everyday Plant-Based Cheeze Recipes

GOOD TO KNOW FOR THIS CHAPTER

THERE IS AN INGREDIENT PRIMER. I have more helpful details on the unique ingredients used in this chapter beginning on page 152.

USE "RAW" NUTS AND SEEDS. Nuts are usually processed in some manner for health reasons, so they aren't usually raw by the strictest definition. But for all the recipes in this chapter, I use unsalted, unroasted nuts, which may be referred to on packaging as raw nuts.

IT ISN'T REALLY CHEESE. No two foods are ever alike, which means the recipe results in this chapter aren't absolutely identical to dairy cheese. However, they all provide cheesy flavors and consistencies that are delicious and pleasing. And they can be enjoyed in place of dairy cheese in recipes or for everyday enjoyment. Don't be surprised if you even like some of them better!

MIXED NUTS ARE AN OPTION. For the nut-based soft cheeses, I use cashews or almonds due to their consistencies, flavors, availability, and affordable prices. However, you can swap some or all of the cashews or almonds for other nuts to mix up the flavor profile. See the milk beverage section starting on page 130 for my nutty notes on flavor.

NUTS CAN BE MEASURED BY WEIGHT. If you prefer to use a scale, most whole tree nuts weigh about 5 ounces per cup, give or take a quarter ounce. This includes cashews, almonds, Brazil nuts, hazelnuts, macadamia nuts, and pine nuts. The notably lighter exceptions are pistachios (4.4 ounces per cup), walnuts (4.2 ounces per cup), and pecans (3.5 ounces per cup).

DAIRY-FREE FETA-ISH

MAKES 1½ CUPS

This cheese alternative takes on flavor and firms slightly as it chills. Despite its simplicity, it works wonderfully in place of dairy-based feta in most recipes.

1 (16-ounce) package firm tofu
½ cup red or white wine vinegar
¼ cup olive oil
¼ cup water
2 teaspoons dried basil
1½ to 2 teaspoons salt, to taste
1 teaspoon dried oregano
¼ to ½ teaspoon black pepper, to taste
¼ teaspoon garlic powder

1. Drain and press the tofu, using a tea towel or paper towels, to remove any excess water.
2. Crumble the tofu or cut it into ½-inch cubes.
3. In a medium bowl, whisk together the vinegar, oil, water, basil, salt, oregano, black pepper, and garlic powder. Add the tofu and stir to thoroughly coat it.
4. Cover and refrigerate for at least 2 hours, but preferably overnight.
5. Drain any excess liquid prior to use.
6. Store in an airtight container in the refrigerator for up to 3 days.

ALMOND RICOTTA OR BAKED FETA

MAKES 1⅓ CUPS

This versatile recipe has a pleasantly mild cheesy taste and texture. Use it unbaked in recipes as a dairy-free ricotta, bake it for a mild spread, or bake and chill it for a more crumbly feta.

1 cup almonds (preferably blanched)
1 teaspoon + 1 teaspoon salt, divided
½ cup water, plus additional for soaking and as needed
3 tablespoons lemon juice
3 tablespoons grapeseed, olive, or rice bran oil
1 teaspoon white miso (gluten free or soy free, if needed)
¼ teaspoon baking powder

1. Put the almonds and 1 teaspoon salt in a container and cover with a few inches of water. Cover and place in the refrigerator to soak for 8 to 24 hours.
2. Drain and rinse the almonds (this should remove most of the salt). If the almonds aren't blanched, I recommend peeling them for optimum flavor and creaminess. It's easy to peel a soaked almond, but there are a lot of them! I do this while watching TV or listening to music. If you don't have time to peel them, the flavor will be a little deeper and more rustic.

3. Put the soaked almonds, ½ cup water, lemon juice, oil, remaining 1 teaspoon salt, miso, and baking powder in your blender or food processor. Blend until relatively smooth and creamy, about 2 minutes. It's okay if it looks slightly coarse. If the mixture is too thick, blend in more water as needed, 1 tablespoon at a time.

4. Line a fine-mesh sieve with a double layer of cheesecloth and place the sieve over a bowl to catch any liquid. Scrape the nut mixture into the center of the cheesecloth. Bring the corners of the cheesecloth together, twist to tighten the nut mixture into a packed ball, and set it back down into the sieve. Place the bowl in the refrigerator for 8 to 24 hours. The nut mixture will set up and release just a little bit of moisture. It's ready when the cheesecloth pulls away without the cheese alternative sticking to it.

5. Use as a ricotta in recipes, or continue with the steps that follow to bake it for a spread or feta crumbles.

6. Preheat your oven to 300°F and line a baking sheet with parchment paper or a silicone baking mat.

7. Remove the slightly firm almond wheel from the cheesecloth and place it on the baking sheet. If needed, pat it into a disk that's about ¾ inch thick.

8. Bake for 45 minutes, or until lightly browned and slightly crackled on top.

9. Use immediately as a warm spread or cool completely and refrigerate for 2 hours or more to create feta crumbles.

10. Store in an airtight container in the refrigerator for up to 1 week.

TOFU RICOTTA

MAKES 2½ CUPS

This makes a soft ricotta, ideal for VERY VEGGIE LASAGNA (page 330), PORTOBELLO-RICOTTA RAVIOLI (page 318), and stuffed shells. I like the texture of firm silken tofu combined with regular tofu, but you can experiment with whatever type and firmness you have on hand.

> 1 (12-ounce) package firm silken tofu
> 8 ounces firm tofu
> 2 tablespoons grapeseed or olive oil
> 1 to 2 tablespoons nutritional yeast flakes, to taste
> 4 teaspoons lemon juice
> 1½ teaspoons salt, or to taste
> ¼ teaspoon black pepper
> 1 teaspoon dried oregano, basil, thyme, or parsley, *or* 1 tablespoon chopped
>   fresh oregano, basil, thyme, or flat-leaf parsley (optional)

1. Drain and gently press each tofu, using a tea towel or paper towels, to remove any excess water.

2. Put the pressed tofus, oil, nutritional yeast, lemon juice, salt, and black pepper in a medium bowl. Mash with a fork or potato masher until all ingredients are well incorporated and the mixture takes on a ricotta-like texture, about 3 minutes.

3. Stir in the herbs (if using).

4. Store in an airtight container in the refrigerator for up to 3 days.

RICH & NUTTY RICOTTA

MAKES ¾ CUP

This cheese alternative is incredibly rich and luxurious. It creates dishes worthy of entertaining when used in recipes like my PALEO EGGPLANT CANNELLONI (page 333).

> ½ cup pine nuts or macadamia nuts
> ½ cup raw cashews
> 1½ tablespoons water, plus additional as needed
> 1 tablespoon lemon juice
> 2 teaspoons nutritional yeast flakes
> 1½ teaspoons grapeseed or olive oil
> ¼ to ½ teaspoon salt, to taste
> ⅛ teaspoon onion powder

1. Put the nuts in your spice grinder or food processor. Process until finely ground, about 1 minute. It's okay if a paste begins to form.
2. Put the ground nuts, water, lemon juice, nutritional yeast, oil, salt, and onion powder in your blender or food processor. Blend until relatively smooth and creamy, about 2 minutes. If the mixture is too thick, blend in more water as needed, 1 teaspoon at a time.
3. Store in an airtight container in the refrigerator for up to 1 week. It will thicken as it chills.

CASHEW CHEEZE WHEEL

MAKES 1⅓ CUPS

This is one of my go-to recipes for a relatively firm dairy-free cheese round that's soft and spreadable. It's mild but deliciously savory, with a slight tang. I recommend serving it cold, as it will gradually soften at room temperature.

> 1 cup raw cashews
> 3 to 4 tablespoons water, plus additional for soaking
> 3 tablespoons lemon juice
> 3 tablespoons grapeseed, rice bran, or other neutral-tasting oil (see page 146)
> 1 teaspoon white miso (gluten free or soy free, if needed)
> ¾ teaspoon salt

1. Put the cashews in a container and cover with a few inches of water. Cover and place in the refrigerator to soak for 6 hours or overnight. Drain and rinse the cashews.
2. Put the soaked cashews, 3 tablespoons water, lemon juice, oil, miso, and salt in your blender or food processor. Process until smooth and creamy, about 2 minutes. If it becomes too thick to blend, add 1 tablespoon water and blend again.
3. Line a fine-mesh sieve with a double layer of cheesecloth and place the sieve over a bowl to catch any liquid. Scrape the nut mixture into the center of the cheesecloth. Bring the corners of the cheesecloth together, twist to tighten the nut mixture into a packed ball, and set it back down into the sieve. Place the bowl in the refrigerator for 8 to 24 hours. The nut mixture will set up and release just a little bit of moisture. It's ready when the cheesecloth pulls away without the cheese alternative sticking to it.

4. Carefully peel away the cheesecloth from the cashew wheel.

5. Store in an airtight container in the refrigerator for up to 1 week.

FLAVOR VARIATIONS

CHEESIER: Add 2 tablespoons nutritional yeast before blending.

SMOKY: Add 2 to 4 tablespoons nutritional yeast and ¾ to 1 teaspoon smoked paprika before blending. You are adding both to taste, but keep in mind that the flavor will intensify a bit as the cashew wheel sits.

BAKED: Place the semi-firm round on a baking sheet lined with parchment paper or a silicone baking mat. Bake it at 300°F for 35 minutes. Let cool for 5 minutes before serving. This will give the cheese alternative a slightly fluffier consistency and delicious crust.

HERB BAKED: Before baking as noted above, drizzle a little olive oil on the wheel and lightly rub to evenly spread it on the exposed surface. Generously sprinkle with chopped fresh herbs, and lightly press them in to adhere.

CASHEW CREAM CHEEZE

MAKES ¾ CUP (8 OUNCES)

Mimicking cream cheese is no easy task. Just one look at the dozens of test jars in my refrigerator is evidence enough. However, I found that I actually prefer the mild and slightly sweet flavor of this alternative. It isn't exactly like the dairy stuff, but it is pretty tasty in its own right. And it works well as a substitute in most cream cheesy recipes.

1 cup raw cashews
2 tablespoons lemon juice
2 tablespoons water, plus additional as needed
1 tablespoon grapeseed, rice bran, or other neutral-tasting oil (see page 146)
¼ teaspoon salt, or to taste

1. Put the cashews in your spice grinder (in batches) or food processor. Process until they pass the powdered stage and begin to clump a bit, about 1 minute.

2. Put the ground cashews, lemon juice, water, oil, and salt in your blender or food processor. Blend until very smooth and creamy, about 3 minutes.

3. Scrape the cashew mixture into a container, cover, and chill in the refrigerator for 12 to 24 hours. It will thicken quite a bit, achieving a nice spreadable consistency.

4. If it thickens up too much, whisk in more water, 1 tablespoon at a time, until it reaches your desired consistency.

5. Store in an airtight container in the refrigerator for up to 1 week.

INSTANT CHEEZE VARIATION

If you would prefer to use this cheeze immediately, reduce the water to 1 tablespoon. Add more water only as needed to get a smooth, creamy consistency.

SEEDY CHEEZE

MAKES APPROXIMATELY 1¼ CUPS

This soft cheese alternative has a ricotta-like consistency and a somewhat pronounced flavor from the seeds. It's a great option for sunflower seed fans and those with nut allergies, but even my nut-loving husband thought this was a tasty spread.

> 1 cup hulled sunflower seeds
> ½ cup water, plus additional for soaking and rinsing
> ¼ cup nutritional yeast, or to taste
> 3½ tablespoons lemon juice
> 2 tablespoons grapeseed, rice bran, or other neutral-tasting oil (see page 146)
> 1¼ teaspoons salt
> 1 teaspoon white miso (gluten free or soy free, if needed)
> ½ teaspoon onion powder
> ½ teaspoon paprika

1. Put the seeds in a container and cover with a few inches of water. Cover and place in the refrigerator to soak for 12 to 24 hours.

2. Rub the soaked seeds between your fingers to release most of the skins. They will tend to float to the top. Drain the water slowly, along with most of the skins. Add more water, and repeat. You can repeat this again, but don't worry if there are still some remaining skins; they won't significantly affect the outcome.

3. Put the drained seeds, ½ cup water, nutritional yeast, lemon juice, oil, salt, miso, onion powder, and paprika in your blender or food processor. Blend until relatively smooth and creamy, about 2 minutes.

4. Line a fine-mesh sieve with a double layer of cheesecloth and place the sieve over a bowl to catch any liquid. Scrape the seed mixture into the center of the cheesecloth. Bring the corners of the cheesecloth together, twist to tighten the seed mixture into a packed ball, and set it back down into the sieve. Place the bowl in the refrigerator for 12 to 24 hours. The seed mixture will set up and release a few tablespoons of liquid. It's ready when the cheesecloth pulls away without the cheese alternative sticking to it.

5. Preheat your oven to 300°F and line a baking sheet with parchment paper or a silicone baking mat.

6. Carefully peel away the cheesecloth from the cheeze wheel. Place the cheeze on your prepared baking sheet.

7. Bake for 40 to 45 minutes, or until it is a little cracked on top and a lightly golden crust has formed. Let cool for 5 minutes before serving.

8. Store in an airtight container in the refrigerator for up to 1 week.

COTTAGE-STYLE CHEEZE

MAKES 1¾ CUPS

Don't let the odd combination of ingredients fool you. This quick, easy, flavorful, and protein-rich recipe is a crowd-pleaser. It even won over a family of cheese lovers. It's not identical to cottage cheese, but it's the closest dairy-free version you will find. And it is delicious in lasagna and casseroles, as a toast topper, or just about any other way you would enjoy cottage cheese.

> 12 ounces organic firm tofu
> ½ cup regular, vegan, or light mayonnaise
> 2 tablespoons water
> 1 tablespoon white miso (gluten free, if needed)
> ⅜ teaspoon salt, or to taste

1. Drain and press the tofu, using a tea towel or paper towels, to remove any excess water. Put the drained tofu in a medium bowl.
2. In a small bowl, whisk together the mayonnaise, water, and miso until smooth. Whisk in the salt.
3. Scrape the mayonnaise mixture onto the tofu and thoroughly mash it together. It is ready when you have small tofu chunks and a cottage cheese–like appearance.
4. Store in an airtight container in the refrigerator for up to 3 days.

. . . .

SAVORY-STYLE VARIATION

Whisk ¾ teaspoon onion powder and ¼ teaspoon garlic powder into the mayonnaise mixture. Optionally stir in 1 to 2 tablespoons minced fresh herbs after the tofu is mashed.

. . . .

PINE NUT PARMA SPRINKLES

MAKES 1 CUP

I tested ten different nuts and seeds, plus several blends, but pine nuts stood out as our favorite for homemade dairy-free Parmesan sprinkles. And though they may seem like a pricey splurge, this small batch yields a lot of flavor. My second-favorite blend is a 50/50 mix of walnuts and cashews used in place of the pine nuts, but you can swap in another nut in a pinch. Just keep in mind that your choice will affect the flavor profile.

> ½ cup raw or toasted pine nuts
> ¼ cup nutritional yeast flakes
> ⅜ to ½ teaspoon sea salt, to taste

1. Put the pine nuts, nutritional yeast, and salt in your spice grinder or small food processor. Process just until powdered, about 30 seconds. It's okay if they clump slightly, but if you process the nuts for too long, they'll begin to clump heavily and turn into nut butter.
2. Store in an airtight container at room temperature for up to 3 days, in the refrigerator for up to 3 weeks, or in the freezer to enjoy later.

SUNFLOWER GRATED PARMA

MAKES 1½ CUPS

Sunflower seeds aren't as rich as pine nuts, so they require an extra boost of flavor. This dairy-free Parmesan version retains a fine, powder-like, grated consistency that's practically foolproof.

> ½ cup sunflower seed kernels
> ½ cup nutritional yeast flakes
> ½ to ¾ teaspoon salt, to taste

1. Put the sunflower seeds, nutritional yeast, and salt in your spice grinder or food processor. Process just until powdered, about 30 seconds.
2. Store in an airtight container at room temperature for up to 3 days, in the refrigerator for up to 3 weeks, or in the freezer to enjoy later.

SNEAKY CHEESY SAUCE

MAKES 2 CUPS

This recipe is loaded with vegetables that work in harmony for a creamy, cheesy, comforting sauce. Enjoy it atop vegetables or grain bowls, or make one of the Mac & Cheeze Recipes below.

½ cup raw cashews
1½ cups unsweetened plain dairy-free milk beverage, plus additional as needed
1 cup cooked, peeled, and diced yellow potatoes (see Vegetable Cooking Tip below)
⅓ cup cooked diced carrots (see Vegetable Cooking Tip below)
¼ to ⅓ cup nutritional yeast flakes, to taste
3 to 4 teaspoons lemon juice, to taste
1¼ teaspoons salt, or to taste
½ teaspoon paprika
Pinch cayenne pepper
1 tablespoon grapeseed, olive, or rice bran oil

1. Put the cashews in your spice grinder or small food processor. Process until powdered, about 30 seconds.
2. Put the ground cashews, milk beverage, potatoes, carrots, nutritional yeast, lemon juice, salt, paprika, and cayenne in your blender. Blend until smooth, about 1 minute.
3. Pour the mixture into your saucepan and place the pan over medium heat. Whisk often until it just begins to boil. Reduce the heat to medium-low and let it bubble, whisking occasionally, for about 3 minutes. If it thickens too much for your liking, whisk in more milk beverage as needed.
4. Remove the pan from the heat and whisk in the oil until smooth.
5. Store in an airtight container in the refrigerator for up to 1 week.

VEGETABLE COOKING TIP: *This recipe is a great way to use up leftover cooked vegetables. But if you don't have any on hand, you can steam peeled carrots and unpeeled halved potatoes together for 10 to 15 minutes, or until quite tender. Once cooked, the potatoes are very easy to peel by hand.*

MAC & CHEEZE RECIPES

STOVETOP MAC & CHEEZE: Cook 12 ounces dry macaroni (gluten free, if needed) according to the package directions. Stir the cooked macaroni into the sauce, while still warm.

BAKED MAC & CHEEZE: Prepare the Stovetop Mac & Cheeze above. Transfer the mixture to a baking dish and cover with salted dairy-free bread crumbs (gluten free, if needed) or cover with a lid. Bake at 350°F for 15 to 20 minutes.

EASY ORANGE CHEESY SAUCE

MAKES 2¼ CUPS

This is my go-to cheesy sauce base since it's so darn easy to make, and it's easily adaptable to taste. The carrots add a wonderful orange hue, a touch of body, and just the right amount of natural sweetness to brighten the flavors without overpowering. The smoked paprika adds a "barbecue" vibe, as my husband puts it, and is completely optional.

2 cups water
¾ cup chopped soft-cooked carrots (see Cooked Carrots Tip on page 283)
6 tablespoons grapeseed, rice bran, or other neutral-tasting oil (see page 146)
¼ to ⅓ cup nutritional yeast flakes, to taste
¼ cup cornstarch or arrowroot starch *or* ⅓ cup all-purpose flour
1 tablespoon lemon juice
1½ teaspoons salt, plus additional as needed
½ teaspoon paprika
¼ teaspoon onion powder
¼ teaspoon garlic powder
¼ teaspoon smoked paprika (optional)
Pinch cayenne pepper
½ to ¾ cup unsweetened plain dairy-free milk beverage

1. Put the water, carrots, oil, nutritional yeast, starch or flour, lemon juice, salt, paprika, onion powder, garlic powder, smoked paprika (if using), and cayenne in your blender. Blend until all of the carrot bits have vanished and the mixture is smooth, about 2 minutes.

2. For the smoothest results, pour the liquid through a fine-mesh sieve (to remove any little carrot bits) into a medium saucepan.

3. Place the saucepan over medium heat and whisk continuously until the sauce begins to thicken, about 3 to 5 minutes.

4. Slowly whisk in the milk beverage as needed to reach your desired consistency.

5. Add more salt, to taste, if needed. I often add another ⅛ teaspoon.

6. This sauce is best used immediately, but it can be cooled completely and stored in an airtight container in the refrigerator for up to 2 days. Gently reheat the sauce when ready to use, but do not bring it to a boil. Whisk in water, if needed, to reach your desired consistency.

STOVETOP MAC & CHEEZE RECIPE

Cook 16 ounces dry macaroni (gluten free, if needed) according to the package directions. Stir the cooked pasta into the sauce while still warm. For a more complete meal that serves 4 to 6 people, stir in steamed cauliflower or broccoli florets and a favorite cooked protein.

MELTY MOZZA CHEESE

MAKES ABOUT ¾ CUP

Is it exactly like mozzarella cheese? Now, that would be a very bold claim. But does it stand in nicely for mozzarella atop pizzas, vegetables, and more? Yes, it really does. It's got that creamy, sticky mouthfeel of mozzarella and it's already melted! If you want a more pungent topper, you can add a little more nutritional yeast, lemon juice, and salt, to taste.

½ cup raw cashews
1 cup unsweetened plain dairy-free milk beverage (see Ingredient Notes below)
2 tablespoons tapioca starch (see Ingredient Notes below)
1 tablespoon nutritional yeast flakes
2 teaspoons lemon juice
¾ teaspoon tahini
¾ teaspoon salt
¼ teaspoon garlic powder
Water, as needed (optional)

1. Put the cashews in your spice grinder or small food processor. Process until powdered, about 30 seconds.

2. Put the ground cashews, milk beverage, starch, nutritional yeast, lemon juice, tahini, salt, and garlic powder in your blender. Blend until smooth, about 1 minute.

3. For the smoothest results, pour the sauce through a fine-mesh sieve (to remove any little nut bits) into a medium saucepan.

4. Place the saucepan over medium heat and whisk the sauce as you bring it to a low boil. Reduce the heat to medium-low and cook while whisking for 2 to 3 minutes. The sauce will become very thick and sticky. If a thinner consistency is desired, whisk in water, as needed.

5. This sauce is best used immediately, but it can be cooled completely and stored in an airtight container in the refrigerator for up to 2 days. Gently reheat the sauce when ready to use, but do not bring it to a boil. Whisk in water, if needed, to get the best consistency.

INGREDIENT NOTES:

STARCH OPTIONS: *Tapioca starch is what makes this more of a sticky, melty cheese alternative. You can substitute cornstarch or arrowroot starch, but the consistency will be less stretchy.*

MILK BEVERAGE OPTIONS: *I use coconut milk beverage because it combines well with the flavor of cashews. You can use another type, but do not use a milk beverage with protein added.*

SLICEABLE SANDWICH CHEEZE

MAKES 2 (6 × 3-INCH) MINI LOAVES OR 3 CUPS

These unique cheeze blocks slice easily for a mild cheesy addition to sandwiches or crackers. The blocks can also be shredded, but the cheeze doesn't readily melt. For a melty cheeze sauce, omit the agar-agar, skip steps 1 and 4 through 7, and add the water in step 3.

    1½ cups water
    1 tablespoon agar-agar powder (can substitute ⅓ cup agar-agar flakes)
    ½ cup raw cashews
    ⅓ cup almonds (preferably blanched) (can substitute more cashews)
    6 tablespoons nutritional yeast flakes
    ⅓ cup unsweetened plain dairy-free milk beverage
    3 tablespoons lemon juice
    1 tablespoon grapeseed, rice bran, or other neutral-tasting oil (see page 146)
    1 tablespoon white miso (gluten free or soy free, if needed)
    1 tablespoon Dijon mustard
    1 teaspoon onion powder
    ¾ teaspoon garlic powder
    ½ to ¾ teaspoon salt, to taste

1. In a small saucepan over medium heat, whisk together the water and agar-agar powder. When it just begins to bubble, reduce the heat to low and simmer for 4 minutes, or until the agar-agar is fully dissolved (this will take closer to 10 minutes if using agar-agar flakes).

2. Put the cashews and almonds in your spice grinder or food processor. Process until powdered, about 30 seconds.

3. Put the ground nuts, nutritional yeast, milk beverage, lemon juice, oil, miso, mustard, onion powder, garlic powder, and salt in your blender or food processor. Blend until smooth and creamy, about 2 minutes.

4. When the agar-agar mixture is ready, add it to the mixture in your blender or food processor. Blend until smooth, about 1 minute.

5. Pour the cheesy mixture into two greased 6 × 3-inch mini loaf pans, a silicone mold, or a lightly greased plastic container. Tap the pans, mold, or container on the counter to level out the cheeze.

6. Let cool to room temperature, and then refrigerate the cheeze for at least 1 hour.

7. Once set, unmold the cheeze and store in an airtight container or plastic wrap in the refrigerator for up to 1 week.

POWDERED CHEEZE MIX

MAKES 3½ CUPS

This powder takes minutes to throw together and is a great convenience to have o...
it to flavor and thicken casseroles, to make the Instant Cheeze Sauce Recipe below, or to w...
up a quick batch of COMPANY'S COMING NACHO DIP (page 283) or GRILLED CHEEZE SANDWICHES
(page 342).

1½ cups raw cashews
1 cup nutritional yeast flakes
¼ cup tapioca starch (can substitute cornstarch)
1 tablespoon paprika
1 tablespoon salt
2 teaspoons garlic powder
2 teaspoons onion powder
¼ teaspoon cane sugar

1. Put the cashews, nutritional yeast, starch, paprika, salt, garlic powder, onion powder,
   and sugar in your spice grinder (in batches) or food processor. Process until powdered or
   finely ground, about 1 minute.

2. Store in an airtight container in the refrigerator for up to 1 month.

NUT-FREE OPTION

Substitute sunflower seeds for the cashews. The seeds are slightly bitter when compared
to the sweetness of cashews, and create their own unique cheesy flavor. For a more pungent flavor punch, use 1¼ cups sunflower seeds plus ¼ cup sesame seeds.

INSTANT CHEEZE SAUCE RECIPE

In a small saucepan, whisk together ½ cup of the powdered cheeze mix and ¾ cup cold
water. Place the pan over medium heat. Cook, while whisking continuously, until the
sauce thickens, about 3 minutes. Whisk in more water as needed if it thickens too much.
Remove from the heat and whisk in ½ teaspoon lemon juice.

CHAPTER 19

BLENDS TO BREWS
Hot, Cold & Creamy Drink Recipes

GOOD TO KNOW FOR THIS CHAPTER

SMOOTHIES LOVE SUPPLEMENTS. Powdered minerals (like calcium or magnesium citrate) and probiotics blend seamlessly into creamy smoothies, and vitamin C crystals can add potent tang. Omega 3–rich oils add body and vitamin D drops can easily sneak in.

BUT PROTEIN POWDERS HAVE THEIR LIMITS. For the best taste, consistency, and balanced nutrition, I typically add just 1 to 2 tablespoons of dairy-free protein powder per smoothie serving. You can add more, but regardless of the type, it will start taking on a powdery vibe. See page 76 for the lowdown on dairy-free protein powders.

GO SLOWLY WITH GREENS. When adding spinach or kale to smoothies, start with just a handful and move up from there. Their mild flavors can easily become more pronounced if too much is added. Also, start with as little liquid as possible when blending. Once creamy, you can blend in more liquid. If you add too much liquid at first, pieces of green might just spin and spin rather than blending in.

BANANAS AREN'T ABSOLUTELY ESSENTIAL. They're easy, sweet, and creamy, but in a pinch, you can substitute a smoothie banana with ⅓ to ½ cup dairy-free yogurt or half of a ripe avocado plus 1 or 2 soft pitted Medjool dates or your favorite sweetener to taste. If a fruity flavor is suitable, you can swap ⅔ cup papaya chunks or low-fiber mango chunks for the banana.

PURE VANILLA FLAVORING IS SOMETIMES PREFERRED. Pure vanilla extract is typically sold in an alcohol solution. Pure vanilla that isn't in alcohol is often called "vanilla flavoring" even if it isn't imitation. For smoothies, icings, and other uncooked preparations, I typically use pure vanilla flavoring. But in recipes where most of the alcohol cooks or bakes off, I use pure vanilla extract. Nonetheless, you can use either extract or flavoring if you keep only one on hand.

THE HOT BEVERAGES ARE MICROWAVE-FRIENDLY. The directions for all of the warm drinks in this chapter are for the stovetop. But if you prefer the speed and ease of your microwave, simply prepare the recipe in a microwave-safe mug and then warm it in the microwave for about 1 minute on high. It should be hot, but not boiling.

WILD BLUE SMOOTHIE

MAKES 1 TO 2 SERVINGS

This was our daily, go-to smoothie for years. We love the beautiful purple hue and the naturally sweet flavor, and my husband was simply enamored by the fact that you can't see or taste the spinach. Trust me, not even your green-hating kids will know it's in there.

> 1 medium very ripe banana, broken into chunks
> 1 cup frozen wild blueberries
> ½ to 1 cup unsweetened plain or vanilla dairy-free milk beverage
> ½ cup baby spinach leaves
> 1 tablespoon packed ground flaxseed or chia seeds
> ¼ teaspoon ground cinnamon (optional)
> ½ cup ice (optional)
> Honey, agave nectar, or pure liquid stevia, to taste (optional)

1. Put the banana, frozen blueberries, ½ cup milk beverage, spinach, seed meal or seeds, and cinnamon (if using) in your blender. Blend until smooth, about 1 minute.
2. For a thinner smoothie, blend in up to ½ cup more milk beverage. For a frostier treat, blend in the ice.
3. Taste test and blend in sweetener, if desired.
4. Pour into 1 or 2 glasses and serve immediately.

BANANA-FREE OPTION

Use the full 1 cup milk beverage, increase the frozen wild blueberries to 1¼ cups, and add 2 soft pitted Medjool dates. Swap 2 tablespoons almond butter or sunflower seed butter for the seeds for a richer, creamier finish.

THE BIG SQUEEZE SMOOTHIE

MAKES 1 SERVING

A few years ago, we discovered a wonderful organic juice company that spikes their fresh-squeezed orange juice with turmeric. The combination is delicious brilliance! I add a pinch of black pepper to help increase turmeric's bioavailability dramatically (by 2,000 percent according to some studies). I like to make this sweet blend with fresh-squeezed orange juice for its natural bone-building abilities and amazing taste, but you can use a calcium-fortified variety, if preferred.

> 1 cup mango chunks (see Mango Note below)
> ⅔ cup frozen pineapple chunks
> ½ cup orange juice, preferably fresh squeezed (about 2 medium oranges)
> ¼ teaspoon ground turmeric
> Small pinch black pepper

1. Put the mango, frozen pineapple, orange juice, turmeric, and pepper in your blender. Blend until smooth, about 1 minute.
2. Pour into a glass and serve immediately.

> *MANGO NOTE:* *Some varieties of mangoes have fibers, which can produce unwanted textures in creamy smoothies. If you can, seek out mangoes with no fibers, such as Honey/Ataulfo. Ones with limited fibers, like Keitt, Kent, and Palmer, should also work well in smoothies. But try to avoid Francis and Tommy Atkins varieties, which are quite fibrous.*

SUMMER BERRY VARIATION

Substitute ⅔ cup fresh or frozen strawberries or blackberries for the pineapple chunks. Blackberries have seeds that don't easily blend. If this bothers you, then you can pre-blend the blackberries and press them through a fine-mesh sieve to remove the seeds.

GINGERSNAP SUPER SMOOTHIE

MAKES 1 SERVING

This creamy blend has a warm spiced finish that you can enjoy year-round. I find fresh ginger a little too potent in smoothies like this one, so I opt for good-quality powdered ginger. If you prefer fresh, start with ½ teaspoon minced and move up from there. I also enjoy this mineral-rich smoothie with the full 2 teaspoons of blackstrap molasses, but since the flavor can be bold, you might want to start with the lesser amount.

> 1 medium to large very ripe frozen banana, broken into chunks
> ½ cup unsweetened plain almond milk beverage, lite coconut milk, or water
> 1½ tablespoons almond butter
> 2 teaspoons blackstrap molasses
> ¼ teaspoon pure vanilla flavoring or extract

⅛ to ¼ teaspoon ground ginger, to taste
⅛ teaspoon ground cinnamon
Pinch salt
1 teaspoon honey or maple syrup *or* 5 drops pure liquid stevia (optional)

1. Put the frozen banana, milk alternative or water, almond butter, molasses, vanilla, ginger, cinnamon, and salt in your blender. Blend until smooth, about 1 minute.
2. Taste test and blend in sweetener, to taste, if desired.
3. Pour into a glass and serve immediately.

NUT-FREE OPTION

Substitute sunflower seed butter for the almond butter and use lite coconut milk or water for the liquid.

JUST PEACHY POWER SMOOTHIE

MAKES 1 SERVING

Peaches provide a creamy base for making healthy banana-free smoothies. However, their flavor can be bland or sour if they aren't ripe enough. If your peaches aren't at their peak, you can swap in another sweet stone fruit, like nectarines, apricots, or dark sweet cherries.

1 cup fresh or frozen ripe peach slices (about 1 medium peach)
¾ cup unsweetened plain dairy-free milk beverage, plus additional if needed
1 tablespoon almond butter or sunflower seed butter
¼ teaspoon pure vanilla flavoring or extract
⅛ teaspoon ground ginger *or* ¼ teaspoon ground cinnamon
Pinch salt (omit if using salted nut or seed butter)
2 teaspoons honey or agave nectar, or to taste
3 to 5 drops pure liquid stevia, or to taste
½ cup ice (optional)

1. Put the peaches, milk beverage, nut or seed butter, vanilla, ginger or cinnamon, and salt (if using) in your blender. Blend until smooth, about 1 minute. If using frozen fruit, you may need to pulse your blender at first to break it up.
2. Blend in the honey or agave nectar and stevia.
3. For a thinner smoothie, blend in more milk beverage as needed. For a frostier treat, blend in the ice.
4. Pour into a glass and serve immediately.

PROTEIN SHAKE VARIATION

Add 1 to 2 tablespoons vanilla dairy-free protein powder (like pea protein) and omit the vanilla. Sweeten to taste, if needed.

PUMPKIN PIE PROTEIN SHAKE

MAKES 1 SERVING

This creamy shake recipe emerged when I had leftover canned pumpkin from the holidays. These days I stock up on pumpkin in the winter so I can enjoy this healthy, cool shake in the summer, too. Please note that the stevia in this recipe isn't purely for adding sweetness. It also helps brighten the spices and other flavors.

   1 medium to large very ripe frozen banana, broken into chunks
   ½ cup lite coconut milk or unsweetened plain dairy-free milk beverage, plus
      additional if needed
   ⅓ to ½ cup pumpkin puree, to taste
   2 tablespoons plain dairy-free protein powder (such as pea protein)
   2 teaspoons maple syrup, or to taste
   ¼ teaspoon pure vanilla flavoring or extract
   ¼ teaspoon pumpkin pie spice (store-bought or Pumpkin Pie Spice Recipe below)
   ¼ teaspoon ground cinnamon (or more pumpkin pie spice)
   2 to 4 drops pure liquid stevia (optional)
   Generous pinch salt

1. Put the banana, coconut milk or milk beverage, pumpkin, protein powder, maple syrup, vanilla, pie spice, cinnamon, stevia (if using), and salt in your blender. Blend until smooth, about 1 minute.
2. If the shake is too thick, blend in more lite coconut milk or milk beverage as needed.
3. Pour into a glass and serve immediately.

PROTEIN VARIATION

If you don't have a favorite protein powder handy, you can substitute 1 to 2 tablespoons of nut or seed butter. This will result in a slightly richer and very delicious shake.

PUMPKIN PIE SPICE RECIPE

In a small bowl, whisk together 2 tablespoons ground cinnamon, 1 tablespoon ground ginger, 1 tablespoon ground nutmeg, and 1 tablespoon ground allspice. You can optionally add up to ¾ teaspoon ground cloves for a spicier kick. This makes about ⅓ cup.

CHOCOLATE FROSTEE

MAKES 2 SERVINGS

The consistency of this cool shake is just like a Wendy's Frosty, but it's made with much healthier ingredients. Don't worry—it's still kid approved!

1 cup lite coconut milk
½ small ripe avocado, pitted and peeled
3 to 4 tablespoons agave nectar, honey, or cane sugar, or to taste
2 tablespoons cocoa powder (can substitute carob powder)
¾ teaspoon pure vanilla flavoring or extract
2 drops pure liquid stevia (optional)
Pinch salt
1 to 1½ cups crushed ice

1. Put the coconut milk, avocado, sweetener, cocoa powder, vanilla, stevia (if using), and salt in your blender. Blend until smooth, about 30 seconds.
2. Blend in the ice until smooth and creamy, about 30 seconds.
3. Pour into 2 glasses and serve immediately.

FLAVOR & FUNCTION VARIATIONS

MINT CHOCOLATE: Add ⅛ teaspoon peppermint extract.

PROTEIN POWER: Add 2 tablespoons of your favorite dairy-free protein powder. Omit the stevia and reduce the sweetener if it is a sweetened powder.

LOWER ADDED SUGARS: Substitute a frozen medium to large very ripe banana, broken into chunks, for half or all of the ice. Add the liquid sweetener or sugar only as needed, to taste.

MOCHA FRAPPÉ-CCINO

MAKES 2 SERVINGS

Since I'm not a coffee drinker, I asked my associate editor, Sarah Hatfield, to whip up this blend using my easy homemade chocolate syrup recipe. It's an allergen-safe alternative that's every bit as good as what you'd get at the coffee shop—and far less expensive!

2 cups ice
½ cup unsweetened plain dairy-free milk beverage or lite coconut milk
⅓ cup cold strong coffee
3 tablespoons CHOCOLATE SYRUP (page 215)
3 tablespoons cane sugar, or to taste

1. Put the ice, milk beverage or coconut milk, coffee, chocolate syrup, and sugar in your blender. Pulse to crush the ice, and then blend until relatively smooth.
2. Pour into 2 glasses and serve immediately.

VANILLA MYLKSHAKE

MAKES 2 SERVINGS

Soaked cashews and frozen rich coconut milk combine to make the perfect sweet and creamy base for this very vanilla treat. Do not be tempted to swap in coconut milk beverage; it won't yield the same indulgent results.

¼ cup full-fat coconut milk
¼ cup raw cashews
½ cup water, plus additional for soaking
2 tablespoons cane sugar or agave nectar
1½ teaspoons pure vanilla flavoring or extract
1 cup crushed ice

1. Pour the coconut milk into ice cube trays and freeze.
2. Meanwhile, put the cashews in a container and cover with a few inches of water. Cover and place in the refrigerator to soak for 4 to 6 hours. Drain and rinse the cashews.
3. Put the soaked cashews, ½ cup water, sweetener, and vanilla in your blender. Blend until smooth, about 1 minute.
4. Blend in the frozen coconut milk cubes and ice until smooth and creamy, about 1 minute.
5. Pour into 2 glasses and serve immediately.

STRAWBERRY MYLK

MAKES 1 SERVING

Strawberry syrup pales in comparison to this fresh strawberry beverage. Since the sweetness of this recipe can vary quite a bit, depending on the flavor of your strawberries and milk beverage, it is important to sweeten to taste.

1 cup plain or unsweetened plain dairy-free milk beverage
½ cup fresh or frozen strawberries
2 to 4 teaspoons cane sugar, agave nectar, or honey, to taste
¼ teaspoon pure vanilla flavoring or extract

1. Put the milk beverage, strawberries, sweetener, and vanilla in your blender. Blend until smooth, about 1 minute.
2. If desired, strain the mylk through a fine-mesh sieve, nut milk bag, or a double layer of cheesecloth to remove any lingering seeds.
3. Store in an airtight container in the refrigerator for up to 2 days.

CHOCOLATE MYLK

MAKES ABOUT 24 SERVINGS OF SYRUP

This recipe is multipurpose. The chocolate syrup not only makes delicious mylk, but it also works as a chocolate topping on ice cream or other desserts, and for whipping up Mocha Frappé-ccinos (page 213). This syrup is deep and dark. I prefer it with the lesser amount of sugar, but if you would like a sweeter sauce, feel free to use the higher amount.

CHOCOLATE SYRUP
1½ to 1¾ cups cane sugar
1 cup cocoa powder
Pinch salt
1 cup cold water
2 teaspoons pure vanilla flavoring or extract

CHOCOLATE MYLK
1 cup plain or unsweetened plain dairy-free milk beverage
1 tablespoon Chocolate Syrup, or to taste

1. **To make the chocolate syrup**, whisk together the sugar, cocoa powder, and salt in a large saucepan until no cocoa clumps remain. Gradually whisk in the water until smooth.
2. Place the pan over medium heat. Whisk continuously as the mixture comes to a boil. Reduce the heat to medium-low and let it bubble for 3 minutes, whisking often.
3. Remove the pan from the heat and stir in the vanilla. Let cool to room temperature.
4. If desired, strain the syrup through a fine-mesh sieve for a very smooth consistency.
5. Store in an airtight container in the refrigerator for up to 3 weeks.
6. **To make 1 serving of chocolate mylk**, pour the milk beverage into a glass and drizzle in the chocolate syrup while stirring.

FLAVOR VARIATIONS

Mylk Chocolate Syrup: Use plain milk beverage, unsweetened milk beverage, or lite coconut milk in place of the water in the chocolate syrup.

Carob Syrup: Substitute carob powder for half or all of the cocoa powder.

INSTANT VANILLA CHAI LATTE

MAKES 2 SERVINGS

Traditional masala chai involves simmering whole spices, but I like having a ground spice mix on hand to heat up my own coffeehouse drinks on a whim. Chai does sometimes contain black pepper, but I prefer it without. If you like the extra kick that black pepper provides, add a pinch or more to your mix.

⅔ cup hot water
1½ teaspoons chai spice mix (see Chai Mix Recipes below), or to taste
1 black, white, or rooibos tea bag
1⅓ cups unsweetened plain dairy-free milk beverage or lite coconut milk
2 to 3 tablespoons honey or your favorite sweetener, or to taste
1 teaspoon pure vanilla flavoring or extract
Pinch salt

1. Pour the hot water into a small saucepan and whisk in the spice mix.
2. Add the tea bag to the hot spiced water and let it brew for 3 to 5 minutes. Remove the tea bag.
3. Whisk the milk beverage, sweetener, vanilla, and salt into the spiced tea.
4. Place the pan over medium-low heat. Heat, while whisking, until the latte is hot and steaming but not boiling.
5. Pour into 2 small mugs and serve immediately.

DRINK VARIATIONS

Spiced Mylk: Omit the water and tea bag and increase the milk beverage to 2 cups. Skip steps 1 and 2, but add the spice mix to the milk beverage in the saucepan in step 3.

Chai Café Latte: Substitute ⅔ cup strong-brewed coffee (regular or decaf) for the hot water and omit the tea bag. Skip step 2.

CHAI MIX RECIPES

Cinnamon-Spice Chai Mix: In a small bowl, whisk together 2 teaspoons ground cinnamon, 1 teaspoon ground ginger, 1 teaspoon ground cardamom, ½ teaspoon ground allspice, and ¼ teaspoon ground cloves. This makes about 1½ tablespoons.

Spicy Chai Mix: In a small bowl, whisk together 1½ teaspoons ground cinnamon, 1¼ teaspoons ground cardamom, ¾ teaspoon ground ginger, ¾ teaspoon ground allspice, and ½ teaspoon ground cloves. This makes about 1½ tablespoons.

HOT DRINKING CHOCOLATE

MAKES 2 SERVINGS

This rich beverage boasts a double dose of chocolate, for a sweet, dessert-like treat. It's perfect for those cold, damp evenings when you are chilled to the bone. For a less indulgent drink, start with 2 tablespoons sweetener and add the remaining 2 tablespoons sweetener only as desired. Or to up the creaminess, use lite coconut milk in place of the milk beverage.

> 2 cups plain or unsweetened plain dairy-free milk beverage
> ¼ cup cane sugar, agave nectar, or sweetener of choice
> 2 tablespoons cocoa powder
> 2 ounces dairy-free semi-sweet chocolate chips or chopped dark chocolate
> ¼ teaspoon pure vanilla flavoring or extract
> Pinch salt
> Regular or vegan marshmallows, for garnish (optional)
> COOL WHIPPED COCONUT CREAM (page 424), for garnish (optional)

1. Put the milk beverage, sweetener, and cocoa powder in a medium saucepan over medium heat. Bring the mixture just to a simmer while whisking continuously to break up any clumps of cocoa.
2. Add the chocolate and continue whisking until melted and smooth.
3. Remove the pan from the heat and whisk in the vanilla and salt.
4. Pour into 2 small mugs and top with marshmallows (if using) or whipped coconut cream (if using).

....

FLAVOR VARIATIONS

SPICED: In step 1, whisk in ¼ teaspoon ground cinnamon, ¼ teaspoon ground cardamom, ¼ teaspoon ground ginger, and a pinch ground nutmeg.

MOCHA: In step 1, whisk in 1 tablespoon instant coffee powder.

PEPPERMINT: Serve with a peppermint candy cane as a stir stick, or stir in ¼ to ½ teaspoon peppermint extract or 2 ounces peppermint schnapps (adults only!) with the vanilla extract.

....

CLASSIC HOT COCOA

MAKES 1 SERVING

Maple syrup adds delicious depth to this warm, comforting beverage. Hot cocoa is typically mellower than hot chocolate, but you can increase the cocoa powder to 1 tablespoon if you like a bolder hit of cacao.

> 1 cup plain or unsweetened plain dairy-free milk beverage
> 2 teaspoons cocoa powder
> 1½ teaspoons maple syrup
> 1½ teaspoons cane sugar, or to taste
> ⅛ teaspoon pure vanilla flavoring or extract
> Pinch salt
> Regular or vegan marshmallows, for garnish (optional)

1. Put the milk beverage, cocoa powder, maple syrup, and sugar in a small saucepan over medium heat. Bring the mixture just to a simmer while whisking continuously to break up any clumps of cocoa.
2. Remove the pan from the heat and whisk in the vanilla and salt.
3. Pour into a small mug and top with marshmallows (if using).

TOASTY CAROB MYLK

MAKES 1 SERVING

This is a nice variation for those who are seeking to cut caffeine or who, like me, enjoy the sweet earthy taste of carob.

> 1 cup plain or unsweetened plain dairy-free milk beverage
> 1 tablespoon carob powder
> 2 teaspoons cane sugar, agave nectar, or maple syrup, or to taste
> ¼ teaspoon pure vanilla flavoring or extract
> Pinch salt
> Regular or vegan marshmallows, for garnish (optional)

1. Put the milk beverage, carob powder, and sweetener in a small saucepan over medium heat. Bring the mixture just to a simmer while whisking continuously to break up any clumps of carob.
2. Remove the pan from the heat and whisk in the vanilla and salt.
3. Pour into a small mug and top with marshmallows (if using).

WARMING UP TO MOLASSES MYLK

MAKES 1 SERVING

It's great to hear that foods like blackstrap molasses are high in dairy-free calcium, but how do you use such an intense sweetener? This comforting warm milk beverage is an instant way to enjoy this mineral-rich ingredient. And the recipe is both adult and kid approved!

1 cup water
1 tablespoon creamy almond butter (can substitute sunflower seed butter for nut free)
1 tablespoon blackstrap molasses
1½ teaspoons maple syrup *or* 3 to 5 drops pure liquid stevia, to taste
½ teaspoon pure vanilla flavoring or extract
⅛ teaspoon ground cinnamon
Pinch salt

1. Put the water, almond butter, molasses, maple syrup or stevia, vanilla, cinnamon, and salt in your blender. Blend until smooth, about 1 minute.
2. Pour the molasses mixture into a saucepan over medium-low heat and warm, while whisking, until it reaches your desired temperature.
3. Pour into a mug and serve immediately.

CHAPTER 20
RISE & DINE!
Nutritious Any Day Breakfast Recipes

GOOD TO KNOW FOR THIS CHAPTER

MANY OF THESE OPTIONS FREEZE WELL. The waffles, pancakes, and French toast sticks in this chapter can be flash frozen. Simply place them in a single layer on a silicone baking mat or parchment paper in the freezer for 2 to 4 hours. Once frozen, store them in airtight plastic freezer bags in the freezer. For a quick breakfast, pop a couple in your toaster or toaster oven to reheat from frozen.

MANY MORNING MIXES CONTAIN DAIRY. You might be wondering why I'm covering basics like pancakes, oatmeal, and even granola in this chapter. Many store-bought varieties actually contain dairy, or are at relatively high risk for cross-contamination with dairy. Allergy-friendly brands are available, but often expensive. My homemade versions are affordable, easy, delicious, and fresh!

QUICK OATS ARE WHOLE GRAIN, TOO. I use rolled oats (also called whole or old-fashioned oats) where a heartier texture is desired, or when the oats will just be ground (rolled oats are often cheaper than quick). Quick oats retain the nutrition of rolled oats, but they have been pre-cooked, dried, and pressed thinner for a shorter cooking time. They work better in recipes where the oats won't have as much time or moisture to "tenderize" or when a creamier consistency is desired.

EASY EVERYDAY BLENDER WAFFLES

MAKES 4 TO 6 SERVINGS

These incredibly simple waffles are modeled after a favorite waffle mix. I love their ease, nutrition, and wholesome taste. Plus, they freeze quite well for a quick and healthy toaster breakfast any morning.

4 cups rolled oats (certified gluten free, if needed)
3 cups water, plus additional as needed
2 small very ripe bananas
2 tablespoons grapeseed, rice bran, or other neutral-tasting oil (page 146), plus additional for greasing
2 teaspoons vanilla extract
¼ to ½ teaspoon salt, to taste
Optional toppings: maple syrup, cut fresh fruit, COOL WHIPPED COCONUT CREAM (page 424), nut butter, or chopped nuts

1. Put the oats, water, bananas, oil, vanilla, and salt in your blender. Blend until relatively smooth, about 1 minute.
2. Let the batter sit to thicken while you grease and preheat your waffle iron.
3. When the waffle iron is ready, give the batter another quick pulse in your blender. If it becomes too thick to pour, blend in more water, 1 tablespoon at a time, until it is pourable but still quite thick.
4. Pour the batter onto your waffle iron and cook according to the waffle iron directions without lifting the lid. Some waffle makers may indicate "done" when the waffles are still a bit soft. I typically wait for the waffles to stop steaming as a more accurate indicator.
5. Serve the waffles with your toppings of choice.
6. Store leftover waffles in an airtight container in the refrigerator for up to 2 days, or freeze to enjoy later. Reheat in your toaster or toaster oven before serving.

FLAVOR VARIATIONS

SWEET CINNAMON: Add 1½ to 2 teaspoons ground cinnamon and 2 tablespoons of your favorite sweetener in step 1.

COCONUT: Substitute 6 tablespoons unsweetened coconut (shredded or grated) for the banana and add 2 to 3 tablespoons of your favorite sweetener in step 1. For an extra dose of coconut, replace the vanilla extract with coconut extract and add ¼ cup plain or vanilla coconut-based dairy-free yogurt in step 1.

PUMPKIN: Use ⅔ cup pumpkin puree in place of the banana, and add ¼ cup brown sugar or coconut sugar and 2 teaspoons pumpkin pie spice (store-bought or recipe on page 212) in step 1.

ESSENTIAL CINNAMON-RAISIN GRANOLA

MAKES 7 CUPS

Since discovering the ease and amazing taste of homemade granola, I haven't needed to scour the ingredient label of another box! My husband loves the fresher texture, and we both love the lower price, especially when I purchase the ingredients in bulk. Plus, this is a very versatile recipe. You can customize the flavor with your favorite nuts, dried fruit, and/or spices.

3½ cups rolled oats (certified gluten free, if needed)
1 cup sliced, slivered, or chopped almonds
1 cup raw cashews, coarsely chopped
⅓ cup firmly packed brown sugar or coconut sugar
1 teaspoon ground cinnamon
¼ teaspoon salt
⅓ cup maple syrup
¼ cup grapeseed, rice bran, or other neutral-tasting oil (see page 146)
1 teaspoon vanilla extract
¾ to 1 cup raisins, to taste

1. Preheat your oven to 250°F.
2. In a large bowl, stir together the oats, almonds, cashews, sugar, cinnamon, and salt. Add the maple syrup, oil, and vanilla, and stir until the dry ingredients are evenly coated.
3. Spread the mixture into 2 large ungreased glass baking dishes (see Baking Note below).
4. Bake for 1 hour, stirring the mixture every 15 minutes.
5. Immediately transfer the cooked granola to a large bowl and stir in the raisins. Let cool completely.
6. Store in an airtight container at room temperature for up to 2 weeks, or in the freezer to enjoy later.

BAKING NOTE: If you have only metal pans or cookie sheets, line them with a silicone baking mat or reduce the oven temperature by 25°F and keep a close eye. Dark metal pans will cause the granola to brown (and consequently burn) very quickly. In a pinch, you can make this entire batch in one 9 × 13-inch baking dish. But it will brown more evenly if divided between 2 dishes.

NUT-FREE OPTION

Substitute any combination of additional oats, sunflower seeds, pumpkin seeds, or unsweetened coconut flakes for the almonds and cashews.

CULTURED COCONUT YOGURT

MAKES 4 CUPS

Though you can purchase dairy-free yogurt in many stores, making your own gives you control over the ingredients, quality, and taste. It's also cost-effective for those who eat yogurt daily. Homemade yogurt can be tricky at first, but after a few batches you'll be customizing flavors and tweaking the texture with ease. The brilliant creator behind this particular yogurt recipe is my good friend Alexa Croft. She runs my favorite health and wellness website for women, **FloAndGrace.com**.

> 2 cups + ½ cup water, divided
> ¾ teaspoon agar-agar powder (for vegan) *or* 2 teaspoons gelatin
> 3 tablespoons tapioca starch (can substitute cornstarch)
> 2 tablespoons sweetener of choice
> 2 (14-ounce) cans full-fat coconut milk
> Dairy-free probiotic powder (the amount equivalent to 30 billion live active cultures) (see Probiotic Note on page 224)

1. Sterilize all of the cooking utensils, bowls, and fermentation containers you will be using by dousing them in boiling water. You want to prevent the risk of any "bad" bacteria growth.

2. Add the 2 cups water to a large pot over medium heat. Sprinkle in the agar-agar or gelatin and bring the liquid to a boil. Reduce the heat to medium-low and gently simmer for 3 to 5 minutes, or until the agar-agar or gelatin is completely dissolved.

3. In a small bowl, whisk together the remaining ½ cup water and starch.

4. Whisk the starch slurry and sweetener into the agar-agar or gelatin mixture. Bring it back to a simmer, and cook, while whisking, for 2 minutes. Add the coconut milk and whisk to combine. Continue cooking just until steam rises from the surface.

5. Remove the pan from the heat and let the coconut mixture cool to 95°F to 100°F.

6. Once the yogurt mixture hits that magic temperature range, whisk in the probiotic powder.

7. Transfer the yogurt mixture to fermentation containers and place them in your yogurt maker. Let the yogurt ferment for 8 to 10 hours.

8. Refrigerate the yogurt containers for 6 to 8 hours. The yogurt will thicken as it cools.

HOW TO SPOT AND PREVENT A BAD BATCH: If there are any hints of pink, gray, or black, throw out the batch and start again. This suggests some "bad" bacteria got in and colonized the batch. This can happen if your equipment was not thoroughly sterilized, if your probiotics were "dead," and/or if the coconut milk mixture was too hot when you added the probiotics.

INSTANT BERRY-BANANA YOGURT

MAKES 1 SERVING

This sweet, unique flavor blend has the consistency and probiotic power of yogurt, but without the dairy or long fermenting times. It also packs in loads of natural prebiotic fiber to aid in the absorption of the good bacteria.

½ medium banana
⅓ cup frozen wild blueberries
¼ cup unsweetened plain or vanilla dairy-free milk beverage
2 ounces avocado flesh (about ½ small to medium ripe avocado, pitted and peeled)
1 tablespoon fresh-squeezed lemon juice
1 serving dairy-free probiotic powder (see Probiotic Note below)
Pinch salt
7 drops pure liquid stevia or your favorite sweetener, to taste

1. Put the banana, blueberries, milk beverage, avocado, lemon juice, probiotic powder, and salt in your blender or food processor. Blend until a smooth puree forms, about 1 minute.
2. Add the stevia or sweetener and blend just to combine.
3. Enjoy the yogurt immediately, or chill it in the refrigerator and enjoy within a few hours. Freeze any leftovers into cubes to blend into smoothies.

PROBIOTIC NOTE: *You can break open a probiotic capsule and empty the contents into the recipe or use a powdered probiotic. For some dairy-free probiotic brands, along with the lowdown on dairy-free yogurt starter cultures, see* **GoDairyFree.org/probiotics**.

BAKED FRENCH TOAST STICKS

MAKES 4 SERVINGS

These easy slices are both mom and kid approved! They're fun for dipping, and a great way to use up leftover bread or gluten-free bread that is less than tender.

8 slices (½ to ¾ inch thick) stale bread (white, wheat, or gluten free)
⅔ cup lite coconut milk
2 tablespoons maple syrup
2 teaspoons vanilla extract
1 teaspoon ground cinnamon
⅛ teaspoon salt
4 large eggs (see Vegan Option on the next page for egg free)
Optional dips: maple syrup, melted dairy-free buttery spread, or
    Nutty Maple-Cinnamon Dip (recipe follows)

1. Preheat your oven to 350°F and line 1 large or 2 medium baking sheets wi̇̇̇̇̇̇̇̇̇̇̇̇̇̇̇̇̇̇̇̇̇̇̇̇ paper or silicone baking mats.

2. Cut each bread slice into 3 or 4 long pieces. For quick, even cutting, stac̈̈ a time and cut in a sawing motion with a bread knife through all of the̊̊̊

3. Put the coconut milk, maple syrup, vanilla, cinnamon, and salt in a glass̊ baking dish. Whisk until the spice is evenly distributed. Add the eggs and whisk un̊ combined.

4. Place as many bread sticks as will fit in a single layer in the egg mixture, and let them sit for 30 to 60 seconds per side. The more thick, hearty, and/or stale your bread is, the longer the bread sticks can sit and soak. Remove the bread sticks, shaking off any excess, and place them on your prepared baking sheets about 1 inch apart. Repeat until all of the slices are lightly saturated with the egg mixture, but not so much that they fall apart. If you have excess egg mixture, you can lightly drizzle it on top of the slices or cut and soak another slice of bread.

5. Bake for 10 minutes. Flip the sticks and bake for 10 more minutes, or until they are sturdy, baked through, and just starting to brown.

6. Serve the toast sticks with your choice of dip.

7. Store leftover sticks in an airtight container in the refrigerator for up to 2 days, or freeze to enjoy later. Reheat in your toaster or toaster oven before serving.

VEGAN OPTION

Increase the coconut milk to 1 cup, and mix ¼ cup mashed banana, 2 tablespoons buckwheat flour, 1 tablespoon oil, and 1 teaspoon baking powder into the wet ingredients. Follow the directions above, but bake for 15 minutes, then gently flip with a spatula (they like to stick, but can be peeled away) and bake for 5 to 7 more minutes. For firmer, crispier toast, increase the oil to 2 tablespoons and the buckwheat flour to 3 tablespoons.

NUTTY MAPLE-CINNAMON DIP RECIPE

In a small bowl, whisk together ¼ cup almond, hazelnut, or sunflower seed butter; ¼ cup unsweetened dairy-free milk beverage; 2 to 4 tablespoons maple syrup (to taste); ½ teaspoon ground cinnamon; and ⅛ teaspoon salt (omit if using salty nut or seed butter).

ACK TO SCHOOL BREAKFAST COOKIES

MAKES 40 COOKIES

Each bite of these kid- and husband-approved delights is packed with whole grains, seeds, and other nutritious goodies. They are fantastic for grabbing on the go, popping into lunch boxes, or serving as an afternoon snack. And they can easily be baked into muffin tins for perfectly portioned cookie cups. The gentle pumpkin flavor, fall spices, and quick convenience of these rustic oat cookies remind me of that exciting yet hurried time of year.

1 cup + 1½ cups rolled oats (certified gluten free, if needed), divided
⅔ cup coconut sugar or lightly packed brown sugar
2 tablespoons flax seeds
¾ teaspoon pumpkin pie spice (store-bought or recipe on page 212)
½ teaspoon baking powder
¼ teaspoon baking soda
¼ teaspoon ground cinnamon
¼ teaspoon salt
¼ cup grapeseed, rice bran, or melted coconut oil
¼ cup pumpkin puree
2 tablespoons maple syrup
1½ teaspoons vanilla extract
⅔ cup dried cranberries
½ cup chopped pecans or pumpkin seeds (for nut free)

1. Preheat your oven to 350°F and line 2 baking sheets with parchment paper or silicone baking mats.
2. Put the 1 cup oats, coconut sugar (if using), and flax seeds in your spice grinder or food processor. Process until powdered, about 1 minute.
3. Transfer the ground oat mixture to a large mixing bowl. Stir in the brown sugar (if using), pie spice, baking powder, baking soda, cinnamon, and salt until well combined. Add the oil, pumpkin, maple syrup, and vanilla and stir until well combined. Fold in the remaining 1½ cups oats, cranberries, and nuts or seeds. It will be a thick, chunky mixture.
4. Drop the dough by the tablespoonful onto your prepared baking sheets and shape the cookie dough with slightly damp hands. The cookies won't spread much.
5. Bake for 10 to 12 minutes, or until the cookies are lightly browned around the edges.
6. Let cool on the baking sheets for 10 to 15 minutes (they will firm up and be easier to handle) before removing the cookies to a wire rack to cool completely.
7. Store in an airtight container at room temperature for up to 3 days, or in the freezer to enjoy later.

....

COOKIE CUPS VARIATION

Line 20 muffin cups with cupcake liners or use silicone muffin cups. With slightly damp hands, press 2 tablespoons of dough into each cup. Bake for 15 minutes, or until the cookie cups are lightly browned around the edges. This makes 20 cookie cups.

....

DUKKAH AVOCADO TOAST

MAKES 2 SERVINGS AND 1 CUP SEASONING

Dukkah (also spelled dukka or duqqa) is a Middle Eastern toasted nut and spice blend that is typically paired with olive oil and crusty bread. But I recently discovered that creamy avocado heightens the whole experience for a hearty, savory breakfast.

DUKKAH SEASONING
⅓ cup hazelnuts (can substitute pumpkin seeds or sunflower seeds for nut free)
¼ cup sesame seeds
1 tablespoon coriander seeds
1 tablespoon cumin seeds
1 teaspoon freshly ground black pepper
½ teaspoon sea salt

AVOCADO TOAST
2 large slices whole-grain bread
½ medium ripe avocado, pitted and peeled
1 teaspoon fresh-squeezed lemon juice (optional)
2 tablespoons Dukkah Seasoning, or to taste
Extra-virgin olive oil, for garnish (optional)

1. **To make the dukkah seasoning**, preheat your oven to 350°F.

2. Spread out the hazelnuts on a baking sheet. Bake for 3 to 4 minutes, or until toasted.

3. Rub the hazelnuts in a clean tea towel to remove as much of the skins as possible.

4. Put the toasted hazelnuts in your spice grinder or small food processor and pulse to finely chop them. Put the chopped nuts in a small container.

5. Heat a dry medium skillet over medium heat. Add the sesame seeds and sauté until golden, about 1 to 2 minutes. Put the toasted seeds in the container with the hazelnuts.

6. Add the coriander seeds and cumin seeds to the skillet and sauté until aromatic and the seeds begin to pop, about 1 to 2 minutes. Put the seeds in your spice grinder and pulse to finely crush them. Put the crushed seeds in the container with the hazelnuts.

7. Add the pepper and salt to the hazelnut mixture, cover, and shake well to thoroughly combine the ingredients.

8. Store the dukkah in an airtight container at room temperature for up to 1 week, or in the refrigerator for up to 1 month.

9. **To make the avocado toast**, toast the bread.

10. Top the toast with the avocado, and smash it on like a thick layer of spread.

11. Drizzle lemon juice (if using) on top of the avocado. Sprinkle with the dukkah seasoning and drizzle on a little olive oil (if using).

PILLOWY WHOLESOME PANCAKES

MAKES 16 PANCAKES

For years, my whole-grain pancake efforts were heavy flops. But I eventually came across an inspiring batch of vegan pancakes. With that recipe as my guide, I was able to create these perfectly fluffy pancakes, which are picky husband approved!

1¾ cups plain or unsweetened plain dairy-free milk beverage

¼ cup grapeseed, rice bran, or other neutral-tasting oil (see page 146), plus additional for the skillet

2 tablespoons ground flaxseed

2 tablespoons agave nectar or honey

2 teaspoons apple cider vinegar

1 teaspoon vanilla extract

2 cups spelt flour (can substitute whole wheat, white whole wheat, or white spelt flour)

1 tablespoon baking powder

½ teaspoon baking soda

¼ teaspoon salt

Optional toppings: maple syrup, cut fresh fruit, or Cool Whipped Coconut Cream (page 424)

1. Measure the milk beverage in a glass measuring cup. Whisk in the oil, flaxseed, sweetener, vinegar, and vanilla.
2. Sift the flour, baking powder, baking soda, and salt into a large bowl. Add the milk beverage mixture and stir until thoroughly combined.
3. Heat a drizzle of oil in a large skillet over medium heat.
4. Using roughly ¼ cup per pancake, pour the batter into the pan. Cook the pancakes until the outside edge begins to look dry and bubbles break on the surface of the batter, about 3 minutes. Flip and cook until both sides are light golden brown, about 2 minutes.
5. Serve with your choice of toppings.

FLATTER OR FLUFFIER STACK VARIATIONS

If you like really thick pancakes, reduce the milk beverage by up to ¼ cup (1½ cups total). If you prefer thinner pancakes, increase the milk beverage by up to ¼ cup (2 cups total).

EGGS BENEDICT WITH BLENDER HOLLANDAISE SAUCE

MAKES 8 SINGLE MUFFINS AND 1 CUP SAUCE

This rich and buttery dairy-free hollandaise sauce is amazingly quick and easy. And believe it or not, I even have an egg-free version to share with you, too.

½ cup coconut oil
3 large egg yolks + 8 whole eggs, divided (see Vegan Option below for egg free)
2 tablespoons water, plus additional for poaching and as needed
1 tablespoon lemon juice
½ teaspoon salt
⅛ teaspoon paprika (for mild) or cayenne pepper (for spicy)
2 teaspoons white vinegar or apple cider vinegar
4 English muffins (gluten free, if needed)
8 slices Canadian bacon (pork or vegan)
2 tablespoons chopped fresh flat-leaf parsley, for garnish (optional)

1. Put the oil in a glass measuring cup and heat in your microwave on high until melted and quite hot, about 1 minute.
2. Put the egg yolks, 2 tablespoons water, and lemon juice in your blender. Blend until emulsified and pale yellow, about 1 minute.
3. With the blender motor running on low speed, very slowly drizzle in the hot oil to temper the eggs. The sauce should thicken to a very rich yet still pourable consistency. If the sauce fails to thicken, the base of your blender jar may be too big. Pour the emulsified mixture into a smaller blender attachment and blend until it reaches your desired thickness. If the sauce becomes too thick, whisk in 1 teaspoon of water at a time, until it reaches your desired consistency.
4. Add the salt and paprika or cayenne to the sauce in your blender. Blend until just combined.
5. To poach the whole eggs, fill a large skillet with 2 inches of water. Bring the water to a rapid simmer and stir in the vinegar. Crack an egg into a small bowl and slide it into the water in one corner of the pan. Repeat this process with remaining eggs (in 2 batches if needed), and cook for 3 to 4 minutes for a runny yolk, 5 to 6 minutes for a firm yolk.
6. Toast the English muffin halves while you poach the eggs. Once toasted, place them, cut side up, on serving plates and top each with a slice of Canadian bacon.
7. Remove each poached egg with a slotted spoon and place them atop the Canadian bacon on the English muffin halves.
8. If the hollandaise sauce has broken, blend it briefly to emulsify. Drizzle it over the poached eggs. Optionally sprinkle each muffin with chopped parsley to serve.

VEGAN OPTION

For the hollandaise sauce, omit the egg yolks, but add ½ cup cooked cannellini beans, 1 tablespoon nutritional yeast, and ¼ teaspoon turmeric or red palm oil (for color) to your blender. You can add all of the oil at once; there's no need to temper it in.

For the eggs Benedict, top the muffins with baked tofu slices or baked portobello mushrooms instead of poached eggs. As noted, you can use a vegan Canadian bacon or bacon slices. But another delicious option is to swap in some lightly cooked greens.

IN AN INSTANT OATMEAL PACKETS

MAKES 12 SERVINGS (ABOUT 6 CUPS)

I grew up on convenient oatmeal packets, but one was never quite enough, and many of the enticing flavors contained dairy. To solve both problems, I came up with my own customizable quick oat formula, along with some fun dairy-free flavors to mix things up.

> 1 cup + 4 cups quick oats (certified gluten free, if needed), divided
> ½ cup firmly packed brown sugar, cane sugar, or coconut sugar
> ¾ teaspoon salt

1. Put the 1 cup oats in your spice grinder or food processor. Pulse until the oats are mostly ground. This creates a more authentic "packet" consistency.
2. In a large bowl, stir together the ground oats, remaining 4 cups oats, sugar, and salt until the ingredients are evenly distributed.
3. Scoop about ½ cup of the oat mixture into a plastic bag or small jar and seal. Repeat until all of the oat mixture is used up.
4. Store the individual servings at room temperature for up to 1 month, or in the freezer for optimal freshness and to enjoy later.
5. **To prepare 1 serving**, pour the contents of 1 packet into a bowl and stir in ⅓ to ½ cup boiling water. Optionally cover, and let sit for 3 to 5 minutes to soften before eating.

FLAVOR VARIATIONS

Banana Bread: Grind 1¼ cups freeze-dried bananas in your spice grinder or blender until powdered. Stir the banana powder, 1 cup chopped walnuts or pecans (omit for nut free), and 1 teaspoon ground cinnamon into the recipe above.

PB & Berry: Stir 1 cup peanut butter powder and 1⅓ cups freeze-dried strawberries or blueberries (can substitute dried berries) into the recipe above.

Almond Joy: Stir 1 cup unsweetened shredded coconut, ⅔ to 1 cup mini dairy-free chocolate chips, ½ cup sliced almonds, and ½ cup dairy-free coconut milk powder (can substitute almond flour) into the recipe above. This flavor works best with cane sugar or coconut sugar.

Cinnamon Roll: Grind ½ cup raw cashews in your spice grinder or food processor until powdered. Stir the ground cashews, 2 teaspoons ground cinnamon, and 1 teaspoon vanilla powder (can substitute the seeds scraped from 1 to 2 inches of vanilla bean) into the recipe above. This flavor works best with brown sugar, but coconut sugar is also good.

BEST DARN BISCUITS & GRAVY

MAKES 4 TO 6 SERVINGS

This sneaky "milk" gravy is perfectly creamy, flavorful, and fulfilling. And when drizzled atop homemade fluffy biscuits, it's comfort food bliss.

2 cups steamed cauliflower florets
2 cups water, plus additional if needed
1 teaspoon nutritional yeast
2 tablespoons olive oil
¾ pound EASY HOMEMADE BREAKFAST SAUSAGE (recipe below) or vegan breakfast sausage
¼ cup all-purpose flour (can substitute a gluten-free all-purpose flour blend)
½ to ¾ teaspoon salt, to taste
¼ teaspoon black pepper
4 to 6 FOUR-INGREDIENT BAKING POWDER BISCUITS (page 258)

1. Put the cooked cauliflower, 1 cup of the water, and nutritional yeast in your blender. Blend until smooth, about 1 minute. Add the remaining 1 cup water and blend to combine.

2. Heat the oil in a large skillet over medium heat. Add the sausage and sauté, while breaking it up into small pieces, until cooked through, about 5 minutes (2 minutes for vegan sausage).

3. Reduce the heat to medium-low and whisk in the flour. Cook while whisking for 2 to 3 minutes. The flour should absorb into the sausage and oil and become slightly golden.

4. Slowly whisk in the cauliflower mixture and cook, whisking often, for 5 minutes, or until it is a rich gravy consistency. If it thickens too much, whisk in a little more water, as needed.

5. Whisk in the salt and black pepper.

6. Cut the biscuits in half horizontally with a serrated knife. Place them, cut side up, on serving plates. Top the biscuits with generous amounts of the gravy.

7. Store leftover sausage gravy in an airtight container in the refrigerator for up to 2 days.

EASY HOMEMADE BREAKFAST SAUSAGE RECIPE

Put ¾ pound lean ground turkey or pork in a medium bowl. Add ¾ teaspoon salt, ¾ teaspoon ground sage, ¾ teaspoon marjoram, ¼ teaspoon black pepper, and a pinch nutmeg. Stir well to evenly distribute the spices.

For a homemade vegan option, substitute 12 ounces firm or extra-firm tofu for the ground meat. Firmly press the tofu with paper towels or a tea towel to drain excess water, and then crumble it with your fingers.

CRUSTLESS CONFETTI MINI QUICHE

MAKES 4 SERVINGS

These personal-size quiches taste remarkably like scrambled eggs! It's hard to believe they're made with calcium- and protein-rich tofu and without an ounce of milk, cream, or cheese. If you prefer eggs, you can substitute 4 large eggs for the silken tofu.

1½ teaspoons grapeseed, olive, or rice bran oil
½ to ¾ cup diced red or orange bell pepper (about 1 small pepper)
2 cups chopped baby spinach leaves
½ teaspoon dried thyme
1 (12-ounce) package firm or extra firm silken tofu, drained
¼ cup unsweetened plain dairy-free milk beverage
2 tablespoons nutritional yeast flakes
2 tablespoons cornstarch or potato starch
1 teaspoon tahini
1 teaspoon salt
¼ teaspoon onion powder
¼ teaspoon turmeric
⅛ teaspoon paprika
⅛ teaspoon garlic powder
⅛ to ¼ teaspoon black pepper, to taste

1. Preheat your oven to 350°F. Grease and optionally flour four 3-inch ramekins.
2. Heat the oil in a medium skillet over medium-low heat. Add the bell pepper and sauté until slightly softened, about 3 minutes. Add the spinach and thyme, and sauté just until wilted, about 1 minute.
3. Drain and press the tofu, using a tea towel or paper towels, to remove any excess water.
4. Put the pressed tofu, milk beverage, nutritional yeast, starch, tahini, salt, onion powder, turmeric, paprika, and garlic powder in your blender. Blend until smooth, about 2 minutes.
5. Add the black pepper and cooked vegetable mixture to your blender. Stir to combine (do not blend).
6. Divide the batter with vegetables between your prepared ramekins.
7. Bake for 30 to 35 minutes, or until golden on top and set. Let cool for 10 minutes before serving.
8. Leftovers can be covered and stored in the refrigerator for up to 2 days.

....

MUFFIN-SIZE MINI QUICHE VARIATION

Use extra firm silken tofu and preferably silicone muffin cups for easiest release. Divide the mixture between 12 muffin cups and bake as directed.

....

CHAPTER 21

BAKESHOP BITES

Single-Serve Pastry Recipes

GOOD TO KNOW FOR THIS CHAPTER

CLIMATE MATTERS. If you live in a very humid climate, muffins and quick breads can come out heavier. On the other hand, if it's quite arid, your baked goods may come out a little too dry. Keep an eye on the moisture level of your batter, and adjust the baking time up or down as needed.

SUNKEN MUFFINS CAN BE SOLVED. Look in the oven (but do not open it!) at about the halfway mark when making muffins, baked donuts, or quick bread. If they have already risen a fair bit, but you end up with slightly indented or fully sunken muffins, then your recipe has too much leavener (baking soda and/or baking powder) for your kitchen. This is common at higher altitudes, where baked goods rise quickly. Reduce the leavener a little or up to half, depending on how caved in your pastries are. If they never fully rose (which is more common at sea level), then you may need to increase or add some baking powder.

EGG-FREE BATTER IS USUALLY THICKER. Thinner batters tend to have less structure. In most cases, egg substitutes don't provide as much liquid, structure, and lift as eggs do. So a thicker, more naturally structured batter can help compensate.

WHITE WHOLE WHEAT FLOUR IS 100 PERCENT WHOLE WHEAT. The "white" in this kind of flour refers to the type of wheat berry it's milled from; it's still whole grain. It just has a lighter, milder taste and color than regular whole wheat flour. In any recipe I call for white whole wheat flour, regular whole wheat flour will technically work. The results will just be a little darker in color and may be heartier in taste.

MAKE IT GLUTEN FREE. For the most part, the quick bread recipes (those made without yeast) in chapters 21 and 22 will work with your favorite 1:1 gluten-free all-purpose flour blend in place of the flour. But if egg is an option in the recipe, I recommend using it unless you need an egg-free baked good specifically. Egg will almost always provide more structure than an egg replacer. See **GoDairyFree.org/gdf-ingredients** for the gluten-free flour blends I currently test with.

CINN-FULL OVERNIGHT CINNAMON ROLLS

MAKES 12 ROLLS

You won't be able to taste the difference between these vegan sweet buns and fluffy store-bought cinnamon rolls. In fact, my husband swears that these are much better.

½ cup warm plain or unsweetened plain dairy-free milk beverage
2¼ teaspoons (one ¼-ounce package) active dry yeast
3 cups bread flour or all-purpose flour, plus additional as needed
1 teaspoon + 2 teaspoons ground cinnamon, divided
1 teaspoon salt
¾ cup mashed ripe banana (can substitute pumpkin puree)
¼ cup rice bran, grapeseed, or melted coconut oil
1 tablespoon cane sugar
½ cup firmly packed brown sugar (can substitute coconut sugar)
3 tablespoons + 1½ teaspoons dairy-free buttery spread or BAKEABLE BUTTER
   (page 192), divided
1 cup powdered confectioners' sugar
½ teaspoon vanilla extract
1 to 2 tablespoons water, or as needed

1. Put the warm milk beverage in a large mixing bowl and sprinkle in the yeast. Let sit for 5 minutes to proof and ensure the yeast is active (see page 250).

2. In a large bowl, whisk together the flour, 1 teaspoon cinnamon, and salt.

3. Add the banana, oil, cane sugar, and half of the flour blend to the yeast mixture and whisk to combine. Gradually stir in the rest of the flour until soft dough forms.

4. Turn out the dough onto a lightly floured surface and knead it for 10 minutes, or until smooth and elastic. Add more flour when needed to keep the dough from sticking to your hands. You should end up with fairly soft dough that is just slightly sticky.

5. Return the dough to the mixing bowl, lightly cover the bowl, and let the dough rise in a warm, draft-free place for 45 minutes, or until doubled in size.

6. Grease a 9 × 9-inch or 11 × 8-inch baking pan.

7. Punch down the dough. Cover and let it rest for 5 minutes.

8. In a small bowl, whisk together the brown sugar, 3 tablespoons buttery spread, and remaining 2 teaspoons cinnamon.

9. Turn out the dough onto a floured surface. Roll the dough into a 12 × 10-inch rectangle. Sprinkle the brown sugar mixture evenly over the dough, leaving a 1-inch margin on one of the long sides. Starting from the other long side, tightly roll up the dough, pinching the seam to seal.

10. Turn the roll seam side down, and slice it into 12 equal-size rolls.

11. Place the slices cut side down in your prepared baking pan. Lightly cover the rolls with plastic wrap. Place the pan in the refrigerator overnight.

12. In the morning, pull the cinnamon rolls from the refrigerator, and place them on top of the stove while you preheat your oven to 375°F.

13. Bake for 20 to 25 minutes, or until the cinnamon rolls are lightly golden brown.

14. Let cool for 10 minutes in the pan.

15. Sift the powdered sugar into a medium bowl. Melt the remaining 1½ teaspoons buttery spread and add it to the bowl, along with the vanilla and 1 tablespoon water. Whisk to combine, adding more water, if needed, to get a drizzly icing.

16. Pull apart the cinnamon rolls and individually drizzle them with icing just before serving.

17. Store un-iced cinnamon rolls covered at room temperature for up to 2 days, or individually wrap them and freeze to enjoy later. Once iced, the rolls are best if eaten the same day. The icing will keep in an airtight container in the refrigerator for up to 1 week, but whisk it again before using.

BAKERY-STYLE BLUEBERRY MUFFINS

MAKES 12 MUFFINS

Beautiful domes and a perfectly tender moist crumb are well within reach. Initially baking the muffins at a higher heat lets them rise and set more quickly. Reducing the heat then allows the muffins to finish baking through without burning. One of the taste testers said these were the best homemade blueberry muffins he's ever had!

> 2 cups all-purpose flour
> 1 tablespoon baking powder (reduce to 2 teaspoons above 4,000 feet)
> ¾ teaspoon salt
> 1 cup + 1 teaspoon cane sugar, divided
> 1 cup unsweetened plain dairy-free milk beverage
> ⅓ cup grapeseed, rice bran, or other neutral-tasting oil (see page 146)
> 1 large egg (see Vegan Option below for egg free)
> 1 teaspoon vanilla extract
> 1¼ cups frozen wild blueberries

1. Preheat your oven to 425°F and line 12 muffin cups with cupcake liners. Grease the rims of the muffin cups if you aren't using silicone.

2. In a medium bowl, whisk together the flour, baking powder, and salt.

3. In a large bowl, whisk together the 1 cup sugar, milk beverage, oil, egg, and vanilla. Add the flour mixture and stir until just combined. Do not overmix; some small lumps are okay. Fold in the blueberries.

4. Divide the batter between your prepared muffin cups. They should be filled up to just ⅛ inch from the top. Sprinkle the batter with the remaining 1 teaspoon sugar.

5. Bake for 10 minutes. Reduce the oven temperature to 350°F and bake for 20 to 22 more minutes. The muffins should feel set when touched.

6. Let cool for 5 minutes in the cups before removing the muffins to a wire rack to cool completely.

7. Store in an airtight container at room temperature for up to 2 days, or individually wrap the muffins and freeze to enjoy later.

VEGAN OPTION

Substitute 3 tablespoons dairy-free yogurt alternative for the egg and increase the baking powder by ⅛ teaspoon.

THE MOST VERSATILE MUFFINS

MAKES 12 MUFFINS

If you only have one muffin recipe on hand, this should be it. This simple formula will allow you to quickly churn out whatever flavor of fluffy pastry your heart desires. See the Flavor Variations below for some possibilities.

2 cups all-purpose flour, whole wheat pastry flour, or a combination of the two
¾ cup cane sugar
1 tablespoon baking powder (reduce to 2 teaspoons above 4,000 feet)
½ teaspoon salt
1 cup plain or unsweetened plain dairy-free milk beverage
¼ cup grapeseed, rice bran, or other neutral-tasting oil (see page 146)
1 large egg *or* ¼ cup unsweetened applesauce *or* 3 tablespoons dairy-free yogurt alternative

1. Preheat your oven to 400°F and grease 12 muffin cups or line them with cupcake liners.
2. In a large bowl, whisk together the flour, sugar, baking powder, and salt. Make a well in the center of the dry ingredients.
3. Measure the milk beverage in a glass measuring cup. Add the oil and egg, applesauce, or yogurt and whisk to combine.
4. Pour the liquid mixture into the well of the dry mixture. Gently stir the ingredients together, just until moistened. Some small lumps are okay; you do not want to overmix.
5. Divide the batter between your prepared muffin cups.
6. Bake for 20 to 24 minutes, or until the tops are golden and a toothpick inserted into the center of a muffin comes out clean.
7. Let cool for 5 minutes in the cups before removing the muffins to a wire rack to cool completely.
8. Store in an airtight container at room temperature for up to 2 days, or individually wrap the muffins and freeze to enjoy later.

FLAVOR VARIATIONS

BERRY: Fold 1 to 1½ cups fresh berries into the batter just after you stir in the liquids. If using frozen berries, toss them in with the flour mixture to help prevent "bleeding" and sinking.

TRAIL MIX: Fold in ½ to ¾ cup chopped nuts and/or chocolate chips just after you stir in the liquids.

SPICE: Whisk 1 teaspoon ground cinnamon, chai spice (page 216), or pumpkin pie spice (page 212) with the dry ingredients.

ESSENCES: Stir 1 teaspoon vanilla, maple, almond, or coconut extract into the wet ingredients.

ZEST: Stir 1 teaspoon grated orange, lemon, or lime zest into the wet ingredients.

BROWN SUGAR: Substitute packed brown sugar, coconut sugar, maple sugar, or date sugar for the cane sugar.

BREAKFAST CUPCAKES: "Frost" the muffins with your favorite nut or seed butter, FRESH STRAWBERRY CHIA JAM (page 284), or ROCKIN' RASPBERRY CHIA JAM (page 284).

CHUNKY MONKEY MUFFINS

MAKES 12 MUFFINS

These lightly sweet banana muffins get an extra hit of indulgence from mini chocolate chips. They have a more rustic and hearty texture than your average banana muffins, and are naturally gluten free due to the use of ground oats.

2 cups rolled or quick oats (certified gluten free, if needed)
2 tablespoons chia seeds or flax seeds
2½ teaspoons baking powder (reduce to 2 teaspoons above 4,000 feet)
½ teaspoon salt
1⅓ cups mashed banana (about 3 medium very ripe bananas)
⅓ cup honey or agave nectar
⅓ cup grapeseed, rice bran, or melted coconut oil
1 teaspoon vanilla extract
½ cup lite coconut milk or unsweetened plain dairy-free milk beverage
½ cup dairy-free semi-sweet or dark chocolate chips
½ cup chopped walnuts (omit for nut free)

1. Preheat your oven to 425°F and line 12 muffin cups with cupcake liners.
2. Put the oats and seeds in your spice grinder or food processor. Process until powdered, about 1 minute.
3. Put the ground oat mixture in a medium bowl. Add the baking powder and salt and whisk to combine.
4. Put the mashed banana, sweetener, oil, and vanilla in a large mixing bowl. Beat with a hand mixer until relatively smooth, about 1 minute. Stir in the coconut milk or milk beverage, and then stir in the oat mixture until relatively smooth. Fold in the chocolate chips and walnuts.
5. Divide the batter between your prepared muffin cups. They will be filled quite high.
6. Bake for 10 minutes. Reduce the oven temperature to 350°F and bake for 12 to 14 more minutes, or until a toothpick inserted into the center of a muffin comes out clean.
7. Let cool for 5 minutes in the cups before removing the muffins to a wire rack to cool completely.
8. Store in an airtight container at room temperature for up to 2 days, or individually wrap the muffins and freeze to enjoy later.

OAT FLOUR & GROUND FLAXSEED VARIATION

Substitute 2 cups (6.2 ounces) oat flour for the oats and 3 tablespoons ground flaxseed for the seeds and skip step 2.

ANY DAY PUMPKIN MUFFINS

MAKES 12 MUFFINS

I love making these tender muffins in the evening, as the flavors soften and infuse overnight. They have a slightly cakey texture, avoiding the overly moist and dense downfalls of many pumpkin muffins.

> 1½ cups all-purpose flour, white whole wheat flour, or a combination of the two
> 2 teaspoons ground cinnamon
> 1 teaspoon baking soda (reduce to ½ teaspoon above 4,000 feet)
> ¾ teaspoon salt
> ¼ teaspoon ground ginger
> ⅛ teaspoon ground allspice or nutmeg
> ⅛ teaspoon ground cloves
> 1 cup pumpkin puree
> 1 cup packed brown sugar or coconut sugar (for less sweet)
> 2 large eggs (see Vegan Option below for egg free)
> ¼ cup grapeseed, rice bran, or other neutral-tasting oil (see page 146)
> ¼ cup orange juice

1. Preheat your oven to 350°F and grease 12 muffin cups or line them with cupcake liners.
2. In a medium bowl, whisk together the flour, cinnamon, baking soda, salt, ginger, allspice or nutmeg, and cloves.
3. Put the pumpkin, sugar, eggs, oil, and orange juice in a large mixing bowl. Beat with a hand mixer until creamy, about 1 minute. Add the flour mixture and stir until just combined. Do not overmix; some small lumps are okay.
4. Divide the batter between your prepared muffin cups. They should each be about two-thirds full. Level the batter out with a spoon or by tapping the muffin pan on the counter.
5. Bake for 25 to 30 minutes, or until a toothpick inserted into the center of a muffin comes out clean.
6. Let cool for 10 minutes in the cups before carefully removing the muffins to a wire rack to cool completely.
7. Store in an airtight container at room temperature for up to 2 days, or individually wrap the muffins and freeze to enjoy later.

VEGAN OPTION

Substitute ½ cup applesauce for the eggs and add ¼ teaspoon baking powder to the dry ingredients (⅛ teaspoon above 4,000 feet).

PEAR-FECTLY GOOD VANILLA MUFFI

MAKES 12 MUFFINS

These muffins received the breakfast treat seal of approval from my extended family. They use a bit less sugar than your average muffin, but compensate with a light sugary topping that pops.

- 2 cups all-purpose flour, whole wheat pastry flour, or a combination of the two
- ½ cup + 2 teaspoons cane sugar, divided
- 2 teaspoons baking powder
- ½ teaspoon baking soda (omit if using egg and/or above 4,000 feet)
- ½ teaspoon salt
- ½ teaspoon ground cardamom
- 1 cup + 2 tablespoons vanilla dairy-free milk beverage
- 1 large egg *or* ¼ cup unsweetened applesauce
- ¼ cup grapeseed, rice bran, or other neutral-tasting oil (see page 146)
- 1 teaspoon vanilla extract
- 1 cup peeled and diced pear (about 1 medium firm but ripe pear)
- ½ cup chopped walnuts (optional)

1. Preheat your oven to 350°F and grease 12 muffin cups or line them with cupcake liners.
2. In a large bowl, whisk together the flour, ½ cup sugar, baking powder, baking soda (if using), salt, and cardamom. Make a well in the center of the dry ingredients.
3. Measure the milk beverage in a glass measuring cup. Add the egg or applesauce, oil, and vanilla and whisk to combine.
4. Pour the liquid mixture into the well of the dry mixture. Gently stir the ingredients together, just until moistened. Some small lumps are okay; you do not want to overmix. Fold in the diced pear and walnuts (if using).
5. Divide the batter between your prepared muffin cups. Sprinkle the batter with the remaining 2 teaspoons sugar.
6. Bake for 18 to 22 minutes, or until the muffin tops are lightly golden and a toothpick inserted into the center of a muffin comes out clean.
7. Let cool for 5 minutes in the cups before carefully removing the muffins to a wire rack to cool completely.
8. Store in an airtight container at room temperature for up to 2 days, or individually wrap the muffins and freeze to enjoy later.

APPLE CINNAMON VARIATION

Substitute 1 teaspoon ground cinnamon for the cardamom, ½ cup firmly packed brown sugar or coconut sugar for the cane sugar, and 1 cup peeled and diced apple for the pear.

MY FAVORITE MAPLE BRAN MUFFINS

MAKES 12 MUFFINS

Most recipes for bran muffins call for white flour and loads of sugar. In my opinion, this defeats the purpose of the healthy bran. So I created this delicious version, which is lighter on the sugar and made with whole wheat flour.

   1¼ cups plain or unsweetened plain dairy-free milk beverage
   1 tablespoon apple cider vinegar or white vinegar
   1⅓ cups wheat bran
   2 tablespoons ground flaxseed
   1 cup whole wheat flour or white whole wheat flour
   1½ teaspoons baking soda (reduce to 1 teaspoon above 4,000 feet)
   1 teaspoon ground cinnamon
   ½ teaspoon salt
   ⅓ cup grapeseed, rice bran, or other neutral-tasting oil (see page 146)
   ⅓ cup maple syrup
   ¼ cup lightly packed brown sugar or coconut sugar
   1 teaspoon vanilla extract
   ⅔ cup raisins

1. Preheat your oven to 350°F and grease 12 muffin cups or line them with cupcake liners.
2. In a large mixing bowl, whisk together the milk beverage and vinegar. Add the bran and flaxseed and stir until fully moistened. Let soak for 5 minutes.
3. In a medium bowl, whisk together the flour, baking soda, cinnamon, and salt.
4. Add the oil, maple syrup, sugar, and vanilla to the bran mixture and whisk to combine. Add the flour mixture and stir just to combine. Some small lumps are okay; you do not want to overmix. Fold in the raisins.
5. Divide the batter between your prepared muffin cups.
6. Bake for 18 to 22 minutes, or until a toothpick inserted into the center of a muffin comes out clean.
7. Let cool for 5 minutes in the cups before removing the muffins to a wire rack to cool completely.
8. Store in an airtight container at room temperature for up to 2 days, or individually wrap the muffins and freeze to enjoy later.

BAKED CAKE DONUTS WITH MAPLE ICING

MAKES 12 TO 16 DONUTS

These donuts puff up perfectly and have the wonderful taste and texture of old-fashioned cake donuts. As a complement, I created a maple icing that's reminiscent of classic maple bars.

CAKE DONUTS
   2 cups white whole wheat flour (can substitute all-purpose flour or an all-purpose gluten-free flour blend)

⅔ cup cane sugar or coconut sugar

2 tablespoons tapioca starch or cornstarch

2 teaspoons baking powder

¾ teaspoon salt

⅓ cup dairy-free buttery spread or Bakeable Butter (page 192)

1 cup lite coconut milk

2 large eggs (see Vegan Option below for egg free)

2 teaspoons vanilla extract *or* 1 teaspoon maple extract or flavoring

MAPLE ICING

1 cup powdered confectioners' sugar

¼ cup maple syrup

1 tablespoon dairy-free buttery spread or Bakeable Butter (page 192), melted

½ teaspoon vanilla extract

¼ teaspoon maple extract or flavoring (optional)

½ teaspoon unsweetened plain dairy-free milk beverage, if needed

1. **To make the donuts,** preheat your oven to 350°F and grease 12 to 16 donut pan wells (see Donut Pan Alternatives below).

2. In a large bowl, whisk together the flour, sugar, starch, baking powder, and salt. Add the buttery spread and whisk until a coarse meal forms.

3. Heat the coconut milk for 30 seconds on high in the microwave, or until quite warm but not hot or boiling.

4. Add the warmed coconut milk, eggs, and vanilla to the flour mixture. Stir until just combined with no flour streaks remaining. Do not overmix; some small lumps are okay.

5. Fill the donut pan wells with batter right up to the top of the center hole, but do not cover the center.

6. Bake for 10 to 12 minutes, or until just set. They will still be fairly light in color.

7. Let cool for 10 minutes in the pan. If needed, run a butter knife around the edge of each donut to loosen, and remove them to a wire rack to cool completely.

8. **To make the icing,** sift the powdered sugar into a medium bowl. Add the maple syrup, melted buttery spread, vanilla, and maple extract (if using) and whisk until smooth. If the icing is too thick, whisk in the milk beverage.

9. Just before serving, dip the tops of the cooled donuts in the maple icing. Place them on a wire rack (icing side up) for a few minutes to set.

10. Store un-iced donuts in an airtight container at room temperature for up to 2 days, or individually wrap them and freeze to enjoy later. Once iced, the donuts are best if eaten the same day. Store the maple icing in an airtight container in the refrigerator for up to 1 week, but whisk it again before using.

DONUT PAN ALTERNATIVES: Pour the batter into small greased ramekins (3 to 4 inches in diameter) until just 1 inch high. Bake as directed to make hole-free donut cakes. Or you can divide the batter between the wells of a mini muffin pan to make baked "donut holes."

VEGAN OPTION

Substitute 2 powdered egg replacer equivalents (usually 1 tablespoon powdered egg replacer plus 2 tablespoons water per egg) for the eggs to keep the nice fluffy texture of these donuts.

GLAZED DONUTS

4 DONUTS + DONUT HOLES

...I know it is probably a blessing in disguise, I become a bit sad whenever I stroll by a donut shop and realize that those soft and squishy indulgences aren't an option. Yes, most bakery varieties are infused with dairy milk. But luckily, homemade dairy-free donuts are a reality for those special occasions.

½ cup warm water (about 105°F)
1 tablespoon active dry yeast
½ cup warm plain or unsweetened plain dairy-free milk beverage
3 tablespoons organic palm shortening or coconut oil, melted
3 tablespoons cane sugar
1½ teaspoons apple cider vinegar or white vinegar
2½ to 3 cups all-purpose flour
1 tablespoon baking powder
1 teaspoon salt
3 to 4 cups high-heat oil (see page 148)
Glaze or topping (see Glaze & Topping Variations following)

1. Put the warm water in a large bowl and sprinkle in the yeast. Let sit for 5 minutes to proof and ensure the yeast is active (see page 250).

2. Add the milk beverage, shortening or coconut oil, sugar, and vinegar to the yeast mixture and whisk to combine. Add 1 cup of the flour, baking powder, and salt and whisk to thoroughly combine. Gradually stir in the remaining 1½ to 2 cups flour as needed to make a soft ball of dough.

3. Turn out the dough onto a lightly floured surface and knead it for 5 minutes, or until smooth and somewhat elastic. Let the dough rest for 5 minutes.

4. Roll out the dough to a ½-inch thickness and cut out donut shapes with a 2½-inch donut cutter. If you don't have a donut cutter, use a large biscuit cutter or the mouth of a drinking glass and, if desired, cut donut holes from the center using a smaller round cutter. Bring any remaining scraps together, reroll, and cut again.

5. Place the donuts on a lightly floured surface, cover, and let rise for about 1 hour, or until doubled in size.

6. Add 3 inches of oil to an electric deep fryer or deep stockpot and heat until the oil reaches 360° to 380°F.

7. Slowly and carefully place each donut into the hot oil. Cook for about 1 to 2 minutes, or until the donuts take on a light golden color. Flip them and cook for 1 minute more.

8. Remove the donuts with a slotted spoon and allow them to drain on paper towels.

9. While still warm, dip the donuts in one of the glaze or topping options. Place them on a wire rack (glaze or topping side up) to set. Serve warm.

10. Store unglazed donuts in an airtight container at room temperature for up to 2 days, or individually wrap them and freeze to enjoy later. Once glazed, the donuts are best if eaten the same day. Store the glaze in an airtight container in the refrigerator for up to 1 week, but whisk it again before using.

GLAZE & TOPPING VARIATIONS

VANILLA GLAZE: Sift 2½ cups powdered confectioners' sugar into a medium bowl. Add ¼ cup plain or unsweetened plain dairy-free milk beverage and ½ teaspoon pure vanilla flavoring or extract and whisk to combine. If needed, whisk in more milk beverage, 1 teaspoon at a time, to thin the glaze. Optionally top the glazed donuts with sprinkles before the glaze sets.

CHOCOLATE GLAZE: Melt ½ cup dairy-free semi-sweet chocolate chips (see page 417) and whisk the melted chocolate into the Vanilla Glaze.

CINNAMON-SUGAR: In a small bowl, whisk together ¼ cup cane sugar and 4 teaspoons ground cinnamon. After dipping or rolling the donuts in the cinnamon-sugar, tap them to shake off excess.

GRANULATED OR POWDERED CONFECTIONERS' SUGAR: Put the sugar in a small bowl. After dipping or rolling the donuts in the sugar, tap them to shake off excess.

BLE CHOCOLATE SCONES WITH
.LA GLAZE

MAKES 8 SCONES

These breakfast treats are an addictive cross between a cookie and a scone. The natural cocoa powder version is a bit cookie-like and crumbly. When made with Dutch-processed cocoa, the texture is more reminiscent of traditional scones. They're different, but equally delicious—our tasters couldn't pick a favorite!

DOUBLE CHOCOLATE SCONES

1½ cups all-purpose flour or white whole wheat flour, plus additional as needed
½ cup natural cocoa powder
⅓ cup cane sugar (can substitute coconut sugar)
1 teaspoon baking powder
1 teaspoon baking soda
½ teaspoon salt
½ cup coconut oil, solid or semi-solid
½ cup dairy-free semi-sweet mini chocolate chips
⅓ cup lite coconut milk, plus additional as needed
2 teaspoons vanilla extract

VANILLA BEAN GLAZE

½ cup powdered confectioners' sugar
2 to 3 teaspoons unsweetened dairy-free milk beverage
½ teaspoon pure vanilla flavoring or extract *or* ½-inch piece vanilla bean

1. **To make the scones**, preheat your oven to 400°F and line a baking sheet with parchment paper or a silicone baking mat.

2. In a large bowl, whisk together the flour, cocoa powder, sugar, baking powder, baking soda, and salt until all of the cocoa clumps are dispersed. Add the coconut oil and whisk until coarse crumbs form. Stir in the chocolate chips.

3. Make a well in the center of the crumb mixture and pour in the coconut milk and vanilla. Gently fold the ingredients together into crumbly dough. Divide the dough in half and bring each half together with your hands into 2 equal-size balls. If the dough is too crumbly, add more lite coconut milk, about 1 teaspoon at a time, until it comes together. If it's sticky, add a little flour, as needed. Try to avoid overworking the dough.

4. Press each dough ball into a 1-inch-high round on your prepared baking sheet. Carefully cut each into fourths (do not cut your baking mat!). Gently pull the quarters about an inch apart.

5. Bake for 15 to 17 minutes, or until the scones appear dry on top.

6. Immediately remove the scones to a wire rack to cool completely.

7. **To make the glaze**, sift the powdered sugar into a medium bowl. Add 2 teaspoons milk beverage and the vanilla (if using vanilla bean, scrape the seeds from the inside of the bean piece into the bowl and discard the pod) and whisk until smooth. Whisk in more milk beverage if needed to get a slightly thick but dippable consistency.

8. Just before serving, dip the tops of the cooled scones in the glaze. Place them on a wire rack (glaze side up) for a few minutes to set.

9. Store unglazed scones in an airtight container at room temperature for up to 2 days, or individually wrap them and freeze to enjoy later. Once glazed, the scones are best if eaten the same day. The glaze will keep in an airtight container in the refrigerator for up to 1 week, but whisk it again before using.

....

DUTCH-PROCESSED COCOA VARIATION

If using Dutch-processed (alkalized) cocoa powder, omit the baking soda and increase the baking powder to 2½ teaspoons. The scones will be just a touch less sweet than the natural cocoa powder version.

....

STRAWBERRY DANISH SCONES

MAKES 14 SCONES

These thumbprint-style scones are a very special treat. Make them with the strawberry icing for a teatime dessert or use whole wheat flour and omit the icing for a heartier breakfast pastry. Either way, I prefer to use homemade chia jam in the holes for a touch of added nutrition and to reduce the risk of bubbling over. Chia jam can be slightly mounded since it tends to hold its shape when cooked. On the contrary, store-bought jam can melt, run over the sides, and even burn.

THUMBPRINT SCONES
2 cups all-purpose flour (can substitute whole wheat pastry flour for part or all)
⅓ cup cane sugar (can substitute coconut sugar)
2 teaspoons baking powder
⅝ teaspoon salt
1 cup full-fat coconut milk, or as needed (see Coconut Milk Note following)
1½ teaspoons vanilla extract
Scant ½ cup FRESH STRAWBERRY CHIA JAM (page 284)

STRAWBERRY ICING
¼ cup freeze-dried strawberries (can substitute 1 tablespoon strawberry powder)
⅔ cup powdered confectioners' sugar
4 teaspoons unsweetened plain dairy-free milk beverage, or as needed
¼ teaspoon vanilla extract

1. **To make the scones,** whisk together the flour, sugar, baking powder, and salt in a large bowl.
2. Make a well in the center of the flour mixture and pour in the coconut milk and vanilla. Gently fold the ingredients together into crumbly dough, using your hands as needed to bring it together and kneading it just a few times. If the dough is too crumbly, add a little more coconut milk, but try to avoid overworking the dough.
3. Place the dough in your freezer, uncovered, for 10 minutes.
4. Preheat your oven to 400°F and line a baking sheet with parchment paper or a silicone baking mat.
5. Turn out the chilled dough onto a lightly floured surface and pat it down to about ¾-inch thickness. Cut the dough with a lightly floured 2-inch biscuit cutter (cut straight down; do not twist the cutter), and place the rounds on your prepared baking sheet. Bring the scraps together, pat the dough out, and cut more rounds with the biscuit cutter. Repeat one more time, if needed, to use up the dough.
6. Using the back of a round 1-tablespoon measuring spoon dipped in flour, press a well firmly into the center of each scone. Add ½ tablespoon chia jam to each well.
7. Bake for 16 to 18 minutes, or until you just barely see a few golden spots, for more tender scones, or until lightly browned, for drier scones.
8. Let cool completely on the baking sheet.
9. **To make the icing,** put the freeze-dried strawberries in your spice grinder and process them into a powder, about 30 seconds.
10. Sift the powdered sugar into a medium bowl. Whisk in the strawberry powder, milk beverage, and vanilla, until smooth. If the icing is too thick to drizzle, whisk in a little more milk beverage, 1 teaspoon at a time, as needed.

11. Just before serving, drizzle the icing over the cooled scones.

12. Store un-iced scones in an airtight container at room temperature for up to 2 days, or individually wrap them and freeze to enjoy later. Once iced, the scones are best if eaten the same day. The icing will keep in an airtight container in the refrigerator for up to 1 week, but whisk it again before using.

COCONUT MILK NOTE: *Coconut milk should be rich and thick, like heavy cream. But it is possible to get a batch that is watered down a little too much. If it appears a bit thin, and doesn't have notable amounts of thick coconut cream, add the coconut milk slowly to the flour, using only as much as needed to get cohesive dough that is lightly moist, but workable and not sticky. Leftover thin coconut milk can be used in place of the milk beverage in the icing.*

FLAKY FRENCH CROISSANTS

MAKES 12 CROISSANTS

My associate editor, Sarah Hatfield, tested numerous batches of croissants to create the perfect dairy-free recipe. The result was these well-loved buttery croissants that taste and feel like authentic French pastries. Sarah was very specific about the ingredients used in this recipe. For example, regular shortening didn't work well at all, but natural palm-coconut blend shortening produced spot-on results.

3 tablespoons + 1 tablespoon warm water, divided
1¼ teaspoons active dry yeast
1 teaspoon + 2 teaspoons cane sugar, divided
⅔ cup warm plain or unsweetened plain dairy-free milk beverage
2 tablespoons grapeseed, rice bran, or other neutral-tasting oil (see page 146)
1½ teaspoons salt
1¾ to 2 cups all-purpose flour, plus additional as needed
⅔ cup organic palm shortening or palm-coconut shortening
1 large egg (see Vegan Option following for egg free)

1. Put the 3 tablespoons warm water in a large mixing bowl. Sprinkle in the yeast and 1 teaspoon sugar. Let sit for 5 minutes to proof and ensure the yeast is active (see page 250).

2. Add the remaining 2 teaspoons sugar, warm milk beverage, oil, and salt to the yeast mixture and whisk to combine. Sift in 1¾ cups flour and stir to combine. If the dough is too wet to knead, add up to ¼ cup additional flour.

3. Knead the dough for 5 to 7 minutes, or until smooth and elastic.

4. Cover the dough and let it rise until it has tripled in size, 60 to 90 minutes.

5. Gently punch down the dough, cover, and let it rise again until doubled, about 60 minutes.

6. Gently punch down the dough and let it rest for 20 minutes.

7. Pat the dough into a 14 × 8-inch rectangle. Spread the shortening over the top two-thirds of the dough, leaving a ¼-inch margin all around. Fold the ungreased third over the middle third, and the greased top third down over that. Turn the dough 90 degrees, so that folds are to the left and right.

8. Roll the dough into a 14 × 6-inch rectangle. Fold the dough into thirds again. Sprinkle lightly with flour, and put the dough in a plastic bag. Refrigerate it for at least 2 hours.

9. Unwrap the dough, sprinkle it with flour, and gently punch it down.

10. Roll the dough into a 14 × 6-inch rectangle. Fold the dough in thirds again. Turn it 90 degrees, and repeat the rolling and folding. Put the dough back in the plastic bag. Refrigerate it for at least 2 hours.

11. Line a baking sheet with parchment paper or a silicone baking mat.

12. Unwrap the dough and roll it into a 20 × 5-inch rectangle. Cut it in half crosswise, and chill one half while shaping the other half.

13. Roll the half into a 15 × 5-inch rectangle. Cut it into three 5 × 5-inch squares. Cut each square in half diagonally to make 6 triangles. Roll each triangle lightly to elongate it and make it 7 inches long. Hold the outer two points of the triangle, and stretch them out slightly as you roll it up. Place each croissant on your prepared baking sheet. Curve the croissants slightly.

14. Repeat step 13 with the other half of the dough.

15. Let the shaped croissants rise until puffy and light, about 60 minutes.

16. Preheat your oven to 475°F.

17. In a small bowl, whisk together the egg and remaining 1 tablespoon water. Brush the glaze on the croissants.

18. Bake for 12 to 15 minutes, or until golden brown.

19. Immediately remove the croissants to a wire rack to cool completely.

20. Store in an airtight container at room temperature for up to 2 days.

VEGAN OPTION

In a small bowl, whisk together 1 tablespoon plain or unsweetened plain dairy-free milk beverage, 1 tablespoon maple syrup, and ⅛ teaspoon baking soda. Substitute this blend for the egg wash.

CHAPTER 22

FRESH BREAD

Quick Yeast & Bun Recipes

GOOD TO KNOW FOR THIS CHAPTER

PROOFING HAS A PURPOSE. When you add active yeast to warm water (around 105°F), it should form little bubbles or foam in the first 5 minutes. If it doesn't, then your yeast might be "dead." If so, it won't properly leaven your bread. It's best to start over with fresh yeast.

YOU CAN FREEZE YEAST. If you buy yeast in a multi-serving package, freezing helps preserve it. Chilled yeast may not proof, since it lowers the temperature of the water. But if you know your yeast was active when you froze it, it should be fine for at least a year or more. If concerned, bring the yeast to room temperature before adding warm water to proof.

USE THE OVEN FOR RISING. Turn on the light in your oven but leave the heat off. Place the covered dough in the oven, close it, and let the dough rise. It's a draft-free space and the light keeps the oven just warm enough. Just be sure to remove the dough from the oven before preheating it!

I USUALLY WHISK RATHER THAN SIFTING OR CUTTING. A simple whisk will combine dry ingredients with ease, quickly breaking up any clumps. The one exception is natural powdered sugar. It tends be more stubborn with clumps, so I usually sift it through a fine-mesh sieve. A whisk also works very efficiently for "cutting" in buttery spread, shortening, or oil to create dough crumbs.

HIGH-ALTITUDE ADJUSTMENTS AREN'T ALWAYS NEEDED. You'll note that I've included ingredient modifications for baking above 4,000 feet in many of the recipes in this book. If you don't see an adjustment, it's because the recipe works well as is regardless of altitude.

ICED LEMON LOAF

MAKES ONE 8 × 4-INCH LOAF (ABOUT 8 SERVINGS)

I'm not usually lured in by the Starbucks pastry case, but something about their iced lemon pound cake always catches my eye. It's loaded with dairy, so I've never had the chance to try it. But I created this loaf recipe to taste exactly how I think their cake *should* taste. It's a perfectly moist, wonderfully sweet citrus quick bread.

LEMON LOAF

1½ cups all-purpose flour
1¼ teaspoons baking powder (reduce to 1 teaspoon above 4,000 feet)
½ teaspoon salt
2 large eggs (see Vegan Option below for egg free)
⅞ cup cane sugar
⅔ cup lite coconut milk
⅓ cup grapeseed, rice bran, or other neutral-tasting oil (see page 146)
2 tablespoons fresh-squeezed lemon juice
2 teaspoons lightly packed grated lemon zest

LEMON ICING

¾ cup powdered confectioners' sugar
1 tablespoon fresh-squeezed lemon juice *or* 1½ teaspoons lemon juice +
    1½ teaspoons unsweetened plain dairy-free milk beverage
¼ teaspoon pure vanilla flavoring or extract

1. **To make the lemon loaf**, preheat your oven to 350°F and grease and flour an 8 × 4-inch baking pan.
2. In a medium bowl, whisk together the flour, baking powder, and salt.
3. Put the eggs, sugar, coconut milk, oil, lemon juice, and zest in a large mixing bowl. Beat with a hand mixer or whisk until combined, about 1 minute. Add the dry ingredients and stir just until combined. Some small lumps are okay; you do not want to overmix.
4. Scrape the batter into your prepared loaf pan and even it out.
5. Bake for 50 to 60 minutes, or until a toothpick inserted into the center of the bread comes out clean.
6. Let cool in the pan on a wire rack for 15 to 20 minutes. Run a knife around the edge of the bread and carefully remove it to the wire rack to cool completely.
7. **To make the lemon icing**, sift the powdered sugar into a medium bowl. Add the lemon juice—or lemon juice plus milk beverage for less pucker—and vanilla. Whisk until smooth.
8. Immediately scrape the icing onto the cooled bread, spreading it out to the sides.
9. Store the iced or un-iced bread in plastic wrap or an airtight container at room temperature for up to 2 days. Leftover bread slices can be individually wrapped and frozen to enjoy later. The icing will keep in an airtight container in the refrigerator for up to 1 week, but warm and whisk it again before using.

VEGAN OPTION

Omit the eggs, but add ⅓ cup plain dairy-free yogurt with the wet ingredients, increase the lite coconut milk to ¾ cup, and increase the baking powder to 1½ teaspoons (1⅛ teaspoons above 4,000 feet).

GLAZED ZUCCHINI-PINEAPPLE BREAD

MAKES ONE 9 × 5-INCH LOAF (10 TO 12 SERVINGS)

I've made this bread so often that I've had the chance to test it with eggs, applesauce, bananas, and yogurt. My husband likes it best with banana, I like it best with yogurt, and our friends like it best with applesauce. In other words, they all work great! The glaze makes this bread a nice sweet treat, but you can omit it if you will be enjoying the loaf for breakfast.

ZUCCHINI-PINEAPPLE BREAD
2 cups all-purpose flour or whole wheat pastry flour
1 teaspoon ground cinnamon
1 teaspoon baking powder
1 teaspoon baking soda (reduce to ½ teaspoon above 4,000 feet)
½ teaspoon salt
¼ teaspoon ground allspice
¾ cup firmly packed brown sugar (can substitute coconut sugar)
½ cup grapeseed, rice bran, or other neutral-tasting oil (see page 146),
     or softened dairy-free buttery spread
2 large eggs or ½ cup unsweetened applesauce or mashed ripe banana
     (about 1 medium banana) or ⅓ cup plain dairy-free yogurt
1 (8-ounce) can crushed pineapple with juice (do not drain)
1 cup grated zucchini
½ cup chopped pecans or walnuts (optional)

PINEAPPLE GLAZE
½ cup powdered confectioners' sugar
1 tablespoon pineapple juice (reserved from the crushed pineapple)
1 teaspoon honey, agave nectar, or corn syrup
¼ teaspoon ground cinnamon

1. **To make the bread,** preheat your oven to 350°F and grease and flour the bottom of a 9 × 5-inch loaf pan.

2. In a large bowl, whisk together the flour, cinnamon, baking powder, baking soda, salt, and allspice.

3. Put the brown sugar; oil or buttery spread; and eggs, applesauce, banana, or yogurt in a large mixing bowl. Beat with a hand mixer until relatively smooth, about 1 minute.

4. Reserve 1 tablespoon of the pineapple juice for the glaze. Stir the rest of the pineapple with its juice and the zucchini into the wet ingredients. Add the dry ingredients and stir just to combine. Some small lumps are okay; you do not want to overmix. Fold in the nuts (if using).

5. Pour the batter into your prepared loaf pan and level it out.

6. Bake for 45 to 55 minutes, or until a toothpick inserted into the center of the loaf comes out clean.

7. Let cool in the pan on a wire rack for 10 minutes. Run a knife around the edge of the bread and carefully remove it to the wire rack to cool completely.

8. **To make the glaze,** sift the powdered sugar into a medium bowl. Add the reserved 1 tablespoon pineapple juice, liquid sweetener, and cinnamon and whisk until smooth.

9. For an extra-moist loaf, poke holes in the top of the loaf before pouring on the glaze.

10. Store the iced or un-iced bread in plastic wrap or an airtight container in the refrigerator for up to 3 days. Leftover bread slices can be individually wrapped and frozen to enjoy later.

MINI LOAVES VARIATION

Pour the batter into 4 greased mini-loaf tins (6 × 3 inches) and bake at 350°F for 25 to 30 minutes, or until a toothpick inserted into the center of a loaf comes out clean.

BREAKFAST-WORTHY BANANA BREAD

MAKES ONE 9 × 5-INCH LOAF (10 TO 12 SERVINGS)

Going out on a limb, I decided to create a banana bread recipe that is free of added sugar. The result was this very mildly sweet loaf that my entire family adores. It toasts well and is a perfect medium for your nut or seed butter, buttery spread, or chia jam (recipes on page 284).

½ cup unsweetened plain dairy-free milk beverage
2 tablespoons ground flaxseed
2 cups spelt flour, whole wheat flour, or white whole wheat flour
1½ teaspoons baking soda (reduce to 1 teaspoon above 4,000 feet)
1 teaspoon ground cinnamon
½ teaspoon ground nutmeg
⅜ teaspoon salt
1½ to 2 cups mashed very ripe banana (3 to 4 bananas; see Banana Note below)
¼ cup grapeseed, rice bran, or other neutral-tasting oil (see page 146)
1 teaspoon vanilla extract
½ cup nuts, dried fruit, or dairy-free chocolate chips (optional)

1. Preheat your oven to 350°F and grease and flour a 9 × 5-inch loaf pan.
2. In a large mixing bowl, whisk together the milk beverage and flaxseed.
3. In a medium bowl, whisk together the flour, baking soda, cinnamon, nutmeg, and salt.
4. Add the bananas, oil, and vanilla to the flaxseed mixture. Beat with a hand mixer until relatively smooth, about 1 minute. Add the dry ingredients and stir just until combined. Some small lumps are okay; you do not want to overmix. Fold in the nuts, fruit, or chocolate chips (if using).
5. Scrape the batter into your prepared loaf pan and even it out.
6. Bake for 30 to 35 minutes, or until the top of the loaf is golden brown and resilient to the touch and a toothpick inserted into the center comes out clean.
7. Let the bread cool in the pan on a wire rack for 15 to 20 minutes. Run a knife around the edge of the bread and carefully remove it to the wire rack to cool completely.
8. Store in plastic wrap or an airtight container at room temperature for up to 2 days. Leftover bread slices can be individually wrapped and frozen to enjoy later. They toast well from frozen.

BANANA NOTE: I prefer to use a full 2 cups of mashed banana for the deepest flavor and very moist bread. But using just 1½ cups will allow the bread to rise a bit more.

MINI LOAVES VARIATION

Pour the batter into 4 greased and floured mini-loaf tins (6 × 3 inches) and bake at 350°F for 25 minutes, or until a toothpick inserted into the center of a loaf comes out clean.

SWEETER VARIATION

Add ¼ to ½ cup honey, agave nectar, or maple syrup with the wet ingredients in step 4 and increase the salt to ½ teaspoon.

SARAH'S CINNAMON RAISIN BREAD

MAKES ONE 9 × 5-INCH LOAF (12 TO 16 SERVINGS)

It's still hard to find good dairy-free cinnamon raisin bread in stores, but Sarah Hatfield, my associate editor, was happy to share this recipe. Her husband, the lead baker in their household, makes this loaf for the whole family to enjoy. And because the dough rests overnight, it can be baked up fresh for a special breakfast.

¾ cup warm water (about 105°F)
1½ tablespoons (two ¼-ounce packages) active dry yeast (reduce to 1 tablespoon above 4,000 feet)
5 cups all-purpose flour, plus additional as needed
½ cup + ¼ cup cane sugar, divided
4 teaspoons baking powder
1 teaspoon salt
½ cup organic palm shortening or coconut oil (solid or semi-solid)
2 cups warm plain or unsweetened plain dairy-free milk beverage
2 tablespoons lemon juice
2 teaspoons ground cinnamon
2 tablespoons dairy-free buttery spread or coconut oil, melted
¼ to ½ cup raisins

1. Put the warm water in a large bowl and sprinkle in the yeast. Let sit for 5 minutes to proof and ensure the yeast is active (see page 250).
2. In a large bowl, whisk together the flour, ½ cup sugar, baking powder, and salt. Add the shortening or coconut oil and whisk until the mixture resemble coarse crumbs.
3. Pour the yeast mixture, warm milk beverage, and lemon juice into the flour mixture and stir until the dough comes together. It will be somewhat soft.
4. Place the dough in a lightly greased large bowl, cover it, and refrigerate overnight.
5. In the morning, turn out the dough onto a lightly floured surface. Knead it for 5 to 7 minutes, or until smooth and elastic.
6. Let the dough sit at room temperature for 45 minutes.
7. Preheat your oven to 400°F and lightly grease a 9 × 5-inch loaf pan or a baking sheet.
8. In a small bowl, whisk together the remaining ¼ cup sugar and cinnamon.
9. Roll out the dough into a rectangle. If using a loaf pan, the width should be just a little shorter than the pan length. Brush the surface of the dough with the melted buttery spread or coconut oil. Evenly sprinkle on the cinnamon-sugar mixture and the raisins.
10. Tightly roll up the dough and pinch the seam closed. Place the dough, seam side down, into your prepared loaf pan (tuck the ends under to fit, if needed) or onto your prepared baking sheet.
11. Bake for 25 to 35 minutes, or until golden and the loaf has a slightly hollow sound when tapped on the bottom.
12. Let cool in the pan on a wire rack for 10 minutes. Carefully remove the bread to the wire rack to cool completely.
13. Store in plastic wrap or an airtight container at room temperature for up to 3 days. Leftover bread slices can be individually wrapped and frozen to enjoy later. They toast well from frozen.

WHOLE-GRAIN SANDWICH BREAD

MAKES ONE 9 × 5-INCH OR 8 × 4-INCH LOAF (ABOUT 12 SERVINGS)

When we lived at Lake Tahoe, I couldn't find a single loaf of dairy-free whole wheat bread at the store. So I learned to bake my own and never looked back. The fresh flavor and fulfilling texture of this homemade bread puts preservative-packed brands to shame. And it's much easier than you might think. My niece baked a loaf of this bread for her sandwiches nearly every week of her senior year in high school.

> 1¼ cups warm water (about 105°F)
> 2¾ teaspoons active dry yeast (reduce to 2¼ teaspoons above 4,000 feet)
> 3 cups white whole wheat flour or whole wheat flour, plus additional as needed
> ¾ cup dry 7- or 8-grain hot cereal (optional)
> ¼ cup grapeseed, rice bran, or other neutral-tasting oil (see page 146)
> ¼ cup maple syrup, honey, or agave nectar
> 3 tablespoons vital wheat gluten
> 1½ teaspoons salt

1. Put the warm water in a large bowl and sprinkle in the yeast. Let sit for 5 minutes to proof and ensure the yeast is active (see page 250).

2. Add about 1 cup of the flour and the dry cereal (if using), oil, sweetener, gluten, and salt to the yeast mixture. Stir to combine. Add the remaining 2 cups flour and stir to combine. Bring the dough together with your hands when it becomes too thick to stir.

3. Turn out the dough onto a lightly floured surface. Knead it for 5 to 7 minutes, or until relatively smooth and elastic. If the dough is too sticky to handle, add more flour, 1 tablespoon at a time, until it is still a little tacky but doesn't stick to your hands. The dry cereal, if using, will soak up some of the moisture as it cooks, so you don't want dough that is too dry.

4. Return the dough to the bowl, lightly cover the bowl, and let the dough rise in a warm, draft-free place for 45 to 60 minutes, or until doubled in size.

5. Grease and flour a 9 × 5-inch loaf pan. If omitting the dry cereal, you can use an 8 × 4-inch loaf pan.

6. Punch down the dough and let it rest for 5 minutes.

7. Briefly knead the dough as you shape it into a loaf that will fit in your pan. Fold the dough under as you shape it so that the seam is on the bottom. Put the shaped dough in your prepared pan, lightly cover it with plastic wrap, and let rise in a warm, draft-free place for 45 to 60 minutes, or until the crown of the dough is peaking about an inch above the pan.

8. Preheat your oven to 350°F.

9. Gently uncover the dough and bake for 35 to 45 minutes, or until the crust is golden and relatively firm to the touch.

10. Remove the loaf to a wire rack to cool completely.

11. Store in plastic wrap or an airtight container at room temperature for up to 3 days. Leftover bread slices can be individually wrapped and frozen to enjoy later. They toast well from frozen.

RISING HELP: *If your loaf is hesitating to rise when in the loaf pan on the second rising, place the slightly risen loaf in a cold oven. Turn the oven on to 350°F and bake for 45 minutes. The loaf will rise more as the oven preheats.*

WHITE-WHEAT BREAD VARIATION

If you don't have vital wheat gluten, you can omit it. But reduce the yeast to 2¼ teaspoons and the wheat flour to 1½ cups. Add 1½ cups white bread flour, plus additional as needed. This type of flour will supply more gluten to the recipe.

BREAD MACHINE VARIATION

Use bread machine yeast. If making the bread at high altitude, you may need to reduce the yeast to 1½ teaspoons. This recipe will make a 1½-pound loaf.

FOUR-INGREDIENT BAKING POWDER BISCUITS

MAKES 10 TO 12 BISCUITS

It doesn't get much easier than these beautiful, tender, naturally vegan biscuits. They take mere minutes to make, and just a few more to bake. And since I know some of you will ask—they don't taste like coconut! In fact, not a single taster guessed these were anything but traditional fluffy biscuits.

> **2 cups all-purpose flour, plus additional as needed**
> **1 tablespoon baking powder**
> **¾ teaspoon salt**
> **1¼ to 1⅓ cups chilled coconut cream (see Coconut Cream Note below)**

1. Preheat your oven to 450°F and line a baking sheet with parchment paper or a silicone baking mat.
2. In a large bowl, whisk together the flour, baking powder, and salt.
3. Add 1¼ cups coconut cream and stir until the dough begins to come together. Stir in additional cream as needed, using your hands when necessary to bring everything together into soft dough that isn't sticky. If it gets too moist, add a little more flour.
4. Turn out the dough onto a floured surface and knead just 5 to 10 times by gently pressing the dough out with the heels of your hands, rotating the dough 90 degrees, folding over, and repeating (you are bringing the dough together and gently creating a few layers).
5. Gently press out the dough to a ¾-inch thickness. Cut the dough with a lightly floured 2¼-inch biscuit cutter (cut straight down; do not twist the cutter) and place the rounds on your prepared baking sheet. Bring the dough scraps together, gently pat out, and cut again. Repeat this process if needed to use up the dough.
6. Optionally chill the biscuits in the freezer for 20 minutes, to help improve the rise.
7. Bake for 12 to 15 minutes, or until the tops just begin taking on a lightly golden hue.
8. Store in an airtight container at room temperature for up to 3 days, or individually wrap the biscuits and freeze to enjoy later.

COCONUT CREAM NOTE: Place full-fat coconut milk or coconut cream in the refrigerator to chill for at least 2 hours or overnight. This should yield a layer of very thick, spoonable cream for use in this recipe. If you're short on time or the coconut cream didn't separate and thicken, you can use the full-fat coconut milk as is. Start with 1 cup full-fat coconut milk and add more as needed.

GLUTEN-FREE OPTION

Substitute 1½ cups all-purpose gluten-free flour blend, ½ cup cornstarch or tapioca starch, and ½ teaspoon xanthan gum for the all-purpose flour. Add ½ teaspoon baking soda to the dry ingredients. Whisk 1 tablespoon apple cider vinegar and 1 teaspoon honey or agave nectar with the coconut cream before adding it to the dry ingredients.

FLAVOR VARIATIONS

SWEET: Whisk up to ¼ cup of your favorite granulated sweetener into the dry flour blend.

HERB: Stir up to ¼ cup chopped fresh herbs (such as thyme, rosemary, chives, or flat-leaf parsley) into the dry flour blend just before adding the wet ingredients.

BUTTERY: Brush the unbaked biscuits with 1 to 2 tablespoons melted dairy-free buttery spread or BAKEABLE BUTTER (page 192). If desired, you can brush them with more buttery spread right after they emerge from the oven.

HEAVENLY HONEY WHEAT PULL-APART ROLLS

MAKES 9 ROLLS

These 100 percent whole-grain rolls are wonderfully tender and soft, with bakery-fresh appeal. They're perfect for quick sandwiches or a slather of nut butter, Bakeable Butter (page 192), or chia jam (recipes on page 284).

3¼ cups white whole wheat flour or whole wheat flour, plus additional as needed
1 tablespoon vital wheat gluten
2¼ teaspoons (one ¼-ounce package) active dry yeast
1¼ teaspoons salt
1 cup warm unsweetened dairy-free milk beverage (about 105°F)
⅓ cup grapeseed, rice bran, or other neutral-tasting oil (see page 146)
¼ cup honey or agave nectar
2 tablespoons unsweetened applesauce

1. In a large mixing bowl, whisk together 2 cups of the flour, the gluten, yeast, and salt. Add the warm milk beverage, oil, sweetener, and applesauce and stir to combine. Add the remaining 1¼ cups flour and stir until soft dough forms. Bring the dough together with your hands when it becomes too thick to stir.

2. Turn out the dough onto a lightly floured surface. Knead it for 5 to 7 minutes, or until smooth and elastic. If the dough is too sticky to handle, add more flour, 1 tablespoon at a time, to keep it from sticking to your hands.

3. Return the dough to the bowl, lightly cover the bowl, and let the dough rise in a warm, draft-free place for 1 hour, or until doubled in size.

4. Punch down the dough and let it rest for 5 minutes.

5. Grease a 9 × 9-inch baking pan.

6. Divide the dough into 9 equal-size pieces. Roll each piece into a ball and space them out in your prepared pan.

7. Lightly cover the pan with plastic wrap and let the dough rise in a warm, draft-free place for 1 hour, or until it has doubled in size.

8. Preheat your oven to 400°F.

9. Gently uncover the rolls and bake on a lower rack in your oven for 20 to 24 minutes, or until slightly dark on the tops and starting to brown around the edges of the pan.

10. Let cool in the pan for 15 minutes before serving.

11. Cover and store at room temperature for up to 3 days, or individually wrap the rolls and freeze to enjoy later.

....

WHITE-WHEAT VARIATION

If you don't have vital wheat gluten, you can omit it. But reduce the white whole wheat flour to 2 cups and add 1¼ cups all-purpose flour or white bread flour, plus additional as needed.

....

SPEEDY WHEAT BUNS

MAKES 8 HAMBURGER BUNS

These buns are ready in 40 minutes flat, including rising times, for last-minute burger needs. They remind me quite a bit of kaiser rolls.

1 cup warm water (about 105°F)
2 tablespoons active dry yeast (reduce to 1½ tablespoons above 4,000 feet)
⅓ cup grapeseed, olive, or rice bran oil
¼ cup cane sugar or coconut sugar
1 large egg (see Vegan Option below for egg free)
2 cups all-purpose flour or white bread flour
1 teaspoon salt
1½ to 1¾ cups whole wheat flour or white whole wheat flour

1. Line a baking sheet with parchment paper or a silicone baking mat.
2. Put the warm water in a large bowl and sprinkle in the yeast. Let sit for 5 minutes to proof and ensure the yeast is active (see page 250).
3. Add the oil, sugar, and egg to the yeast mixture and whisk to combine. Add the all-purpose or bread flour and salt and stir to combine. Gradually stir in the wheat flour, as needed, until soft dough forms. Bring the dough together with your hands when it becomes too thick to stir. It should be slightly tacky but should not stick to your hands.
4. Turn out the dough onto a lightly floured surface. Knead it for about 5 minutes, or until smooth and elastic.
5. Divide the dough into 8 equal-size pieces. Shape each piece into a round and place them on your prepared baking sheet. Lightly cover the dough with plastic wrap and let it rest while your oven preheats (about 10 to 15 minutes).
6. Preheat your oven to 425°F.
7. Gently remove the plastic wrap and bake for 10 to 12 minutes, or until lightly golden.
8. Let cool on the baking sheet or a wire rack for 5 to 10 minutes before slicing.
9. Store in an airtight container at room temperature for up to 3 days, or individually wrap and freeze to enjoy later.

VEGAN OPTION

Substitute for the egg with 1 powdered egg replacer (usually 1 tablespoon powder + 2 tablespoons water) or whisk 1 tablespoon ground flaxseed or ground chia seed with 3 tablespoons water and let it gel for 5 minutes before adding.

HOT DOG BUN VARIATION

Divide the dough into 12 equal-size pieces. Roll each piece into a 4- to 5-inch-long roll. Bake as directed above.

SIMPLY SLIDER BUNS

MAKES 8 TO 10 BUNS

I haven't been able to find dairy-free slider buns in my local area, so I thought I'd make my own. These mini breads make mealtime more fun, and are great for building game day sandwiches.

⅔ cup warm water (about 105°F)
1 teaspoon active dry yeast
2 teaspoons olive oil or melted dairy-free buttery spread
1 teaspoon cane sugar or your favorite sweetener
½ teaspoon salt
1¾ cups all-purpose flour, plus additional as needed
2 tablespoons unsweetened plain or unsweetened dairy-free milk beverage

1. Put the warm water in a large bowl and sprinkle in the yeast. Let sit for 5 minutes to proof and ensure the yeast is active (see page 250).

2. Add the oil or buttery spread, sugar, and salt to the yeast mixture and whisk to combine. Gradually stir in the flour. Bring the dough together with your hands when it becomes too thick to stir.

3. Turn out the dough onto a lightly floured surface. Knead it for about 5 minutes, or until smooth and elastic. Add more flour as needed to keep the dough from sticking to your hands, but it should remain slightly sticky to the touch.

4. Lightly cover the bowl and let the dough rise in a warm, draft-free place for 1 hour, or until it has doubled in size.

5. Punch down the dough and let it rest for 5 minutes.

6. Line a baking sheet with parchment paper or a silicone baking mat.

7. Divide the dough into 8 to 10 equal-size pieces. Shape each piece into a round and place them on your prepared baking sheet.

8. Lightly cover the dough with plastic wrap and let them rise for 30 minutes, or until doubled in size. They won't rise much more in the oven.

9. Preheat your oven to 400°F.

10. Gently remove the plastic wrap from the dough balls and brush the tops with the milk beverage.

11. Bake for 12 to 15 minutes, or until lightly golden.

12. Store in an airtight container at room temperature for up to 3 days, or individually wrap the buns and freeze to enjoy later.

WHITE-WHEAT VARIATION

Replace ½ cup of the flour with white whole wheat flour or whole wheat flour for a slightly heartier bun. If you would like to use a higher ratio of whole wheat flour (1 cup or more), add 1 tablespoon vital wheat gluten with the flour.

CHAPTER 23

SNACK ON THIS
Sweet & Savory Light Recipes

GOOD TO KNOW FOR THIS CHAPTER

The recipes in this chapter include great make-ahead options and even some light meals. But for a small snack on the fly, nosh on any of these naturally dairy-free eats:

ANTS ON A LOG: Black (raisins) or red (dried cranberries) ants on a peanut butter- or seed butter-filled celery log.

HOMEMADE TRAIL MIX: Toss together your favorite nuts, seeds, dried fruit, cereal, chopped protein bars, and/or dairy-free chocolate chips.

ORANGE SLICES: They're a favorite as is, but sprinkle on some cinnamon for an elevated, refreshing snack.

BABY CARROTS: They go great with most dips, but are flavorful enough to snack on as is.

NUT BUTTER DIP: Sweeten creamy nut or seed butter with honey, maple syrup, or agave nectar, to taste. Use it as a dip for apple slices or pretzels or spread it on rice cakes or toast.

MELON WEDGES: Fill a honeydew or cantaloupe wedge with a scoop of dairy-free yogurt.

EDAMAME: Boil baby soybean pods in lightly salted water for 3 to 5 minutes, or until bright green. Sprinkle them with coarse sea salt, and eat the beans in the pods.

HUMMUS SLICES: Top cucumber slices with hummus and a dusting of paprika. Most store-bought brands are dairy free, but be sure to verify the ingredients.

TOASTED NUTS OR SEEDS: Scatter nuts or seeds on a baking sheet and bake in a 350°F oven until lightly toasted and fragrant. Season with salt and other spices as desired.

FRUIT SALAD: Toss together a seasonal blend of chopped fresh fruit or berries, and optionally stir in some dairy-free yogurt. When your favorite fresh fruit is not in season, you can defrost firm frozen fruits, such as mango or blueberries.

TORTILLA CHIPS AND SALSA OR GUACAMOLE: This is my husband's go-to snack when the munchies hit. Most brands of plain or salted tortilla chips are dairy free, but of course verify if cross-contamination is a concern for you. Guacamole is typically dairy free, but you should always check the labels for sour cream or other milk additives.

FROZEN GRAPES: Grapes freeze wonderfully in plastic freezer bags, and they make a perfect healthy snack on a hot summer day.

JAMMIN' GRAIN BARS

MAKES 12 BARS

This is my riff on the ever-popular Nutri-Grain bars. They look surprisingly similar, but I think this healthier version tastes better than the original, and they freeze well. Simply wrap a frozen bar in a paper towel and microwave for 30 seconds on high for a nearly fresh baked good.

2 cups white whole wheat flour (can substitute half all-purpose flour)
½ cup wheat bran
6 tablespoons firmly packed brown sugar or coconut sugar
1 teaspoon baking powder
½ teaspoon salt
¼ teaspoon ground cinnamon
¼ cup coconut oil, solid or semi-solid, or organic palm shortening
¾ cup full-fat coconut milk
2 tablespoons unsweetened applesauce or pumpkin puree
1½ teaspoons vanilla extract
1 cup dried blueberries, cherries, cranberries, or a combination
½ cup water, plus additional as needed
Topping of choice (see Topping & Flavor Variations following)

1. In a large bowl, whisk together the flour, bran, sugar, baking powder, salt, and cinnamon. Add the coconut oil or shortening and whisk until coarse crumbs form.

2. In a small bowl, whisk together the coconut milk, applesauce or pumpkin, and vanilla.

3. Add the wet mixture to the crumbly flour mixture and stir until it comes together into thick dough.

4. Divide the dough in half and shape each half into a thick, flat square. Wrap both squares tightly in plastic wrap and refrigerate while you make the filling.

5. Put the dried berries and water in a small saucepan. Bring the fruit to a low boil. Cover, reduce the heat to low, and let the fruit simmer for 15 to 20 minutes. Let cool for 5 minutes.

6. Pour the berries and remaining liquid into your blender or food processor. Pulse or puree the berries for a coarse or blended mixture, respectively. If it's too thick to blend, add a little water, ½ teaspoon at a time, until a thick paste forms.

7. Preheat your oven to 350°F and line a large baking sheet with parchment paper or a silicone baking mat.

8. Unwrap one square of the chilled dough and place it on a lightly floured surface. Roll it out to make an 8 × 12-inch rectangle. Cut the rectangle down the middle vertically to make two 4 × 12-inch rectangles. Note that the dough may tend to break, but it's very forgiving. Just press any broken parts back together as you go.

9. Spread a quarter of the berry mixture down the middle of one rectangle. Fold the uncut long edge over the berry middle. Fold the other long edge over so it overlaps just a little, and press the two sides together with moist fingers. Repeat this process with the second rectangle.

10. Cut each long rectangle into thirds to create 6 long bars. Flip so they are seam side down, and move the bars to your prepared baking sheet.

11. Repeat steps 8 through 10 with the remaining square of dough.

12. Top the bars as desired.

13. Bake for 17 to 20 minutes, or until the bar tops are lightly golden.

14. Let cool for 5 minutes on the baking sheet before removing the bars to a wire rack to cool completely.

15. Store in an airtight container at room temperature for up to 3 days, or individually wrap the bars and freeze to enjoy later.

TOPPING & FLAVOR VARIATIONS

UNSWEETENED: Brush the tops of the uncooked bars with 1 tablespoon unsweetened plain dairy-free milk beverage and sprinkle with 2 to 3 teaspoons wheat or oat bran.

MAPLE: Brush the tops of the uncooked bars with 1 tablespoon maple syrup. Optionally top with 2 to 3 teaspoons wheat or oat bran.

SUGAR: Brush the tops of the uncooked bars with 1 tablespoon unsweetened dairy-free milk beverage and sprinkle with 2 to 3 teaspoons coconut sugar or coarse sugar and 2 to 3 teaspoons wheat or oat bran.

PB&J: For heartier bars, spread ¼ to ⅓ cup peanut butter, sunflower seed butter, or nut butter on the dough before the berry mixture.

CHEWY NO-BAKE GRANOLA BARS

MAKES 16 TO 20 BARS

This is one of those recipes that took me a dozen times to perfect. After many failed attempts at baked granola bars, I realized that the chewy granola bar I was craving required no baking at all. My husband is addicted to these, so I often make a large batch and store them in the refrigerator or freezer.

3 cups crispy rice cereal
2¼ cups quick oats (certified gluten free, if needed)
½ cup sliced almonds
½ cup unsweetened shredded coconut
½ cup agave nectar or honey
¼ cup firmly packed brown sugar (can substitute coconut sugar)
1 cup creamy almond butter or peanut butter
1½ teaspoons vanilla extract
½ teaspoon salt (omit if using salted nut butter)
⅔ cup dairy-free semi-sweet chocolate chips (mini chips if available)

1. Grease a 9 × 13-inch baking dish.

2. In a large bowl, stir together the rice cereal, oats, almonds, and coconut.

3. Put the liquid sweetener and brown sugar in a small saucepan over medium heat. Bring to a boil, and then immediately remove the saucepan from the heat. Whisk in the nut butter, vanilla, and salt until smooth.

4. Pour the hot, gooey mixture into the cereal mix and stir until well combined. Let cool for 2 minutes. Stir in the chocolate chips.

5. Press the mixture very firmly into your prepared baking dish with a piece of plastic wrap, parchment paper, or wax paper to avoid sticking.

6. Place the bars in the freezer for 30 minutes.

7. Cut the mixture into fourths horizontally, and then fourths or fifths vertically to create long bars.

8. Store in an airtight container in the refrigerator for up to 2 weeks, or in plastic freezer bags in the freezer to enjoy later.

NUT-FREE OPTION

Substitute ½ cup more oats, shredded coconut, seeds, or chopped dried fruit for the almonds and use sunflower seed butter in place of the nut butter.

CHOCOLATE, NUTS & SEA SALT NICE BARS

MAKES 16 BARS

Over the years, many chocolate-covered bar varieties have waffled back and forth between containing dairy and not containing dairy. And many of those chocolaty gems are still made on shared lines with milky ingredients. So I decided to whip up my own crispy, chewy, nutty bars, complete with a chocolate dunk on the bottom and a drizzle on the top. They're similar to Kind Bars, but with an even more delicious, homemade twist.

2 cups almonds
¾ cup hazelnuts
¾ cup peanuts or cashews
⅔ cup crispy rice cereal
3 tablespoons ground flaxseed
¾ cup honey or brown rice syrup
1¼ teaspoons vanilla extract
¼ teaspoon + ¼ to ½ teaspoon salt, divided
¾ cup dairy-free semi-sweet or dark chocolate chips
1 teaspoon coconut oil or organic palm shortening

1. Preheat your oven to 350°F, line a 7 × 11-inch baking dish with parchment paper or greased wax paper, and grease a large bowl.

2. Spread out the almonds, hazelnuts, and peanuts or cashews on a baking sheet. Bake for 8 to 12 minutes, or until the nuts are lightly fragrant and beginning to release their oils. Let cool for 5 minutes.

3. Rub the hazelnuts in a paper towel or clean kitchen towel to remove any loose skins.

4. Put the toasted nuts, rice cereal, and ground flaxseed in your greased bowl and stir to combine.

5. Put the sweetener, vanilla, and ¼ teaspoon salt in a small saucepan over medium heat. Cook until the mixture reaches 250°F (it will bubble up; this is the "firm ball" stage). Immediately remove the pan from the heat and pour the hot mixture over the nuts and cereal. Stir to thoroughly combine.

6. Firmly press the sticky mixture into your prepared baking dish using lightly greased hands or a piece of parchment paper. Sprinkle the top with the remaining ¼ to ½ teaspoon salt, to taste. Let cool for 15 minutes.

7. Using the paper, lift the pressed mixture out of your baking dish and invert it onto a cutting board. Peel away the paper. It should still be quite pliable. If it's too soft, let it cool for another 10 minutes. Cut the slab into fourths each way, to create 16 bars. Let cool completely.

8. Melt the chocolate chips with the shortening (see page 417 for How to Melt Chocolate).

9. Dunk the bottoms of the bars in the melted chocolate and place them, chocolate side up, on a cutting board or wire rack. Let the chocolate set at room temperature, or place the bars in the freezer for 15 minutes.

10. Once the chocolate is set, turn the bars chocolate side down and drizzle the tops with the remaining melted chocolate.

11. Store in an airtight container at room temperature for up to 1 week, in the refrigerator for up to 1 month, or in the freezer to enjoy later.

CHOCOLATE PEANUT BUTTER OAT CUPS

MAKES 16 SNACK CUPS

These "bars" are made in muffin cups for perfectly portioned servings and a fun, healthy riff on peanut butter cups. They're sweet and a little dessert-like, but still wholesome in nature.

1 cup creamy peanut butter (can substitute sunflower seed butter for peanut free)
⅔ cup honey or agave nectar
1 teaspoon vanilla extract
⅛ to ¼ teaspoon salt, to taste
3 cups quick oats (certified gluten free, if needed)
¾ cup dairy-free semi-sweet or dark chocolate chips
1½ teaspoons coconut oil, buttery spread, or organic palm shortening
½ cup chopped roasted salted peanuts (omit for peanut free)

1. Put the peanut butter, honey, and vanilla in a large saucepan over medium-low heat. Whisk to combine as the ingredients melt together. Whisk in the salt.

2. Add the oats to your saucepan and stir as the mixture cooks for 3 to 5 minutes. It will become a very thick dough consistency, but keep stirring. Cooking helps remove the "raw" taste of the oats and binds the ingredients. Remove the saucepan from the heat and let cool for 5 minutes.

3. Divide the oat mixture between 16 silicone muffin cups or muffin tins lined with cupcake liners and firmly press it in. Place the oat cups in the refrigerator for 15 minutes.

4. Melt the chocolate chips with the oil, buttery spread, or shortening (see page 417 for How to Melt Chocolate).

5. Dip the bottoms of the cooled oat cups in the chocolate, halfway up the sides. Place the oat cups, chocolate side up, on a cutting board or wire rack. Sprinkle each oat cup with 1½ teaspoons chopped peanuts (if using). Let the chocolate set at room temperature, or place the bars in the freezer for 10 minutes.

6. Store in an airtight container in the refrigerator or freezer for optimal freshness. They can be enjoyed chilled or at room temperature.

OAT SQUARES VARIATION

Press the oat mixture into an 8 × 8-inch baking dish lined with parchment paper. Once completely cooled, invert the oat slab onto a cutting board and peel off the parchment paper. Cut the oat mixture into fourths each way to make 16 squares. Dip in chocolate as instructed above.

PINEAPPLE-COCONUT PROTEIN BITES

MAKES 24 BITES

It's easy to get caught in a chocolate rut with homemade snacks. So I decided to mix things up with these piña colada–inspired snack balls. They're sweet, tangy, and richly fulfilling.

    1 cup freeze-dried pineapple, or as needed
    ¾ cup unsweetened shredded coconut
    ⅓ cup unsweetened plain dairy-free protein powder (preferably pea protein)
    ⅓ cup honey or agave nectar
    ¼ cup coconut butter, softened
    ¼ cup coconut oil, melted
    ½ teaspoon pure vanilla flavoring or extract

1. Put the pineapple in your spice grinder or food processor. Process until powdered, about 30 seconds.

2. Put the pineapple powder, coconut, and protein powder in a medium bowl and whisk to combine.

3. In another medium bowl, whisk together the sweetener, coconut butter, coconut oil, and vanilla. Add the dry pineapple-coconut mixture and stir to combine.

4. If the mixture is too sticky to work with, place it in the refrigerator for 15 minutes.

5. Line a plate with parchment paper.

6. Roll the pineapple-coconut mixture into 1-inch balls and place them on your prepared plate.

7. Refrigerate the bites for 30 to 60 minutes, or until set.

8. Store in an airtight container in the refrigerator or freezer for optimal freshness. They can be enjoyed chilled or at room temperature.

POWER FUDGIES

MAKES 32 FUDGY BALLS

These mighty bites not only provide quick and lasting energy, but they're also little mineral bombs for supporting healthy muscles and bones. Do not be tempted to sub in cocoa powder for the carob. Carob is mellower, sweeter, and caffeine free, and contains more minerals than cocoa.

> ½ cup creamy almond butter (can substitute sunflower seed butter for nut free) (see Nut Butter Note below)
> ½ cup honey or agave nectar
> ½ cup carob powder
> ⅛ teaspoon salt (omit if using salted almond butter)
> ½ cup + ¼ cup sesame seeds, hemp seeds, or unsweetened shredded coconut, divided

1. In a medium bowl, stir together the almond butter, sweetener, carob powder, and salt (if using) until smooth. Add the ½ cup seeds or coconut and stir until the ingredients are evenly dispersed.
2. Refrigerate the mixture for 20 minutes.
3. Put the remaining ¼ cup seeds or coconut in a small dish.
4. Roll the carob mixture into 1-inch balls and roll them in the seeds or coconut to coat.
5. Store in an airtight container in the refrigerator or freezer for optimal freshness. They can be enjoyed chilled or at room temperature.

NUT BUTTER NOTE: I use a thick almond butter for making this recipe. If you're using a somewhat runny nut or seed butter, you may need to add a little oat flour, quick oats, or protein powder to the carob mixture to help the balls set up.

APPLE A DAY "DONUTS"

MAKES 4 TO 6 SNACKS

Cored and sliced apples have a fun donut shape. So I top them with a sweet, creamy topping for a treat-like snack.

> ¾ cup raw cashews (see Nut-Free Option following)
> 1 tablespoon coconut sugar, maple sugar, or brown sugar
> 2 tablespoons coconut oil, softened or melted
> ¼ teaspoon pure vanilla flavoring or extract
> Generous pinch salt
> 3 medium organic apples (preferably refrigerated)
> ¼ cup dried apple pieces
> Ground cinnamon, for sprinkling

1. Put the cashews and sugar in your spice grinder or food processor. Process until finely ground and beginning to clump, about 1 minute.
2. Put the ground cashew mixture, coconut oil, vanilla, and salt in your blender or food processor. Blend until smooth and creamy.
3. Core the apples and slice them horizontally into ½-inch-thick rounds.
4. Drizzle the cashew butter mixture on top of each apple round, and lightly spread it to cover the exposed cut apple. Top it with dried apple pieces and sprinkle lightly with cinnamon.
5. Chill the apple slices in the refrigerator until the "icing" is set, about 30 minutes.

FRESHNESS TIP: If you are concerned about browning, you can toss the apple rounds with citrus juice (lemon, pineapple, orange). But since the tops are coated and the bottoms are resting on a plate, browning is usually minimal.

NUT-FREE OPTION

Substitute ⅓ cup sunflower seed butter or other nut-free "butter" for the cashews.

CHOCOLATE PISTACHIO FIGS

MAKES 30 FIG BITES (6 TO 8 SERVINGS)

I have experimented with several fig recipes, but I find that the simpler, the better with this calcium-rich dried fruit. And although both chocolate and figs are sweet, this combination has a light savory component that tempers the natural sugars and gives it snack-worthy flavor.

⅔ cup dairy-free semi-sweet or dark chocolate chips or chunks
1 teaspoon coconut oil or organic palm shortening
¼ to ½ teaspoon orange extract, to taste (optional)
30 whole dried figs (one 12-ounce package)
½ cup unsalted or lightly shelled pistachios, finely chopped (can substitute hemp, sunflower, or pumpkin seeds for nut free)

1. Line a baking sheet with wax paper or parchment paper.
2. Melt the chocolate chips with the oil or shortening (see page 417 for How to Melt Chocolate). Whisk in the orange extract (if using).
3. Holding a fig by the stem, dip it into the chocolate, about halfway up, then dip the bottom in the chopped nuts. Place it on your prepared baking sheet. Repeat this process with the remaining figs.
4. Refrigerate the chocolate-dipped figs until set, about 30 minutes.
5. Store in an airtight container in the refrigerator for up to 2 weeks.

PINWHEELS

MAKES 6 TO 8 SERVINGS

My associate editor, Sarah Hatfield, has four kids, which means light lunches are in high demand. And since one of her children doesn't like sandwiches, she turned to these protein-packed pinwheels. They were inspired by a bean dip that her kids love to eat with veggies and crackers. The recipe includes two bean spread options to help mix things up throughout the week.

1 (15-ounce) can black beans, drained and rinsed
2 tablespoons olive oil
1 tablespoon apple cider vinegar
¼ teaspoon garlic powder
¼ teaspoon salt
1 tablespoon water, if needed
6 to 8 whole-grain or gluten-free tortillas or wraps
Optional toppings: ½ to 1 cup grated carrot, celery, or cucumber matchsticks, baby spinach leaves, bell pepper strips, roasted red pepper slices, avocado slices, or turkey slices

1. Put the beans, oil, vinegar, garlic powder, and salt in your food processor or blender. Process until the mixture is very smooth. If the mixture is too thick, add the water and process to combine. Alternatively, you can thoroughly mash the ingredients together with a fork or stick blender in a bowl, but it will not be as smooth.

2. Spread the bean mixture on one side of the tortillas or wraps. Top each with your toppings of choice.

3. Roll each tortilla or wrap into a tight cylinder. Individually wrap them in plastic wrap and refrigerate for at least 1 hour, or up to 1 day.

4. When ready to serve, unwrap the roll-ups and slice them into 1-inch rounds.

....

WHITE BEAN SPREAD VARIATION

Substitute cannellini beans for the black beans and lemon juice for the vinegar. Add ½ teaspoon chopped fresh rosemary to the bean mixture.

....

UN-SUSHI SNACKERS

MAKES 12 SNACK ROLLS

I've been known to wrap up all types of sandwich fillings in seaweed wraps, so this slightly cheesy spread and sprinkling of fresh vegetables is really no stretch. These are best eaten immediately, as the nori can get a bit soggy as they sit. If you plan to pack them along for later in the day, I recommend storing the nori separately and assembling them at snack time.

    1 cup raw sunflower seeds
    ¼ cup water
    1 tablespoon apple cider vinegar
    1 teaspoon honey or agave nectar
    ¾ teaspoon salt
    ¼ teaspoon garlic powder
    6 nori sheets, torn in half
    2 large carrots, cut into thin sticks (about 3 to 4 inches long)
    1 cucumber, cut into thin sticks (about 3 to 4 inches long)

1. Put the sunflower seeds in your spice grinder or food processor. Process until powdered, about 30 seconds.

2. Put the ground sunflower seeds, water, vinegar, sweetener, salt, and garlic powder in your blender. Blend until smooth, about 1 minute.

3. Scrape the mixture into an airtight container, cover, and chill for 1 hour or overnight.

4. When ready to eat, slather some of the seed butter mixture on one end of a nori sheet half. Top it with the carrot and cucumber sticks, and roll the seaweed up. Repeat with as many as you would like to eat right away.

5. Store leftover seed mixture in an airtight container in the refrigerator for up to 3 days.

OTHER FILLING VARIATIONS

Leftover roasted sweet potatoes, stir-fried eggplant, or any other cooked vegetables make a great vegan filling for these easy nori snack rolls.

FIVE-MINUTE NACHOS

MAKES 4 SERVINGS

These nachos are not only prepared in 5 minutes, but my husband and I can also devour every last chip in 5 minutes. This cheesy sauce also works well on other Mexican-inspired recipes, including enchiladas.

¼ cup raw cashews
1 cup unsweetened plain dairy-free milk beverage or vegetable broth
2 tablespoons grapeseed, olive, rice bran, or neutral-tasting oil (see page 146)
2 ounces pimientos or roasted red bell peppers, drained
2 tablespoons tapioca starch (can substitute cornstarch or arrowroot starch)
2 tablespoons nutritional yeast flakes
1 tablespoon lemon juice
½ to 1 teaspoon salt
1 (4-ounce) can diced green chiles, drained (optional)
Tortilla chips
Optional toppings: chopped tomato, chopped avocado, and sliced black olives
Salsa, for serving

1. Put the cashews in your spice grinder or food processor. Process until finely ground and beginning to clump, about 1 minute.

2. Put the ground cashews, milk beverage or broth, oil, pimientos or peppers, starch, nutritional yeast, lemon juice, and ½ teaspoon salt in your blender. Blend until smooth, about 2 minutes. Blend in additional salt, to taste.

3. Pour the mixture into a medium saucepan. Cook over medium heat while whisking, until the cheesy sauce is thick but still pourable, about 5 minutes. Stir in the green chiles (if using).

4. Place the tortilla chips on a serving platter and pour the nacho "cheese" sauce evenly over the top. Sprinkle on any of the toppings, if desired.

5. Serve with your favorite salsa.

6. It is best enjoyed immediately, but leftover, cooled cheesy sauce can be stored in an airtight container in the refrigerator for up to 2 days. Gently reheat it and whisk before serving.

MAKE IT A MEAL: Top the nachos with one 15-ounce can black beans (drained and rinsed), ¾ to 1 pound chopped and sautéed vegetables (like onions, zucchini, bell pepper, or mushrooms), diced or shredded cooked chicken, cooked ground beef, or vegan ground round.

PLEASE PASS THE CHEEZE POPCORN

MAKES 10 CUPS

This easy cheesy popcorn is perfect for afternoon snacks or movie nights, and can be customized to your personal tastes. Increase or reduce the salt, as desired, and use curry powder, chili powder, or smoked paprika for slight variations in the flavor vibe.

⅓ cup nutritional yeast flakes
½ to 1 teaspoon curry powder, chili powder, or smoked paprika, to taste
¼ to ½ teaspoon garlic powder, to taste
½ teaspoon onion powder
½ teaspoon salt
10 cups air-popped popcorn (from ⅓ cup popcorn kernels)
3 tablespoons coconut oil or dairy-free buttery spread, melted

1. Put the nutritional yeast, spice, garlic powder, onion powder, and salt in your spice grinder. Process until powdered, about 15 seconds.
2. Put the popcorn in a large bowl. Drizzle the melted oil or buttery spread over the popcorn while tossing the popcorn to evenly coat.
3. Sprinkle the popcorn with about 2 tablespoons of the seasoning blend, or to taste, while tossing the popcorn to evenly coat.
4. Store leftover seasoning in an airtight container at room temperature for up to 1 month.

PERFECT STOVETOP POPCORN RECIPE

If you don't have an air popper, add 3 tablespoons high-heat oil (see page 148) to a large pot with a lid over medium-high heat. Toss a few popcorn kernels into the pot and cover it. Once the kernels pop, add ⅓ cup popcorn kernels, cover the pan, and remove it from the heat for 30 seconds. Return the pan to the heat. Once the popping begins, gently shake the pan by moving it back and forth over the burner. When the popping slows to more than 5 seconds between pops, remove it from the heat. Carefully remove the lid, as some kernels may still pop and the steam is hot. Transfer the popcorn to a large bowl to serve. This makes approximately 10 cups. If you're using this popcorn in the Cheeze Popcorn recipe above, you can omit the drizzle of oil or buttery spread.

EASY CHEESY CRACKERS

MAKES 60 TO 70 CRACKERS

These surprisingly simple crackers are reminiscent of those classic little cheese squares, but they have a fresher, more wholesome taste that's addictive in its own right.

¾ cup all-purpose flour, whole wheat pastry flour, or all-purpose gluten-free flour blend
¼ cup chickpea/garbanzo bean flour
2 to 3 tablespoons nutritional yeast flakes, to taste
¾ teaspoon salt
¼ teaspoon paprika
¼ teaspoon onion powder
⅛ teaspoon garlic powder
3 tablespoons oil
3 tablespoons water, or as needed
½ teaspoon lemon juice

1. Preheat your oven to 350°F and line a large baking sheet with parchment paper.
2. In a medium bowl, whisk together the flours, nutritional yeast, salt, paprika, onion powder, and garlic powder. Add the oil and whisk until coarse crumbs form. Add the water and lemon juice and stir. When it becomes somewhat dry, bring the dough together with your hands. It should be relatively cohesive but not sticky. If it's too dry, splash in more water. If it's too sticky, sprinkle on a little more flour.
3. Turn out the dough onto a lightly floured surface and flour your rolling pin. Roll out the dough into a thin square or rectangle that's about ⅛ inch thick.
4. Using a knife or pizza cutter, cut horizontal lines about 1 inch apart and vertical lines about 1 inch apart to make 1-inch squares. Alternatively, use small cookie cutters to cut out shapes.
5. Transfer the squares or shapes to your prepared baking sheet, spaced out slightly for better air circulation and crisping.
6. Bring the remaining dough scraps together and repeat steps 4 and 5.
7. If you want to avoid air bubbles in your crackers, prick the tops of the dough with a fork.
8. Bake for 15 to 17 minutes, or until the edges of the crackers just begin to look golden.
9. Let cool on the baking sheet; the crackers will crisp up as they cool.
10. Store in an airtight container at room temperature for up to 1 week, or in plastic freezer bags in the freezer to preserve freshness and enjoy later.

FLAVOR VARIATIONS

BUTTERY: Swap dairy-free buttery spread for the oil.

CHEESIER: Use more nutritional yeast for a cheesier flavor (or less for a milder flavor).

SALTED: Increase the salt to 1 teaspoon or sprinkle a little sea salt on the rolled-out dough and do one last light roll to gently press it in.

HEARTY: Substitute white whole wheat flour or spelt flour for the primary flour.

BEAN-LESS: If you don't have chickpea/garbanzo bean flour, omit it and increase the other flour to 1 cup.

GARLIC & HERB BABY CHEEZES

MAKES 18 BABY CHEEZES

These soft little cheezes smell so good while they bake! Enjoy them as a spread on crackers or bread, or crumble them onto salads. I sometimes just nibble on one or two for a delicious hit of savory energy.

1 cup whole almonds (preferably blanched)
3 to 4 tablespoons water, plus additional for soaking
3 tablespoons lemon juice
3 tablespoons olive oil
2 teaspoons white miso (gluten free or soy free, if needed)
1 teaspoon + ⅛ teaspoon (optional) salt, divided
1 teaspoon nutritional yeast flakes
¼ cup almond meal
2 teaspoons dried herbs (thyme, basil, and/or rosemary), crushed between your fingers
½ teaspoon garlic powder

1. Put the almonds in a container and cover with a few inches of water. Cover and place in the refrigerator to soak for 12 to 24 hours.

2. Drain and rinse the almonds. If the almonds aren't blanched, you can optionally peel them for optimum flavor and creaminess. It's easy to peel a soaked almond, but there are a lot of them! I do this while watching TV or listening to music. If you don't have time to peel them, the flavor will be a little deeper and more rustic.

3. Put the soaked almonds, 3 tablespoons water, lemon juice, olive oil, miso, 1 teaspoon salt, and nutritional yeast in your blender or food processor. Process until relatively smooth, about 2 minutes. If it's a little too thick and chunky, add 1 more tablespoon water and process until relatively smooth.

4. Line a fine-mesh sieve with a double layer of cheesecloth and place the sieve over a bowl to catch any liquid. Scrape the almond mixture into the center of the cheesecloth. Bring the corners of the cheesecloth together, twist to tighten the almond mixture into a packed ball, and set it back down into the sieve. Place the bowl in the refrigerator for 8 to 24 hours. The almond mixture will set up and release just a little bit of moisture. It's ready when the cheesecloth pulls away without the cheese alternative sticking to it.

5. Preheat your oven to 300°F and line a baking sheet with parchment paper or a silicone baking mat.

6. In a small bowl, whisk together the almond meal, herbs, garlic powder, and remaining ⅛ teaspoon salt (if using).

7. Remove the almond cheeze from the cheesecloth. Scoop a tablespoon of the almond cheeze and roughly shape it into a ball. It will be a little sticky. You can lightly wet or flour your hands as you work with it or you can freeze the cheeze for about 45 minutes to firm it up before shaping. Roll the ball in the almond meal mixture and place it on your prepared baking sheet. Gently flatten the round into a little disk, about ½ inch high. Repeat with the remaining almond cheeze.

8. Bake for 30 minutes, or until the crust is lightly golden.

9. Let cool for 10 minutes on the baking sheet before serving.

10. The cheezes will hold up for a few hours at room temperature, but store leftovers in the refrigerator for up to 1 week, or freeze them in plastic freezer bags to enjoy later.

CHAPTER 24

LAY IT ON THICK
Dips, Dressings & Spreads

GOOD TO KNOW FOR THIS CHAPTER

NOT ALL MAYONNAISES ARE CREATED EQUAL. As mentioned earlier, most mayos are dairy free. However, natural and organic brands often contain "healthier" oils, which can create different flavor nuances. And vegan mayos, although great egg-free substitutes, can vary quite a bit. Most taste good, but they each provide different flavor nuances. And some thin out more than the norm when stirred with any liquid. Don't be afraid to experiment with different mayonnaises, but do know that they may affect taste and consistency outcomes more significantly in recipes like dressings and dips.

BASIC VINAIGRETTE IS TYPICALLY DAIRY FREE. For this reason, I focus more on complicated or creamy recipes in this chapter. But the basic formula for homemade vinaigrette is oil (about ⅓ cup), vinegar or lemon juice (about ¼ cup), salt, and pepper to taste. You can add Italian seasoning (dry or fresh herbs) and garlic for a quick Italian variation. Keep in mind that some vinaigrette brands do contain cheese or other dairy ingredients.

COCONUT OIL ISN'T GOOD FOR EVERYTHING. Since coconut oil solidifies instantly when it hits cold liquids (creating little chunks), I typically don't recommend using it in dressings. But spreads and dips that are warmed and then cooled can benefit from the thickening power of coconut oil.

PIZZA DIP

MAKES 4 TO 6 SERVINGS

This kid-friendly dip goes very well with crusty French bread, warm pita wedges, chicken fingers, or vegetables (such as lightly steamed cauliflower florets). It's also a great pasta sauce. Simply cook 12 ounces of noodles and optionally double the pepperoni.

1 (15-ounce) can or 2 (8-ounce) cans tomato sauce
2 ounces regular or vegan pepperoni, diced (optional)
½ teaspoon dried oregano
½ teaspoon dried basil
¼ teaspoon garlic powder
Pinch crushed red pepper
¼ cup raw cashews
½ cup water or unsweetened plain dairy-free milk beverage
2 tablespoons nutritional yeast flakes
1 tablespoon tapioca starch (can substitute cornstarch)
¼ cup sliced olives (optional)

1. In a small saucepan over medium-low heat, whisk together the tomato sauce, pepperoni (if using), oregano, basil, garlic powder, and red pepper. Bring the mixture to a simmer, and cook for 5 minutes.

2. Put the cashews in your spice grinder or food processor. Process until powdered, about 1 minute.

3. Put the ground cashews, water or milk beverage, nutritional yeast, and tapioca starch in your blender. Blend until smooth, about 1 minute.

4. Pour the cashew mixture into the tomato sauce mixture and whisk to combine. Bring it back to a simmer and cook, whisking occasionally, for 3 minutes, or until it has thickened to a dip consistency. Stir in the olives (if using). Let the dip cool for 5 minutes before serving.

5. Store in an airtight container in the refrigerator for up to 2 days. If the dip thickens too much as it chills, briefly heat it, whisking in more water, if needed.

NUT-FREE OPTION

Reduce the water or milk beverage to ¼ cup and omit the cashews, tapioca starch, and nutritional yeast. Stir in ¾ cup vegan mozzarella or cheddar shreds and 2 tablespoons bread crumbs (gluten free, if needed) in step 4.

BABA GHANOUSH

MAKES 6 SERVINGS

Hummus is nice, but eggplant takes it up a giant notch in my book. Serve this flavorful Mediterranean dip with French bread, pita wedges, or raw vegetables.

1 large eggplant (about 1½ pounds)
1 teaspoon grapeseed or olive oil
2 tablespoons tahini, plus additional as needed
2 tablespoons lemon juice, plus additional as needed
1 or 2 garlic cloves, crushed or minced (½ to 1 teaspoon)
¼ to ½ teaspoon ground cumin, to taste
½ teaspoon salt, or to taste
2 to 3 teaspoons extra-virgin olive oil
1 tablespoon minced fresh flat-leaf parsley (optional)

1. Preheat your oven to 400°F.
2. Cut the eggplant in half lengthwise. Drizzle the grapeseed or olive oil in a large baking dish. Place the eggplant, cut sides down, in the baking dish, making sure the undersides of the eggplant are coated in the oil to avoid sticking.
3. Bake for 30 to 40 minutes, or until the eggplant is very tender (the skin will be browned). Let cool for 5 minutes.
4. Peel the skin off the eggplant or scoop out the flesh, and put the flesh in a medium mixing bowl.
5. Using a fork or hand mixer, mash or blend the eggplant until it is relatively smooth but retains some of its texture. Add the tahini, lemon juice, garlic, and cumin and stir to combine. Add the salt and stir in more tahini and/or lemon juice, if desired.
6. Transfer the mixture to a serving bowl and spread it with the back of a spoon to form a shallow well.
7. Drizzle the extra-virgin olive oil into the well, and sprinkle the dip with the parsley (if using).
8. Store in an airtight container in the refrigerator for up to 3 days.

RAWESOME NUT DIP

MAKES 8 TO 10 SERVINGS

This wonderfully rich, nutritious, and slightly cheesy dip recipe was created by my friend Dreena Burton. It's from her cookbook *Eat, Drink & Be Vegan*. Dreena is one of the most talented vegan recipe creators that I know, and this versatile spread is proof. You can enjoy it as a sandwich spread, baked potato topping, soup garnish, manicotti stuffing, or simply as a dip with your favorite vegetables.

½ cup chopped red or orange bell pepper
½ cup almonds
½ cup pistachios
¼ cup walnuts
¼ cup pine nuts or more walnuts (see Nut Note below)
¼ cup water, plus additional as needed
3 to 3½ tablespoons lemon juice, to taste
1 small garlic clove, smashed
½ teaspoon salt
½ cup fresh basil
1 to 1½ teaspoons fresh thyme, to taste
Freshly ground black pepper, to taste

1. Put the bell pepper, almonds, pistachios, walnuts, pine nuts (if using), water, lemon juice, garlic, and salt in your blender or food processor. Process until relatively smooth, scraping down the sides as needed. If it is too thick for your machine, add more water, 1 tablespoon at a time, as needed. You can leave the blend a little chunky or puree it until very smooth.
2. Add the basil, thyme, and black pepper to the nut mixture and pulse to combine.
3. Store in an airtight container in the refrigerator for up to 3 days.

NUT NOTE: You can substitute other nuts or seeds, but keep in mind that they each differ in flavor. Cashews, almonds, and pistachios have sweeter flavors, but walnuts and pine nuts have more savory and sometimes bitter notes.

CHEESIER VARIATION

Add 1 to 2 tablespoons nutritional yeast flakes to your food processor or blender in step 1.

SUPER SPINACH & ARTICHOKE DIP

MAKES 12 TO 16 SERVINGS

I like to call this my "Popeye" dip, since it's loaded with spinach and several other powerhouse ingredients. It can easily double as a party appetizer and a healthy lunch box favorite. But keep in mind that spinach doesn't keep for very long. If you would like a dip that keeps for a few days, omit the spinach and simply enjoy this as a nutritious artichoke dip. Either way, it goes well with tortilla chips, potato chips, baguette slices, or cut vegetables.

2 cups cauliflower florets
½ cup raw cashews
⅔ cup cooked cannellini beans
½ cup + 2 tablespoons water
2 to 3 tablespoons nutritional yeast flakes, to taste
4 teaspoons lemon juice
1½ to 1⅝ teaspoons salt, to taste
1½ teaspoons white miso (gluten free or soy free, if needed)
¼ teaspoon onion powder
¼ teaspoon garlic powder
2 cups finely chopped baby spinach leaves
1 (14-ounce) can artichoke hearts, drained and finely chopped
¼ teaspoon black pepper or crushed red pepper (optional)

1. Preheat your oven to 375°F.
2. Steam the cauliflower until quite tender, 10 to 12 minutes.
3. Put the cashews in your spice grinder or food processor. Process until powdered, about 1 minute.
4. Put the cooked cauliflower, ground cashews, beans, water, nutritional yeast, lemon juice, salt, miso, onion powder, and garlic powder in your blender or food processor. Process until very smooth, about 2 minutes.
5. Pour the mixture into an 8 × 8-inch or slightly smaller baking dish. Stir in the spinach, artichokes, and black or red pepper (if using). Level the mixture out.
6. Bake for 35 minutes, or until golden on top. Let cool for 10 minutes before serving.
7. Store in an airtight container in the refrigerator for up to 1 day.

COMPANY'S COMING NACHO DIP

MAKES 4 SERVINGS

This shortcut recipe is a delicious and fast way to use that dairy-free powdered cheeze mix you're now keeping on hand!

½ cup POWDERED CHEEZE MIX (page 207)
¼ cup cold water, plus additional as needed
½ cup salsa

1. In a small saucepan, whisk together the cheeze mix and water until smooth. Stir in the salsa.
2. Place the saucepan over medium heat. Bring the mixture to a low boil. Reduce the heat to low, and cook, while whisking, until it thickens, about 2 minutes. If it becomes too thick, whisk in more water, 1 tablespoon at a time, until it reaches your desired consistency. Let cool for 3 minutes before serving.
3. Store in an airtight container in the refrigerator for up to 3 days. If the dip thickens too much as it chills, briefly heat it, whisking in more water, if needed.

BUTTERY CARROT SPREAD

MAKES 1½ CUPS

This simple spread comes together quickly, and is delicious with vegetables or atop toast. But since the recipe is very carrot heavy, I recommend tasting your carrots before using them in this recipe. Fresh, sweet carrots will result in a wonderful spread, while flat or bitter carrots won't wow as much.

1½ cups chopped soft-cooked carrots (see Cooked Carrots Tip below)
½ cup unsweetened plain dairy-free milk beverage, brought to room temperature
⅓ cup coconut oil
½ teaspoon salt, plus additional to taste
½ teaspoon white miso (gluten free or soy free, if needed) (optional)
¼ teaspoon ground ginger (optional)

1. Lightly mash the carrots and put them in your blender or food processor. Add the milk beverage, coconut oil, and salt. Blend until the mixture is smooth and creamy, about 1 to 2 minutes.
2. Optionally add the miso, ginger, and/or more salt, if desired. Blend to combine, about 30 seconds.
3. Store in an airtight container in the refrigerator for up to 3 days. It will set up more as it cools.

COOKED CARROTS TIP: To make 1½ cups of cooked carrots, peel and slice about 2 large carrots. For soft-cooked carrots that blend well, I steam the slices for about 15 minutes.

FRESH STRAWBERRY CHIA JAM

MAKES ¾ CUP

This versatile sweet topping has a natural little dose of omega-3 fatty acids and dairy-free calcium. I also like that it's quick to prepare, and it sets up fairly thick for versatility in recipes.

1½ cups chopped strawberries
2 to 4 tablespoons honey or agave nectar, to taste
2 tablespoons chia seeds
2 to 3 teaspoons lemon juice, to taste
¼ teaspoon pure vanilla flavoring or extract (optional)

1. Put the strawberries in your blender and pulse a few times to break them up.
2. Put the crushed strawberries and sweetener in a small saucepan over medium heat and whisk to combine. Bring the berries to a low boil. Reduce the heat to medium-low and simmer, stirring occasionally, for about 10 minutes. It should thicken a bit.
3. Remove from the heat and stir in the chia seeds, lemon juice, and vanilla (if using). Let cool completely. The jam will thicken significantly as it sits.
4. Store in an airtight container in the refrigerator for up to 1 week, or in the freezer to enjoy later.

ROCKIN' RASPBERRY CHIA JAM

MAKES ¾ CUP

This is another favorite for infusing calcium-rich chia seeds into our everyday eats. Raspberries have little indigestible seeds and a tarter flavor than strawberries, so the ingredients and preparation to make chia jam are a little different. This recipe also works well with blackberries, but you should start with a reduced amount of sweetener and add more to taste. Ripe blackberries tend to be naturally sweeter and less tart than raspberries.

2 cups raspberries
⅓ cup honey or agave nectar, or to taste
2½ tablespoons chia seeds
2 to 3 teaspoons lemon juice, to taste
½ teaspoon pure vanilla flavoring or extract

1. Put the raspberries and honey or agave nectar in your blender. Blend until smooth, about 1 minute.
2. Strain the raspberry puree through a fine-mesh sieve into a small saucepan to remove the tiny seeds. Press with a spoon to get all of the puree through, and scrape the underside of your sieve for any seedless puree that clings to it.
3. Place the saucepan over medium heat. Bring the berries to a low boil. Reduce the heat to medium-low and simmer, stirring occasionally, for about 10 minutes. It should thicken a bit.
4. Remove from the heat and stir in the chia seeds, lemon juice, and vanilla. Let cool completely. The jam will thicken significantly as it sits.
5. Store in an airtight container in the refrigerator for up to 1 week, or in the freezer to enjoy later.

FIVE-STAR RANCH DRESSING OR DIP

MAKES 1⅓ CUPS

While I do enjoy the lightness of vinaigrette, sometimes a thick and creamy dressing is the only way to go. Luckily, this delicious dairy-free ranch is just a whisk away.

1 cup regular or vegan mayonnaise
⅓ cup unsweetened plain dairy-free milk beverage, plus additional as needed
2 teaspoons dried or chopped fresh flat-leaf parsley
1 teaspoon lemon juice
½ teaspoon garlic powder
½ teaspoon onion powder
⅛ to ¼ teaspoon black pepper, to taste
⅛ teaspoon salt

1. In a medium bowl, whisk together the mayonnaise, milk beverage, parsley, lemon juice, garlic powder, onion power, pepper, and salt. Whisk in more milk beverage if the dressing is too thick.
2. Cover and refrigerate the dressing for at least 30 minutes before serving.
3. Store in an airtight container in the refrigerator for up to 1 week. Shake or whisk the dressing before each use.

QUICK RANCH DIP VARIATION

Substitute the milk beverage with store-bought or homemade dairy-free sour cream alternative (recipes beginning on page 189).

JAPANESE RESTAURANT–STYLE DRESSING

MAKES 1½ CUPS

This light drizzle reminds me of the small salads we receive at our favorite sushi restaurant before each meal. It's got a French dressing meets Asian ginger dressing vibe that somehow works.

½ cup peanut, grapeseed, or rice bran oil
½ cup diced yellow onion (½ small to medium onion)
⅓ cup rice vinegar
2 tablespoons ketchup
2 tablespoons minced fresh ginger (can substitute ¼ teaspoon ground ginger)
4 teaspoons soy sauce (can substitute gluten-free tamari or soy-free coconut aminos)
2 teaspoons agave nectar, honey, brown sugar, or cane sugar
2 teaspoons lemon juice
1 teaspoon sesame oil
1 garlic clove, smashed
¼ to ½ teaspoon salt, to taste
Freshly ground black pepper, to taste (optional)

1. Put the oil, onion, vinegar, ketchup, ginger, soy sauce, sweetener, lemon juice, sesame oil, garlic, and salt in your blender. Blend until smooth, about 1 minute.
2. Add some black pepper (if using), and pulse just to combine.
3. Store in an airtight container in the refrigerator for up to 1 week. Shake or whisk the dressing before each use.

DREAMY HONEY DIJON DRESSING

MAKES 1¾ CUPS

I like to use a generous amount of creamy salad dressing, so I often lean on healthier recipes like this one. It uses cashews for richness, and that amazing combination of honey, lemon, and Dijon for addictive yet wholesome flavor. Beyond cold salads, I also like it as a sauce for steamed vegetables, like broccoli, cauliflower, or carrots.

1 cup raw cashews
¾ cup unsweetened plain dairy-free milk beverage, plus additional as needed
¼ to ⅓ cup lemon juice, to taste
¼ cup Dijon mustard
¼ cup honey or agave nectar
¼ teaspoon salt

1. Put the cashews in your spice grinder or food processor. Process until powdered and beginning to clump, about 1 minute.
2. Put the cashew powder and milk beverage in your blender. Blend until smooth, about 1 minute. Add the lemon juice, mustard, sweetener, and salt and blend until smooth, about 1 minute.

3. Pour the dressing into a container, cover, and refrigerate for 30 minutes before using. It will thicken as it chills.

4. Store in an airtight container in the refrigerator for up to 1 week. Shake or whisk the dressing before each use. If it thickens too much as it chills, whisk in additional milk beverage, as needed.

ALL-IN ASIAN DRESSING OR DIP

MAKES 1½ CUPS

I'm a huge fan of sesame dressings but often find them a bit too oily. So for this version, I added tofu and miso. These ingredients provide even more Asian flavor depth and a creamy consistency with less fat but more dairy-free protein, calcium, and probiotic power.

6 ounces firm silken tofu
¼ cup water, plus additional as needed
¼ cup sesame oil
¼ cup rice vinegar
3 to 4 tablespoons maple syrup, to taste
3 tablespoons white miso
2 tablespoons soy sauce (can substitute gluten-free tamari)
½ teaspoon ground ginger
⅛ teaspoon salt (optional)

1. Put the tofu, water, oil, vinegar, maple syrup, miso, soy sauce, and ginger in your blender. Blend until smooth, about 1 minute.

2. Taste test and blend in the salt if more depth of flavor is desired. For a thinner consistency, blend in more water, as needed.

3. Store in an airtight container in the refrigerator for up to 1 week. Shake or whisk the dressing before each use.

KICKIN' CHIPOTLE DRESSING

MAKES ¾ CUP

This easy, creamy dressing is great on dairy-free tacos or seven-layer salads. It's also a tasty condiment for veggie burgers and a slightly spicy option for homemade potato or pasta salad.

- ⅔ cup regular or vegan mayonnaise
- 2 tablespoons lime juice
- 1 or 2 chipotle peppers in adobo sauce, seeded
- 1 teaspoon adobo sauce (from the canned chipotle peppers)
- 1 teaspoon honey or agave nectar
- ½ teaspoon ground cumin
- ½ teaspoon salt
- Unsweetened plain dairy-free milk beverage, as needed

1. Put the mayonnaise, lime juice, chipotle peppers, adobo sauce, sweetener, cumin, and salt in your blender or food processor. Use 1 chipotle pepper for relatively tame spice and 2 for high heat. Process until smooth, about 1 minute.
2. If the dressing is too thick, blend in a little milk beverage, as needed.
3. Store in an airtight container in the refrigerator for up to 1 week. Shake or whisk the dressing before each use.

BALSAMIC TAHINI DRESSING

MAKES ABOUT ¾ CUP

For some of us, tahini can have an overwhelming bitterness, regardless of the brand used. But this recipe tempers and complements it nicely with a sweet and savory blend of ingredients. This rich dressing is great on my ROASTED SWEET POTATO & GREENS SALAD (page 354), but it also works well on cruciferous vegetables and hearty proteins.

- ¼ cup tahini
- ¼ cup balsamic vinegar
- 2 tablespoons extra-virgin olive oil
- 2 tablespoons honey, maple syrup, or agave nectar
- 1 tablespoon water, plus additional as needed
- ¼ teaspoon salt

1. Put the tahini, vinegar, oil, sweetener, water, and salt in your blender or a medium bowl. Blend or whisk until smooth and creamy, about 1 minute.
2. The dressing will thicken as it sits. If it becomes too thick, whisk in more water, as needed.
3. Store in an airtight container in the refrigerator for up to 1 week. Shake or whisk the dressing before each use.

CHAPTER 25
SOUP FOR THE SOUL
Fulfilling Rich & Hearty Recipes

GOOD TO KNOW FOR THIS CHAPTER

BLEND HOT SOUPS CAUTIOUSLY. If your liquid is too hot, the steam can build pressure as you blend and blow the lid off your blender, or even cause scalding soup to fly out when you remove the lid. Not fun. To ensure safety, remove the plastic insert from the blender lid, then secure the lid on the blender. Firmly hold a kitchen towel over the hole in the lid as you blend. This will allow steam to escape.

AN IMMERSION OR STICK BLENDER IS HELPFUL. This handheld electric tool is relatively compact, and will let you blend or puree soups right in the pot. It doesn't always produce the silken finish that a stand blender can achieve, but it is much easier to clean and avoids the blender volcano concerns mentioned above.

THE CONSISTENCY IS YOUR CALL. Many of these recipes involve pureeing part or all of the soup. Feel free to puree or not puree, depending on how thin and chunky or thick and creamy you like your soup.

MANY COMFORT SOUPS ARE NATURALLY DAIRY FREE. You won't find recipes for certain soups in this book, because there are hundreds of great options for them online. Some of these include gazpacho, vegetable, lentil, chili, split pea, Thai coconut, pho, tortilla, minestrone (hold the Parmesan), chicken noodle, won ton, hot and sour, Manhattan clam chowder, and hamburger soup.

SALT IS KEY. For all my soup recipes, I provide either a specific amount or a range. But either way, you are encouraged to salt to taste, especially since stock and broth, key soup ingredients, can vary in widely in saltiness. Soup is typically high in sodium, because salt is really what makes the flavors pop. But if you are watching your sodium intake, start with a lesser amount and salt just until the soup has that addictive "I can't stop taste testing it" flavor.

MY "CONDENSED CREAM OF . . ." SOUPS ARE IDEAL FOR RECIPES. Please don't pass those recipes up! Beginning on page 290, all three variations will welcome many casseroles back into your life. And they are pretty darn good as straight-up soup, too.

CLASSIC CONDENSED CREAM OF MUSHROOM SOUP

MAKES 1¼ CUPS (EQUIVALENT OF ONE 10¾-OUNCE CAN OF CAMPBELL'S)

Here it is, one of the most requested dairy-free recipes on the planet. My engineer/home chef husband and I dissected the ingredients on the original Campbell's can. We calculated, tested, and finally came up with this version that we believe is as close as you can get without the MSG, "modified" ingredients, and secret spices used in their version. Amazingly, this mock recipe is fairly low in fat and takes just one pan and mere minutes to prepare.

> 1¼ cups unsweetened plain dairy-free milk beverage (do not use one with added protein)
> 2 tablespoons all-purpose flour or white rice flour (for gluten free)
> 1 tablespoon cornstarch
> 1 tablespoon grapeseed, rice bran, or other neutral-tasting oil (see page 146)
> ¾ to 1 teaspoon salt, to taste
> ⅛ teaspoon onion powder
> Generous pinch garlic powder
> ½ cup canned mushrooms (pieces and stems), drained

1. Put the milk beverage, flour, starch, oil, salt, onion powder, and garlic powder in your blender. Blend until smooth, about 30 seconds.

2. Pour the soup mixture into a small saucepan over medium-low heat and add the mushrooms. Cook for about 10 minutes, whisking often. It should reduce to about 1¼ cups of very thick "condensed" cream of mushroom soup, weighing roughly 10¾ ounces.

3. Use this condensed soup in recipes as you would the original.

4. Store in an airtight container in the refrigerator for up to 2 days, or freeze it to enjoy later.

TO PREPARE AS SOUP: *For a quick cream of mushroom or celery soup, whisk 1 cup water into the condensed soup, and warm it over low heat until it reaches your desired temperature. This makes 2 servings.*

CONDENSED CREAM OF CELERY SOUP VARIATION

Sauté 1 cup diced celery in 1 teaspoon oil over medium-low heat for 3 minutes, or until tender. Substitute the cooked celery for the mushrooms.

HEALTHY CONDENSED CREAM OF CHICKEN SOUP

MAKES 1¼ CUPS (EQUIVALENT OF ONE 10¾-OUNCE CAN OF CAMPBELL'S)

This delicious condensed soup isn't exactly like Campbell's, but it still works as a 1:1 substitute. And honestly, we like it better. Even my picky dairy-loving niece was happy to make the switch.

- ½ cup raw cashews
- ¾ cup unsweetened plain coconut milk beverage
- ¾ cup chicken or vegan no-chicken broth
- ⅛ teaspoon onion powder
- ⅛ teaspoon garlic powder
- ⅛ teaspoon black pepper
- ⅛ teaspoon thyme
- ½ teaspoon salt, or to taste

1. Put the cashews in your spice grinder or food processor. Process until powdered, about 1 minute.
2. Put the cashew powder and milk beverage in your blender. Blend until smooth, about 1 minute.
3. Pour the cashew mixture and broth into a medium saucepan over medium heat. Add the onion powder, garlic powder, black pepper, and thyme and whisk to combine. Bring the soup to a boil. Reduce the heat to medium-low and simmer for about 10 minutes, whisking often. It should reduce to about 1¼ cups of very thick "condensed" cream of chicken soup, weighing roughly 10½ ounces.
4. Whisk in the salt.
5. Use this condensed soup in recipes as you would the original.
6. Store in an airtight container in the refrigerator for up to 2 days, or freeze it to enjoy later.

TO PREPARE AS SOUP: For a quick cream of chicken soup, whisk 1 cup water into the condensed soup, and warm it over low heat until it reaches your desired temperature. Optionally stir in about ½ cup diced cooked chicken or vegan "chicken." This makes 2 servings.

ROASTED EGGPLANT & TOMATO SOUP

MAKES 4 TO 6 SERVINGS

The satiny finish of this delicate soup makes it perfect for impressing dinner guests, or for a light summer meal. The addition of coconut or nut cream is optional, but highly recommended. It provides that rich and comforting "cream of . . ." experience. For a lighter indulgence, you can top each bowl with a dollop of SOUR CASHEW CREAM (page 189) instead.

1 pound tomatoes (about 3 medium), halved
1 medium eggplant (1¼ to 1½ pounds), halved lengthwise
6 garlic cloves, peeled
1 tablespoon + 1 tablespoon grapeseed or olive oil, divided
1 small yellow onion *or* 2 large shallots, chopped (½ to ¾ cup)
1 tablespoon chopped fresh thyme *or* 1 teaspoon dried thyme
4 cups chicken or vegan no-chicken broth
½ teaspoon salt, or to taste
⅛ teaspoon crushed red pepper (optional)
1 cup full-fat coconut milk, coconut cream, or nut cream (page 161) (optional)
Freshly ground black pepper, to taste (optional)

1. Preheat your oven to 400°F and grease a large baking dish.
2. Place the tomatoes and eggplant halves, cut sides down, in the baking dish. Set the garlic next to them. Drizzle the vegetables with 1 tablespoon oil and ensure that everything is well coated.
3. Roast for 40 to 45 minutes, or until very tender and the skins are brown in spots. Let cool for 5 minutes.
4. Heat the remaining 1 tablespoon oil in a large pot over medium heat. Add the onion or shallots and sauté until tender and translucent, about 5 minutes.
5. Add the thyme and sauté for 30 seconds. Add the broth, salt, and red pepper (if using) and whisk to combine.
6. Pinch the skins off the tomatoes and remove the flesh from the eggplant shell. Add the eggplant flesh and tomato pulp and the garlic cloves to the pot.
7. Bring the soup to a boil. Reduce the heat to low, cover, and simmer for 5 to 10 minutes. Remove from the heat and let cool for 10 minutes.
8. Transfer the soup to your blender (in batches, if needed) and blend until smooth and creamy, about 2 minutes (see page 289 for tips).
9. Return the soup to your pot, optionally straining it through a fine-mesh sieve to remove any remaining eggplant and tomato seeds.
10. Stir in the coconut milk, coconut cream, or nut cream (if using) and season with more salt, if desired, and black pepper (if using).
11. Store leftover soup in an airtight container in the refrigerator for up to 2 days.

CURRIED CAULIFLOWER BISQUE

MAKES 3 TO 4 SERVINGS

My husband dislikes the flavor of Indian curries and isn't a big fan of cauliflower. But even he admitted that this subtle mix of spices worked nicely with the creamy vegetable base. The fact that he went back for seconds solidified this one as a winner.

    1 tablespoon olive oil or dairy-free buttery spread
    ½ cup chopped sweet onion (½ small to medium onion)
    1 to 2 teaspoons garam masala, to taste (store-bought or GARAM MASALA RECIPE below)
    2 garlic cloves, minced (about 1 teaspoon)
    4 cups chicken or vegetable broth
    ½ to 1 teaspoon salt, to taste
    12 ounces cauliflower florets (roughly 1 small head)
    6 ounces broccoli florets (roughly 1 medium crown)
    1 teaspoon lemon juice (optional)

1. Heat the oil or buttery spread in a large pot over medium-low heat. Add the onion and sauté for 5 minutes, or until it begins to soften.

2. Add the garam masala and garlic and sauté for 1 minute.

3. Stir in the broth and ½ teaspoon salt. Add the cauliflower and broccoli florets and turn the heat up to medium. Bring the soup to a boil. Reduce the heat to medium-low, cover, and simmer for 20 minutes, or until the cauliflower is quite tender. Let cool for 5 minutes.

4. Transfer the soup to your blender (in batches, if needed) and blend until smooth and creamy, about 2 minutes (see page 289 for tips).

5. Return the soup to your pot and season with more salt, if desired, and the lemon juice (if using).

6. Store leftover soup in an airtight container in the refrigerator for up to 2 days.

· ·

EVEN CREAMIER VARIATION

Reduce the broth to 3 cups. When the soup is finished, stir in 1 cup unsweetened plain dairy-free milk beverage or lite coconut milk.

· ·

GARAM MASALA RECIPE

In a small bowl, whisk together ⅝ teaspoon ground coriander, ½ teaspoon ground cumin, ¼ teaspoon ground cardamom, ¼ teaspoon black pepper, ⅛ teaspoon ground cloves, ⅛ teaspoon ground cinnamon, and ⅛ teaspoon ground nutmeg. This makes 2 teaspoons.

LIGHT VICHYSSOISE

MAKES 4 SERVINGS

Despite the French name, many argue that this creamy soup is actually an American invention. It usually contains dairy cream, but that addition isn't necessary. This soup is served cold in summer, but it can also be enjoyed warm in the winter months.

1 cup + 2 cups vegetable broth, divided
4 large leeks (white parts only), thinly sliced
1 garlic clove, minced (about ½ teaspoon)
1 pound Yukon gold potatoes, optionally peeled and cut into ½-inch chunks
2 tablespoons dairy-free buttery spread (can substitute olive oil)
¼ teaspoon salt, or to taste
¼ teaspoon white pepper
Pinch ground nutmeg
4 chives or green onions (green parts only), sliced

1. Put the 1 cup broth, leeks, and garlic in a large pot over medium-high heat. Bring the broth to a boil. Reduce the heat to low, cover, and cook until the leeks just begin to soften, about 6 to 8 minutes.

2. Add the potatoes and remaining 2 cups broth. Cover and cook until the potatoes are soft, about 20 minutes.

3. Remove the soup from the heat. Stir in the buttery spread, salt, pepper, and nutmeg. Let cool for 5 minutes.

4. Transfer the soup to your blender (in batches, if needed) and blend until smooth and creamy, about 2 minutes (see page 289 for tips).

5. Serve the soup warm or allow it to cool to room temperature, pour it into an airtight container, and refrigerate it for at least 3 hours to serve cold.

6. Ladle into bowls and garnish with the sliced chives or green onions.

7. Store leftover soup in an airtight container in the refrigerator for up to 2 days.

COMFORTING CORN CHOWDER

MAKES 4 SERVINGS

This popular soup is usually made with heavy cream, but the delicious blend of cashews and coconut milk in this recipe will make you happy to shun tradition. It's not only rich, but also full of complementary flavors that satisfied even my pickiest tasters.

3 tablespoons dairy-free buttery spread (can substitute olive oil)
1 cup diced yellow onion (1 small to medium onion)
1 teaspoon dried thyme *or* 1 tablespoon fresh thyme
3½ cups chicken or vegetable broth
1½ cups full-fat coconut milk
2 cups diced russet or yellow potatoes, optionally peeled (about 10 ounces)
⅓ cup raw cashews
3 cups fresh (about 4 ears) or frozen (thawed) corn kernels
¾ teaspoon salt, or to taste
¼ teaspoon black pepper

1. Melt the buttery spread in a large pot over medium-low heat. Add the onion and sauté for 5 minutes, or until translucent. Add the thyme and sauté for 1 minute.

2. Add the broth, coconut milk, and potatoes and stir to combine. Increase the heat to medium and bring the mixture to a boil. Reduce the heat to medium-low and simmer for 10 minutes, or until the potatoes are tender.

3. Put the cashews in your spice grinder or food processor. Process until powdered, about 1 minute.

4. Transfer about ½ cup of the cooked potatoes and onion and about 1 cup of the creamy broth to your blender. Add the cashew powder. Blend until smooth, about 1 minute (see page 289 for tips).

5. Return the pureed soup to your pot and stir in the corn. Bring the soup back to a simmer, and cook over medium-low heat for 8 minutes, stirring occasionally.

6. Season the soup with the salt and pepper and cook for 2 more minutes.

7. Store leftover soup in an airtight container in the refrigerator for up to 2 days.

OPTIONAL EXTRAS: Once cooked, add cooked chorizo, vegan chorizo, crumbled cooked bacon, cooked chopped chicken, cannellini beans, hot sauce, a drizzle of extra-virgin olive oil, chopped roasted red bell pepper, chopped fresh parsley, or chopped fresh basil.

NUT-FREE OPTION

Omit the cashews. Add ¼ cup all-purpose flour, wheat flour, or all-purpose gluten-free flour with the thyme. Whisk as it cooks. Continuously whisk as you drizzle in the broth to make a smooth liquid. Continue as directed.

CORN-FREE CHOWDER VARIATION

The base of this chowder lends itself well to other vegetables. Feel free to replace the corn with diced carrot, celery, peas, zucchini, edamame, or other assorted vegetables.

CREAM OF ASPARAGUS SOUP

MAKES 6 TO 8 SERVINGS

When we lived at Lake Tahoe, there was a wonderful restaurant that we liked to visit on special occasions, called Soule Domain. Every night, the chef prepared a soup that was served to every guest. It was always dairy free and vegan, yet incredibly luxurious. One night, I asked the chef's secret. He said it was simple: "Just boil some white rice in broth or water with your vegetable of choice, puree, and season to taste." He was right; it really is that simple!

2 pounds asparagus
2 tablespoons grapeseed or olive oil
3 cups chopped yellow onion (2 medium to large onions)
2 garlic cloves, minced (about 1 teaspoon)
8 cups chicken, vegan no-chicken, or vegetable broth
⅔ cup uncooked white basmati or jasmine rice
1 teaspoon salt, or to taste
2 sprigs fresh thyme *or* ½ teaspoon dried thyme
Freshly ground black pepper, to taste

1. Trim the woody ends from the asparagus and cut the remaining stalks into ½-inch pieces. Set the tips aside.
2. Heat the oil in a large pot over medium heat. Add the onion and sauté for 5 minutes, or until soft and translucent.
3. Add the garlic and sauté for 1 minute.
4. Stir in the broth, asparagus pieces (but not the tips), rice, salt, and thyme. Bring the soup to a boil. Reduce the heat to low, cover, and simmer for 25 to 30 minutes, or until the rice is very tender. If using thyme sprigs, remove them.
5. Transfer the soup to your blender (in batches, if needed) and blend until smooth and creamy, about 2 minutes (see page 289 for tips).
6. Return the soup to your pot. Add the asparagus tips and simmer for about 5 minutes, or until the asparagus tips are bright green and crisp-tender. Season with more salt, if desired, and black pepper.
7. Store leftover soup in an airtight container in the refrigerator for up to 2 days.

CREAM OF BROCCOLI SOUP VARIATION

Substitute 2 pounds of broccoli florets for the asparagus, reserving 1 cup of small florets to stir in when you would be adding the asparagus tips.

AFRICAN PEANUT STEW

MAKES 4 SERVINGS

For years I was intrigued by the comforting sound of African stew. After perusing many recipe ideas, I finally got up the nerve to try my own version. The result was this rich and nourishing recipe that I now turn to often.

2 tablespoons grapeseed, olive, or peanut oil
1 cup diced yellow onion (1 small to medium onion)
4 garlic cloves, minced (about 2 teaspoons)
1 tablespoon minced fresh ginger
1½ pounds sweet potatoes, peeled and cut into ¾-inch chunks (about 4 cups)
1 pound tomatoes, diced
½ to 1 teaspoon seeded and minced jalapeño pepper, to taste
1½ cups water
1 cup vegetable or chicken broth
1 teaspoon salt, or to taste
¾ pound cauliflower florets (about 6 cups)
¼ cup creamy unsalted peanut butter (can substitute sunflower seed butter for peanut free)
4 cups cooked brown rice, couscous, or quinoa
2 cups packed baby spinach leaves
1 small lime, cut into 4 wedges

1. Heat the oil in a large pot over medium heat. Add the onion and sauté until tender and translucent, about 3 to 5 minutes.
2. Add the garlic and ginger and sauté for 1 minute.
3. Stir in the sweet potatoes, tomatoes, and jalapeño and cook for 5 minutes.
4. Add the water, broth, and salt and bring the stew to a boil. Reduce the heat to medium-low, cover, and simmer for 10 minutes.
5. Add the cauliflower, cover, and simmer for 10 to 15 minutes, or until the vegetables are tender.
6. Transfer ½ cup of the soup liquid to a small bowl. Whisk in the peanut butter until smooth.
7. Return the soup with the peanut butter to your pot and continue to cook the stew for 5 minutes, uncovered, stirring often. It should thicken a bit.
8. Divide the brown rice, couscous, or quinoa and spinach between 4 bowls. Ladle the hot stew on top and serve each bowl with a lime wedge.
9. Store leftover soup in an airtight container in the refrigerator for up to 2 days.

MEXICAN BEAN SOUP

MAKES 4 SERVINGS

I like to use pinto beans in this soup, due to the color they impart when cooked with the paprika and tomatoes, but black beans are equally tasty. If you are sensitive to salt, feel free to use low-sodium broth and adjust the salt to taste after cooking. The spices do help flavor this soup quite a bit on their own.

> 2 teaspoons grapeseed, olive, or peanut oil
> 1 cup chopped yellow onion (1 small to medium onion)
> 2 to 4 garlic cloves, minced (1 to 2 teaspoons)
> 1 small jalapeño pepper, seeded and minced
> 1½ teaspoons ground cumin
> 1 teaspoon dried oregano
> ½ teaspoon paprika
> 2 cups vegetable broth
> 2 (15-ounce) cans pinto or black beans, drained and rinsed
> 1 (14-ounce) can diced tomatoes *or* 1 pound tomatoes, chopped
> 1 to 2 teaspoons lime juice (optional)
> ¼ to ½ teaspoon salt, or to taste
> Optional garnishes: dairy-free sour cream alternative (recipes beginning on page 189), chopped avocado, or crushed tortilla chips

1. Heat the oil in a large saucepan over medium-low heat. Add the onion and sauté for 5 minutes, or until it begins to soften.
2. Add the garlic and jalapeño and sauté for 1 minute.
3. Add the cumin, oregano, and paprika and sauté for 1 minute.
4. Slowly stir in the broth. Add the beans, tomatoes, lime juice (if using), and ¼ teaspoon salt. Increase the heat to medium and bring the soup to a boil. Reduce the heat to low, cover, and simmer for 15 minutes. Let cool for 5 minutes.
5. Transfer half (for chunky) or all (for creamy) of the soup to your blender (in batches, if needed) and blend until smooth, about 2 minutes (see page 289 for tips).
6. Return the pureed soup to your pot. Season with more salt, if desired.
7. Divide the soup between 4 bowls and top with your garnishes of choice.
8. Store leftover soup in an airtight container in the refrigerator for up to 2 days.

WARMING WINTER SQUASH SOUP

MAKES 4 SERVINGS

This silky, nutritious soup is loaded with beta-carotene from the combination of carrots and squash. Consequently, it also has a natural light sweetness that complements the warm spices and savory ingredients. But if you prefer this type of soup a little sweeter, you can whisk in up to 2 tablespoons of maple syrup or brown sugar before simmering.

1 tablespoon grapeseed or olive oil
⅔ cup minced yellow onion (about 1 small onion)
2 to 4 garlic cloves, minced (1 to 2 teaspoons)
½ teaspoon ground ginger
¼ teaspoon ground nutmeg
⅛ teaspoon ground cloves
⅛ teaspoon ground cardamom
3 cups vegetable broth
1 cup baby carrots
8 ounces cubed butternut squash (see Butternut Squash Tips below)
¼ teaspoon salt, or to taste
⅔ cup pumpkin puree
1 cup plain or unsweetened plain dairy-free milk beverage
Freshly ground black pepper, to taste (optional)

1. Heat the oil in a large pot over medium-low heat. Add the onion and sauté for 5 to 7 minutes, or until soft and translucent.
2. Add the garlic and sauté for 1 minute.
3. Add the ginger, nutmeg, cloves, and cardamom and sauté for 1 minute.
4. Stir in the broth, carrots, squash, and salt. Increase the heat to medium and bring the soup to a boil. Reduce the heat to low, cover, and simmer until the vegetables are quite soft, about 15 to 20 minutes.
5. Remove the soup from the heat and stir in the pumpkin.
6. Transfer the soup to your blender (in batches, if needed) and blend until smooth, about 2 minutes (see page 289 for tips).
7. Return the soup to your pot. Stir in the milk beverage and heat the soup to your desired temperature. Season with more salt and black pepper, if desired.
8. Store leftover soup in an airtight container in the refrigerator for up to 2 days.

BUTTERNUT SQUASH TIPS: Since butternut squash can be a pain to cut, I often purchase pre-cubed squash for recipes like this. It can be found in the produce or freezer section of many grocers. Alternatively, you can quickly soften a butternut squash by cutting slits in it and microwaving it on high for 3 minutes. Let it cool for a couple of minutes before cutting.

HEARTY MUSHROOM BARLEY STEW

MAKES 2 TO 3 SERVINGS

This earthy soup has delicious umami depth that hits the spot on a cool fall or chilly winter day.

1 tablespoon grapeseed or olive oil
1¼ cups chopped yellow onion (about ½ large onion)
½ cup dry pearl barley, rinsed (can substitute whole-grain sorghum for gluten free)
2 large garlic cloves, minced (about 1 teaspoon)
1 teaspoon dried thyme
8 ounces sliced button or cremini mushrooms
4 cups beef or mushroom broth
1 tablespoon tomato paste
1 teaspoon balsamic vinegar
1 teaspoon white miso (gluten free or soy free, if needed) or more salt to taste
1 bay leaf
¼ to 1 teaspoon salt, to taste
Freshly ground black pepper, to taste

1. Heat the oil in a large pot over medium heat. Add the onion and sauté for 5 minutes, or until translucent.

2. Reduce the heat to medium-low. Add the barley, garlic, and thyme and sauté for 3 minutes.

3. Stir in the mushrooms. Add the broth, tomato paste, vinegar, miso, bay leaf, and ¼ teaspoon salt and stir to combine. Bring the soup to a boil. Reduce the heat to low, cover, and simmer for at least 1 hour, or until the barley is tender. (If using sorghum, it will be soft but slightly chewy once cooked.)

4. Remove the bay leaf. Season to taste with more salt, if desired, and black pepper.

5. Store leftover soup in an airtight container in the refrigerator for up to 2 days.

CREAMY POTATO MISO SOUP

MAKES 2 SERVINGS

This wonderfully simple soup hits all the right notes for flavor, warmth, and ease. It's a personal favorite.

1 teaspoon grapeseed or olive oil
2 garlic cloves, minced (about 1 teaspoon)
3 cups chicken or vegan no-chicken broth
¾ pound Yukon gold potatoes, diced into ½-inch cubes
¼ teaspoon onion powder
1 tablespoon cashew butter (optional, but recommended)
1 tablespoon white miso (gluten free or soy free, if needed)
1 teaspoon dried or chopped fresh chives
Freshly ground black pepper, to taste
Crispy won ton strips, tortilla strips, or crackers, for serving (gluten free, if needed) (optional)

1. Heat the oil in a large saucepan over medium-low heat. Add the garlic and sauté until fragrant, about 3 minutes.
2. Add the broth, potatoes, and onion powder. Increase the heat to medium and bring the soup to a boil. Reduce the heat to medium-low, cover, and simmer for 15 to 20 minutes, or until the potatoes are tender. Let cool for 5 minutes.
3. Transfer the soup to your blender (in batches, if needed) and blend until smooth, about 2 minutes (see page 289 for tips).
4. Return the soup to your pan. Add the cashew butter (if using) and miso and whisk until smooth. Stir in the chives and black pepper.
5. Divide the soup between 2 bowls and top with crunchy strips or crackers (if using).
6. Store leftover soup in an airtight container in the refrigerator for up to 2 days.

CHEESY BROCCOLI SOUP

MAKES 4 SERVINGS

A craving for comfort food led me to create this rich and creamy soup one lazy afternoon. My husband tends to shy away from the notion of cheesy dairy-free items, but this soup received two enthusiastic thumbs up. The taste is full of flavor, yet the cheesy notes are not overstated. It's perfect for timid dairy-free palates.

½ cup raw cashews
1 cup + 3 cups water, divided
1 tablespoon grapeseed, olive, or rice bran oil
1 cup chopped yellow onion (1 small to medium onion)
1 pound cauliflower florets (about 1 medium head)
6 ounces baby carrots or about 3 medium carrots, peeled and sliced
5 tablespoons nutritional yeast flakes
1 tablespoon tahini
2 teaspoons lemon juice
1½ to 2 teaspoons salt, to taste
½ teaspoon paprika
½ teaspoon ground mustard powder
¼ teaspoon garlic powder
Freshly ground black pepper, to taste
½ pound steamed broccoli florets, broken or smashed into small pieces

1. Put the cashews in your spice grinder or food processor. Process until powdered, about 1 minute.

2. Put the cashew powder and 1 cup water in your blender. Blend until smooth, about 1 minute.

3. Heat the oil in a large saucepan over medium heat. Add the onion and sauté for 5 minutes, or until soft and translucent.

4. Add the cauliflower, carrots, and remaining 3 cups water. Bring the mixture to a boil. Reduce the heat to medium-low, cover, and simmer for 20 minutes, or until the vegetables are quite tender.

5. Add the cashew cream, nutritional yeast, tahini, lemon juice, salt, paprika, mustard powder, and garlic powder and whisk until smooth.

6. Transfer the soup to your blender (in batches, if needed) and blend until smooth, about 2 minutes (see page 289 for tips).

7. Return the soup to your pan and season with the black pepper. Stir in the cooked broccoli.

8. Store leftover soup in an airtight container in the refrigerator for up to 2 days.

CHAPTER 26

PIZZA NIGHT
Toppings, Crusts & Whole Pie Recipes

GOOD TO KNOW FOR THIS CHAPTER

TRADITIONAL PIZZA SAUCE AND DOUGH ARE OFTEN DAIRY FREE. There are some brands with cheese, but red pizza sauce brands are often made without dairy. Likewise, don't be surprised to spot fresh pizza dough that happens to be vegan in the refrigerated section of your local grocer. Nevertheless, this chapter provides easy at-home options that can be made in a pinch—and go above and beyond what you can buy at the store.

DOUGH FREEZES WELL. You can make large batches of pizza dough, divide it into single pizza balls, tightly wrap, and freeze for later. To defrost, place the wrapped dough in your refrigerator the night before. Or you can let it defrost at room temperature, which takes around 4 hours.

YOU CAN ALSO MAKE HOMEMADE FROZEN PIZZAS. Once the crust has had an initial baking, the toppings have been added, and the pizza has cooled, double wrap it in plastic wrap and freeze. To bake, unwrap the pizza and place it on a baking sheet. Preheat the oven to the temperature of your initial recipe and bake the pizza until hot, bubbly, and lightly browned. It will take a few extra minutes since you are baking from frozen.

I CUT OUT THE MIDDLEMAN WITH CHEESY PIZZAS. I find it odd that people try to make dairy-free cheese firm up just so they can shred it and then re-melt it. Thick cheesy sauce is easy to drizzle or spread on, and it behaves like melted cheese—some recipes even bubble up and brown. Not to mention, it's far easier to whip up, can be ready almost instantly, and doesn't require specialty thickeners.

BUT CHEESELESS PIZZA IS SOMETHING YOU MUST TRY. I've won many dairy lovers over to the cheese-free side with pizza. Just use extra sauce and pile on the flavorful toppings.

YOU CAN MIX AND MATCH. In this chapter, I've broken out the crust and sauce recipes so that you can easily choose your own toppings when you aren't making one of the full pizza recipes.

WHITE CHEESELESS PIZZA

MAKES ONE 12-INCH PIZZA

You can top this pizza with some dairy-free mozzarella shreds, as they do meld well with the flavors in this recipe. But I think you'll find that the creamy "white" sauce provides enough richness on its own.

> 1 batch CREAMY GARLIC PIZZA SAUCE (page 314)
> 1 (12-inch) pizza crust, prepared as directed (recipes starting on page 310)
> 1 cup chopped cooked chicken, vegan chicken, or diced baked tofu
> 1 cup baby spinach leaves
> 1 small tomato, thinly sliced
> 4 ounces button mushrooms, thinly sliced
> Crushed red pepper, for garnish

1. Spread the creamy garlic sauce on the pizza crust. Top with the chicken, spinach, tomato slices, and mushroom slices.
2. Bake according to the pizza crust directions, or until the crust is golden and the toppings are heated through.
3. Serve the pizza with crushed red pepper for sprinkling.
4. Leftover pizza can be stored in an airtight container in the refrigerator for up to 2 days.

ROASTED RATATOUILLE PIZZA

MAKES ONE 12-INCH PIZZA

One of the most popular varieties of Amy's brand of frozen pizzas is their naturally vegan roasted vegetable. This recipe is a fresh twist on that idea. It uses traditional ratatouille ingredients for a pizza so flavorful and rich that it doesn't need a shred of cheese. The vegetables and sauce for this recipe can be made ahead and stored in the refrigerator for up to 2 days.

> 1 (¾-pound) eggplant, peeled and cut into ½-inch pieces (about 4 cups)
> ¾ pound grape tomatoes (about 2¼ cups)
> 1 small to medium zucchini, ends removed, cut into chunks (about 1½ cups)
> 1 medium red bell pepper, cored and chopped (about 1½ cups)
> 1 small to medium sweet onion, cut into small wedges (about 1 cup)
> 3 tablespoons grapeseed or olive oil
> ¾ teaspoon + ⅛ teaspoon salt, divided
> ½ teaspoon dried oregano, crumbled
> ½ teaspoon dried thyme, crumbled
> ¼ teaspoon fennel seeds
> 1 tablespoon water
> 2 teaspoons honey, agave nectar, or cane sugar, or to taste
> 1 (12-inch) pizza crust, prepared as directed (recipes starting on page 310)
> Other toppings (see Topping Ideas following) (optional)

1. Preheat your oven to 425°F and line a large rimmed baking sheet with a silicone bakin. mat or parchment paper.

2. Put the eggplant, tomatoes, zucchini, bell pepper, and onion on your prepared baking sheet. Drizzle the vegetables with the oil and toss to evenly coat. Sprinkle on the ¾ teaspoon salt, oregano, thyme, and fennel seeds and toss to evenly coat. Spread out the vegetables into a single layer.

3. Bake for 30 minutes. Remove the baking sheet from the oven, stir the vegetables, and spread them back into a single layer. Bake for 10 to 20 minutes, or until the tomatoes are slightly browned and all the vegetables look quite tender.

4. Scoop up all of the tomatoes plus enough of the other vegetables to equal a total of 1½ cups, and put them in your blender or food processor. Add the water and remaining ⅛ teaspoon salt. Pulse or blend for a slightly chunky or smooth sauce, respectively. Blend in the sweetener. The amount needed will depend on the sweetness of your tomatoes, but pizza sauce is typically a little sweeter than marinara.

5. Spread the sauce on your pizza crust. Evenly top the pizza with the remaining roasted vegetables and any other toppings, if desired.

6. Bake according to the pizza crust directions, or until the crust is golden and the toppings are heated through.

7. Leftover pizza can be stored in an airtight container in the refrigerator for up to 2 days.

TOPPING IDEAS: *Crushed red pepper, sliced olives (black or green), mild or hot dairy-free Italian sausage (vegan, chicken, pork, or turkey), and* ALMOND RICOTTA OR BAKED FETA *(page 196) are nice complements to this pizza.*

. . . .

PASTA VARIATION

Cook 8 to 12 ounces of pasta or dairy-free gnocchi. Toss the cooked pasta or gnocchi with the roasted sauce and vegetables. Optionally add cooked dairy-free Italian sausage (vegan, chicken, pork, or turkey) for a heartier meal.

. . . .

Y PEPPERONI PIZZA

-INCH PIZZA

...ck cheesy sauce within this recipe is easy to drizzle or spread on your favorite pizza. It's "pre-melted" and can even bubble and brown for a more traditional feel. For slightly stretchier sauce, use the tapioca starch.

⅔ cup unsweetened plain dairy-free milk beverage, plus additional as needed
3 to 4 tablespoons nutritional yeast flakes, to taste
1½ tablespoons olive oil or neutral-tasting oil (see page 146)
1 tablespoon cornstarch (can substitute 4 teaspoons tapioca starch for a very stretchy sauce)
2 teaspoons lemon juice, or to taste
½ teaspoon salt
½ teaspoon paprika
⅛ teaspoon garlic powder
⅛ teaspoon onion powder
Pinch cayenne pepper (optional)
½ batch ROASTED TOMATO PIZZA SAUCE (page 313)
1 (12-inch) pizza crust, prepared as directed (recipes starting on page 310)
5 ounces dairy-free or vegan pepperoni
Crushed red pepper, for garnish

1. Put the milk beverage, nutritional yeast, oil, starch, lemon juice, salt, paprika, garlic powder, onion powder, and cayenne (if using) in your blender. Blend until smooth, about 1 minute.

2. Pour the mixture into a small saucepan over medium heat. Bring it to a boil and whisk as it bubbles for 2 minutes, or until relatively thick. It will continue to thicken as it cools. If it thickens too much, or you prefer a thinner cheesy drizzle, whisk in additional milk beverage to thin as desired.

3. Spread the tomato sauce on the pizza crust. Top with the pepperoni slices, overlapping them since they will shrink. Drizzle, spread, or pipe on the cheesy sauce. You will probably have some leftover cheesy sauce.

4. Bake according to the pizza crust directions, or until the crust is golden and the toppings are heated through. Optionally broil the pizza for 1 to 2 minutes to brown the cheesy sauce before serving.

5. Sprinkle the cooked pizza with crushed red pepper, as desired, or serve the pepper on the side.

6. Leftover pizza and cooled leftover cheesy sauce can be stored in separate airtight containers in the refrigerator for up to 2 days.

THAI CHICK-UN PIZZA

MAKES ONE 12-INCH PIZZA

This Thai-inspired savory pie is another crowd-pleasing recipe from my friend Dreena Burton. It's a favorite from one of her original cookbooks, *Eat, Drink & Be Vegan*. To round out this boldly flavored meal, she suggests a salad of "cooling vegetables," including celery, cucumber, tomatoes, and jicama.

> 1 cup cooked chickpeas/garbanzo beans or chopped vegan chicken
> ½ batch THAI PEANUT PIZZA SAUCE (page 315)
> 1 (12-inch) pizza crust, prepared as directed (recipes starting on page 310)
> 1 to 1½ cups thinly sliced red bell pepper (about 1 medium to large pepper)
> ¾ cup fresh or canned pineapple chunks, drained
> ½ cup sliced green onions
> ½ cup mung bean sprouts, for garnish
> Chopped peanuts, for garnish (omit for peanut free)
> Fresh cilantro leaves, for garnish

1. Preheat your oven to 425°F.
2. If using chickpeas, put them in a bowl or on a cutting board and lightly smash them with a fork.
3. Spread the peanut sauce evenly on the pizza crust. Sprinkle the flattened chickpeas or chopped vegan chicken, bell pepper slices, and pineapple chunks evenly on the pizza.
4. Bake for 15 minutes, or until the crust is just starting to turn golden and the toppings have heated through. Sprinkle on the green onions and bake for 1 more minute.
5. Sprinkle the pizza with the bean sprouts, peanuts, and cilantro just before serving.
6. Leftover pizza, without the garnishes, can be stored in an airtight container in the refrigerator for up to 2 days.

··

KID-FRIENDLY VARIATION

Reduce the ginger in the peanut sauce to 1½ teaspoons and optionally omit the crushed red pepper and green onions.

··

PESTO POLENTA PIE

MAKES 4 TO 6 SERVINGS

This unique savory pie has a thicker crust than your average pizza, and it is best eaten with a knife and fork. But it still provides the full-flavor Italian experience of more traditional slices.

3 cups water
1 teaspoon salt
1 cup dry polenta (yellow cornmeal)
1 tablespoon extra-virgin olive oil
1 tablespoon nutritional yeast flakes (optional)
1 batch AVOCADO PESTO PIZZA SAUCE (page 314)
½ pound dairy-free Italian sausage (turkey, pork, or vegan), cooked and crumbled or sliced
1 pound cherry or small heirloom tomatoes, sliced (can substitute chopped sun-dried tomatoes)
Sea salt, as needed
Balsamic vinegar, for garnish (optional)
Crushed red pepper, for garnish (optional)

1. Grease two 8- or 9-inch pie pans.
2. Pour the water into a medium saucepan over medium heat and bring it to a boil. Add the salt and slowly pour in the polenta while whisking. Reduce the heat to low and simmer, whisking often, until the polenta is very thick, about 10 minutes.
3. Stir in the oil and nutritional yeast (if using).
4. Divide the cooked polenta between your prepared pie pans and smooth it out.
5. Cover the surface of the polenta with plastic wrap. Refrigerate until the polenta is firm, about 2 hours.
6. Preheat your oven to 350°F.
7. Remove the plastic wrap from the polenta and bake for 10 minutes.
8. Remove the polenta pies from your oven and turn the oven to broil.
9. Spread the pesto atop the polenta crusts. Top with the cooked sausage and tomato slices, and lightly sprinkle with a few pinches of sea salt.
10. Broil for 5 minutes, or until the tomatoes soften and the pesto deepens slightly in color.
11. Serve polenta slices with balsamic vinegar for drizzling and crushed red pepper for sprinkling, if desired.
12. Leftover polenta pie can be covered and refrigerated for up to 2 days.

....

STOVETOP SQUARES VARIATION

Chill the polenta in a 9 × 13-inch or larger baking dish or pan for 2 hours or more. Cut the firm polenta into squares. Pan-fry the squares in a little oil over medium heat until heated through and golden, about 3 to 5 minutes per side. Top each square with the avocado pesto, cooked sausage, and tomatoes. Optionally broil for 5 minutes in your oven, or just serve fresh.

....

PERSONAL PORTOBELLO PIZZAS

MAKES 3 SERVINGS

These plant-based rounds are definitely for mushroom lovers! They aren't identical to classic pies, but they have a pizza vibe that's deliciously healthy in its own right. The tofu topping can be spread on toasted bagels, if preferred. But as is, it's a high-calcium, high-protein, and filling little main dish.

  3 portobello mushrooms
  2 tablespoons + 2 tablespoons grapeseed or olive oil, divided
  8 ounces firm tofu
  3 tablespoons tomato paste
  1 tablespoon soy sauce (can substitute gluten-free tamari)
  1 teaspoon nutritional yeast flakes
  ½ to 1 teaspoon dried oregano, to taste
  ½ teaspoon ground or crushed fennel seeds
  1 garlic clove, crushed (about ½ teaspoon), *or* ⅛ teaspoon garlic powder
  ⅛ teaspoon salt, or to taste
  ¼ teaspoon crushed red pepper
  Optional toppings (see Topping Ideas below)

1. Preheat your oven to 400°F.
2. Remove the stems from the mushrooms (leave the gills) and brush away any dirt with a dry paper towel or cloth.
3. Brush the mushroom tops with 2 tablespoons oil and place them on a baking sheet, tops down. Bake for 5 minutes.
4. Drain and lightly press the tofu, using a tea towel or paper towels, to remove any excess water.
5. Put the tofu, tomato paste, remaining 2 tablespoons oil, soy sauce, nutritional yeast, oregano, fennel seeds, garlic, and salt in a bowl or your food processor. Mash with a fork or pulse in your food processor to thoroughly combine. The mixture should be evenly distributed and fully mashed, but not pureed.
6. Spread the tofu mixture evenly on the gill side of the mushrooms. Sprinkle with the crushed red pepper and additional toppings, if desired.
7. Bake for 15 to 20 minutes, or until the mushrooms have softened and the toppings look baked.

TOPPING IDEAS: *Although we like these portobellos as is, they do go well with traditional Italian toppings, too. I recommend chopped fresh basil, chopped or sliced olives, pepperoni (regular or vegan), caramelized onions, cooked dairy-free Italian sausage (turkey, pork, or vegan), sun-dried tomatoes, roasted red peppers, diced and sautéed bell peppers, a drizzle of balsamic vinegar, or* PINE NUT PARMA SPRINKLES *(page 202). Because the mushrooms do release some juices as they cook, and the tofu is a soft mixture, it's best to avoid fresh toppings like tomatoes or uncooked peppers that will release more moisture as they bake.*

NO-RISE PIZZA CRUST

MAKES ONE 12- TO 14-INCH PIZZA CRUST (6 SERVINGS)

This simple crust benefits from up to 30 minutes of "resting time," especially for thick crust fans. But in a pinch, you can pop the dough in the oven as soon as it is preheated.

1 cup warm water (about 105°F)
2¼ teaspoons (one ¼-ounce package) active dry yeast
1 teaspoon cane sugar (can substitute your favorite sweetener)
1½ cups all-purpose flour, plus additional as needed
1 tablespoon grapeseed, olive, or rice bran oil
1 teaspoon salt
1 teaspoon dried Italian herbs (optional)
1 cup whole wheat flour (can substitute more all-purpose flour)
Cornmeal, for sprinkling (optional)
Dairy-free sauce and toppings

1. Put the warm water in a large bowl and sprinkle in the yeast and sugar. Let sit for 5 minutes to proof and ensure the yeast is active (see page 250).

2. Add the all-purpose flour, oil, salt, and herbs (if using) and stir to combine. Gradually add the wheat flour, bringing the dough together with your hands when you can no longer stir it.

3. Knead the dough for 2 to 3 minutes, adding more flour as needed to prevent sticking, until you have a smooth dough ball.

4. Let the dough rest for 10 to 20 minutes while you prepare your pizza toppings.

5. Preheat your oven to 450°F and grease or line a pizza pan or baking sheet with parchment paper. Sprinkle it with cornmeal (if using).

6. Roll out the dough to your desired size and shape. It will be a thicker crust once baked. Gently transfer it to your prepared pan or baking sheet.

7. Bake for 5 minutes.

8. Top the crust with your desired sauce and toppings. Bake for 10 to 15 more minutes, or until the crust takes on a nice golden hue and the toppings are heated through.

ANCIENT GRAIN PIZZA CRUST

MAKES ONE 12- TO 14-INCH PIZZA CRUST (6 SERVINGS)

While it may sound overly hearty, spelt has a pleasant nutty flavor that I almost prefer to wheat. This crust is a bit "breadier" than your average white or wheat pizza crust, but tasty nonetheless. If you want to experiment with another ancient grain, kamut flour works well in place of the spelt flour in this recipe.

> 1½ cups + 1 cup whole spelt flour, divided, plus additional as needed
> 1 tablespoon active dry yeast (see the Yeast Note below)
> 1 teaspoon salt
> 1 cup warm water (about 105°F)
> ¼ cup grapeseed or olive oil
> Dairy-free sauce and toppings

1. In a large bowl, whisk together 1½ cups flour, the yeast, and salt. Add the warm water and oil and stir well to combine.

2. Gradually add the remaining 1 cup flour, bringing the dough together with your hands when you can no longer stir it.

3. Knead the dough for 2 to 3 minutes, adding more flour as needed. The dough should be very soft and supple, but it shouldn't stick to your hands.

4. Let the dough rest for 10 to 20 minutes while you prepare your pizza toppings.

5. Preheat your oven to 400°F and grease a pizza pan or line a baking sheet with parchment paper.

6. Press the dough into your greased pizza pan or press and shape it on your prepared baking sheet. The dough tends to pull apart a bit because spelt has less gluten than wheat, so carefully press it into shape rather than pulling and stretching. If any breaks off, just press it back in; it's forgiving dough.

7. Top the dough with your desired sauce and toppings. Bake for 20 to 25 minutes, or until the crust is nicely browned and the toppings are heated through.

YEAST NOTE: *Since this recipe doesn't involve proofing the yeast, it's important to know in advance if your yeast is still active. If concerned, sprinkle just a little yeast in warm water (about 105°F) and let it sit for 5 minutes to proof (see page 250).*

Note that 1 tablespoon yeast is a little more than one ¼-ounce package. At higher altitude (above 3,000 feet), one package should be enough.

GLUTEN-FREE CLASSIC PIZZA CRUST

MAKES ONE 12-INCH PIZZA CRUST (6 SERVINGS)

After many years and countless recipe tests, my search for the perfect gluten-free pizza crust ended with the King Arthur Flour Company. After a few tweaks of their formula, I landed on this delicious recipe. It bakes up with a chewy, crispy exterior and tender interior that tastes almost doughy when it melds with the sauce and toppings. And don't be afraid of the unique preparation and very wet dough—it bakes up perfectly!

1 cup millet flour (can substitute brown or white rice flour)
⅔ cup tapioca starch
1 teaspoon baking powder
1 teaspoon xanthan gum
¾ teaspoon salt
¼ teaspoon onion powder
1 cup warm unsweetened plain dairy-free milk beverage
2 tablespoons + 2 tablespoons grapeseed, rice bran, olive, or neutral-tasting oil (see page 146), divided
1 tablespoon cane sugar or your sweetener of choice
1½ teaspoons active dry yeast
Dairy-free sauce and toppings

1. In a large mixing bowl, whisk together the flour, starch, baking powder, xanthan gum, salt, and onion powder.
2. Put the warm milk beverage, 2 tablespoons oil, sweetener, and yeast in a medium bowl. Add ½ cup of the flour mixture and whisk to combine; it's okay if lumps remain. Let sit for 15 minutes, or until the mixture looks a bit bubbly.
3. Scrape the wet mixture into the remaining flour mixture in your mixing bowl. Beat with a hand mixer or stand mixer for 3 to 4 minutes. This helps "activate" the binding powers of the xanthan gum. It will be very thick but somewhat loose, moist, and sticky, like a cross between batter and dough.
4. Cover the bowl and let the dough rest for 30 minutes.
5. Cover a 12-inch round pizza pan with a piece of parchment paper. Drizzle the remaining 2 tablespoons oil onto the center of the parchment paper. Scrape the dough from the bowl onto the puddle of oil.
6. Using wet fingers or a silicone spatula, gently spread or press the dough from the center outward to fill the pizza pan. It will be very sticky. Re-wet your fingers as needed while pressing out the dough, and just patch up any holes that form. Don't worry, in the end it will bake nicely.
7. Let the dough rest, uncovered, while you preheat your oven to 425°F.
8. Bake for 10 minutes. Remove the crust from the oven and top as desired. Bake for 15 more minutes, or until the crust is lightly browned and the toppings are cooked as desired.

ROASTED TOMATO PIZZA SAUCE

MAKES 1 CUP (ENOUGH FOR ONE 15-INCH PIZZA OR TWO 12-INCH PIZZAS)

This sauce does need time to bake and cook, but the hands-on time is only 5 to 10 minutes. And the wonderful depth from roasting ripe tomatoes is well worth the small wait. It's delicious not only atop pizza, but also tossed with your favorite noodles.

1¼ pounds pearl, cherry, small heirloom, or small cluster tomatoes
2 garlic cloves, peeled
1 tablespoon olive oil
½ teaspoon + ⅛ teaspoon salt, divided, or to taste
½ teaspoon dried oregano *or* 1½ teaspoons fresh minced oregano
Freshly ground black pepper, to taste
1 teaspoon honey, agave nectar, or cane sugar, or to taste (optional)

1. Preheat your oven to 375°F.
2. Halve or quarter the tomatoes if using cluster or another medium-size variety.
3. Put the tomatoes and whole garlic cloves on a baking sheet. Drizzle with the oil, sprinkle with ½ teaspoon salt, and toss to evenly coat. Turn any cut tomatoes cut side up.
4. Roast for 40 minutes. Remove the garlic and small tomatoes. If using a larger cluster variety, roast the tomatoes for an additional 20 minutes, or until lightly browned. Let cool for 5 minutes.
5. Put the garlic and tomatoes in your blender. Blend until smooth, about 1 minute.
6. Pour the sauce into a small saucepan over medium-low heat. Whisk in the oregano, remaining ⅛ teaspoon salt, and black pepper. Let the sauce simmer for 10 to 20 minutes, while you prepare a pizza crust or pasta.
7. Taste test the sauce, and if it's too acidic or your tomatoes weren't sweet enough, whisk in the sweetener.
8. This sauce can be made up to 2 days in advance and stored in an airtight container in the refrigerator.

CREAMY GARLIC PIZZA SAUCE

MAKES ½ CUP (ENOUGH FOR ONE 12-INCH PIZZA)

This magical sauce makes vegetables disappear. A few teenage taste-testers inhaled mushroom and spinach toppings whenever this comforting sauce made an appearance.

> 1 small garlic head (the whole bulb)
> 1 teaspoon olive oil
> ½ cup raw cashews
> ¼ cup water, plus additional as needed
> ⅜ to ½ teaspoon salt, to taste

1. Preheat your oven to 400°F.
2. Slice the top off the garlic head to expose the cloves. Place the head, exposed side up, on a piece of aluminum foil and drizzle with the oil. Tightly wrap the foil around the garlic.
3. Roast for 30 minutes, or until the cloves are quite soft. Unwrap the head and let it cool for 5 minutes.
4. Put the cashews in your spice grinder or food processor and process them into a powder, about 1 minute.
5. Put the cashew powder, water, and salt in your blender. Squeeze the roasted garlic cloves out of their skins and into the blender. Blend until thick and creamy, about 2 minutes.
6. This sauce can be made up to 2 days ahead and stored in an airtight container in the refrigerator. It will thicken as it sits, so whisk in more water, as needed, before using.

AVOCADO PESTO PIZZA SAUCE

MAKES 1¼ CUPS (ENOUGH FOR ONE 15-INCH PIZZA OR TWO 9-INCH PIZZAS)

This creamy, rich pesto is a unique mélange of ingredients that meld together deliciously when baked atop a pizza, bagel, or polenta pie (page 308).

> 1½ cups lightly packed fresh basil
> ½ cup lightly packed fresh flat-leaf parsley
> ½ cup mashed avocado (about 1 large ripe avocado, pitted and peeled)
> ¼ cup grapeseed or extra-virgin olive oil
> ⅓ cup lite coconut milk
> 2 garlic cloves, smashed
> 2 to 3 teaspoons lemon juice, to taste
> 1 teaspoon nutritional yeast flakes (optional)
> ½ to ¾ teaspoon salt, to taste

1. Put the basil, parsley, avocado, oil, coconut milk, garlic, 2 teaspoons lemon juice, nutritional yeast (if using), and ½ teaspoon salt in your blender or food processor. Pulse 5 times to chop the herbs, and then blend until relatively smooth.
2. Blend in more salt and lemon juice, if needed.
3. This sauce is best used fresh, but it will keep in an airtight container in the refrigerator for up to 2 days. Just expect the top to oxidize and lose its pretty green hue.

THAI PEANUT PIZZA SAUCE

MAKES 1½ CUPS (ENOUGH FOR ONE 15-INCH PIZZA OR TWO 12-INCH PIZZAS)

This is the thick, spreadable sauce my friend Dreena Burton uses on her THAI CHICK-UN PIZZA (page 307), but it works well with a surprising range of toppings and even atop roasted sweet potato slices.

⅔ cup creamy peanut butter (can substitute sunflower seed butter for peanut free)
⅓ cup ketchup
¼ cup lite coconut milk or unsweetened plain dairy-free milk beverage
2 tablespoons rice vinegar
2 tablespoons soy sauce (can substitute gluten-free tamari or soy-free coconut aminos)
2 large garlic cloves, smashed
1½ tablespoons minced fresh ginger
1½ to 2 teaspoons agave nectar, to taste (optional)
¼ teaspoon crushed red pepper, or to taste
Water, as needed

1. Put the peanut butter, ketchup, coconut milk or milk beverage, rice vinegar, soy sauce, garlic, ginger, agave nectar (if using), and crushed red pepper in your blender or food processor. Blend until smooth, about 1 minute.

2. The sauce should be thick enough to spread on your pizza, but not runny. If needed, blend in water, 1 tablespoon at a time, to thin.

3. This sauce can be made up to 2 days ahead and stored in an airtight container in the refrigerator.

PIZZA TOPPING IDEAS

Beyond the recipes and combinations in this chapter, you might want to try some of the sauce and topping ideas below to mix things up.

DAIRY-FREE SAUCES
Aioli, dairy free or vegan
Barbecue sauce
Bruschetta
Chimichurri sauce
Hummus
Olive oil and crushed garlic
Roasted red pepper puree
Salsa

EVERYDAY TOPPINGS
Artichoke hearts
Bacon, regular or vegan
Bell peppers, any color
Caramelized onions
Chicken, dairy free or vegan
Chorizo, dairy free or vegan
Cooked sausage, dairy free or vegan
Green onions (green part only)
Herbs, fresh or dried
Jalapeño peppers
Mushrooms
Olives (black, green, or kalamata)
Onions (yellow, red, or shallots)
Pepperoni, dairy free or vegan
Roasted red peppers
Salami, dairy free or vegan
Spinach leaves
Sun-dried tomatoes

MEATY NOTE: If you aren't buying vegan "meat" toppings, keep an eye on the label for dairy-based ingredients. It isn't uncommon for cured meat to have some milk derivatives added. See page 106 for the dairy ingredient list.

CHAPTER 27

SO MANY PASTA-BILITIES
Stuffed, Casserole & Quick Noodle Recipes

GOOD TO KNOW FOR THIS CHAPTER

MOST NOODLES ARE DAIRY-FREE. Aside from stuffed pasta, like tortellini, dry pasta (wheat based or gluten free) is typically dairy free. Fresh unfilled pasta is usually dairy free, too, but it's often made with eggs.

PROTEIN-RICH NOODLES ARE GREAT FOR VEGAN PASTA. If you want a well-rounded meal but don't want to add chicken or tofu, seek out high-protein noodles. The ones made purely with beans or lentils perform very well, are rich in plant-based protein, and are sometimes high in calcium, too.

GRAIN-FREE NOODLES DO EXIST. My favorite variety is kelp noodles. They are calcium rich and easy to prepare, but their "crunchy" texture and "from the sea" flavor isn't a match for every recipe. Shirataki noodles are made from the root of the konjac plant and are a bit more flexible with flavors.

SPAGHETTI SQUASH IS A DELICIOUS "NOODLE" STAPLE. This hearty squash will keep at room temperature for a few weeks, and can be cooked with ease. Simply prick holes in the squash with a sharp fork or knife. Then bake it whole at 375°F for 60 to 90 minutes, depending on the size of the squash. Let it cool for 15 minutes. Cut it in half horizontally and scoop out the seeds. Pull out the "noodles" with a fork.

DAIRY-FREE PASTA IS FORGIVING. The vegetables and protein suggestions paired with these recipes are ones that I've tried and enjoyed. But don't be afraid to swap in other vegetables or proteins that you have on hand and think will fit with the flavor profile.

GLUTEN-FREE PASTA IS BEST WHEN RINSED. Many chefs proclaim pasta rinsing unnecessary, but ample blind taste tests with gluten-free pasta have proven to me that rinsing the noodles once cooked is essential. They aren't usually "starchy" like wheat-based pasta, but rather have more of a gummy exterior that needs to be rinsed away for the most appetizing results. Unless specified otherwise in the recipes that follow, you should rinse the noodles if using gluten free.

GREEK PASTA SALAD

MAKES 8 SERVINGS

Tofu soaks up the flavors of the marinade for a mock feta cheese in this somewhat traditional recipe.

> 1 pound rotini or fusilli pasta (gluten free, if needed)
> 6 tablespoons olive oil
> 6 tablespoons red or white wine vinegar
> ¼ cup lemon juice
> 2 tablespoons dried oregano
> 4 garlic cloves, minced (about 2 teaspoons)
> ½ to 1 teaspoon salt, or to taste
> Freshly ground black pepper, to taste
> 8 ounces soft or firm tofu, drained and crumbled or cut into ½-inch cubes
> 1 (14-ounce) can artichoke hearts, drained and quartered
> 1 cup cooked chickpeas/garbanzo beans
> 1 cup chopped yellow onion (1 small to medium onion)
> 1 bell pepper (any color), cored and chopped
> ½ pound tomatoes, halved if small or cut into ½-inch chunks
> 1 (2¼-ounce) can sliced olives, drained

1. Cook the pasta according to the package directions while preparing the tofu and vinaigrette.
2. In a large bowl, whisk together the oil, vinegar, lemon juice, oregano, garlic, salt, and pepper. Add the tofu and toss to coat it with the vinaigrette.
3. Rinse the cooked pasta in cool water. Add the pasta, artichoke hearts, beans, onion, bell pepper, tomatoes, and olives to the tofu and vinaigrette. Toss to evenly coat the ingredients.
4. Cover and refrigerate the salad for at least 1 hour, but preferably overnight.
5. Store leftovers in an airtight container in the refrigerator for up to 3 days.

PORTOBELLO-RICOTTA RAVIOLI

MAKES 70 TO 80 RAVIOLI (6 TO 8 SERVINGS)

There are few dairy foods that I miss these days, but I do have fond memories of one frozen food item, of all things. Our local grocery store kept stock of these simple but delicious portobello mushroom raviolis that we would boil up whenever we didn't feel like cooking. They weren't rich with dairy, but they did unfortunately harbor some cheese. One day I decided it was time to recreate them, in dairy-free fashion. I usually serve them topped with a marinara, a drizzle of olive oil, and some Parmesan substitute (page 202), or a light primavera sauce (page 321).

1 tablespoon grapeseed or olive oil

½ cup diced yellow onion (½ small to medium onion)

4 garlic cloves, minced (about 2 teaspoons)

2 cups diced button or cremini mushrooms

2 cups diced portobello mushrooms

1 batch TOFU RICOTTA (page 197) (can substitute the ALMOND RICOTTA on page 196 for soy free)

Won ton, egg roll, or gyoza wrappers (see Pasta Note below)

1. Heat the oil in a large skillet over medium-low heat. Add the onion and sauté until translucent, about 5 minutes.

2. Add the garlic and sauté for 1 minute.

3. Add the mushrooms and sauté until they are soft and have released most of their juices, about 5 minutes. Drain off any excess liquid.

4. Put the dairy-free ricotta in a medium bowl. Add the mushroom mixture and stir to evenly combine.

5. Set a small bowl of water next to your work surface.

6. Lay some of the wrappers out in a single layer on your work surface. Add a small amount of the mushroom filling to the middle of one half of each wrapper. Err on the side of less filling to ensure a proper seal and to minimize exploding raviolis during the boiling process. Tap your finger in the water and lightly dampen the outer edge of the wrappers. Fold the wrappers over to cover the filling, and squeeze out any excess air as you press to seal each side of the raviolis. Be careful with your fingernails when pressing the dough down; it can be easy to poke holes in the wrappers. Repeat this process until all of the filling is used up.

7. **To cook the ravioli**, bring a large pot of water to a boil. Add the ravioli in batches. They should have ample room to move to avoid sticking. Boil for 3 to 5 minutes, or until the wrappers are tender like cooked noodles. Remove the ravioli to plates with a slotted spoon. Repeat until all the ravioli are cooked.

8. Store cooked leftovers in an airtight container in the refrigerator for up to 1 day.

FREEZING TIPS: Prior to cooking, this ravioli freezes well. As you make them, space them out on baking sheets that will fit in your freezer. Place the baking sheet(s) in your freezer for 1 hour. Flip the ravioli and freeze for 1 hour more. Place the frozen ravioli in airtight freezer bags and return them to your freezer. When ready to eat, pop your desired amount of frozen ravioli in boiling water and cook as instructed above. They may take a few more minutes to cook.

PASTA NOTE: If using won ton or gyoza wrappers, about 70 to 80 wrappers will suffice for this recipe. You will need fewer if using egg roll wrappers. For the best results, I purchase egg roll wrappers and cut them into sixths (in half horizontally and in thirds vertically). Just a teaspoon of filling is needed for each of these smaller ravioli. For vegan and egg free, choose your wrappers carefully. Many Asian wrappers are made with egg. You can also substitute the vegan pasta dough from my HOMEMADE CHEEZE TORTELLINI (page 323).

ALMOST TOO EASY ALFREDO

MAKES 4 SERVINGS

I usually serve salad, steamed broccoli florets, or asparagus on the side to balance this rich, creamy, and oh-so-easy pasta dish.

> 8 ounces dry spaghetti or fettuccine (gluten free, if needed)
> ¾ cup raw cashews
> 1 cup chicken or vegan no-chicken broth
> ¼ cup full-fat coconut milk
> 2 garlic cloves, crushed (about 1 teaspoon) (can substitute ¼ teaspoon garlic powder)
> Water, as needed
> 1½ teaspoons lemon juice
> ¾ teaspoon salt, plus additional to taste
> Freshly ground black pepper, to taste
> Chopped fresh herbs, for garnish (optional)

1. Cook the pasta according to the package directions while preparing the rest of the recipe.
2. Put the cashews in your spice grinder or food processor. Process until powdered, about 1 minute.
3. Put the cashew powder, broth, coconut milk, and garlic in your blender. Blend until smooth and creamy, about 2 minutes.
4. Pour the nut cream through a fine-mesh sieve (to catch any remaining cashew pieces) into a medium pan over medium heat. Bring the sauce to a boil. Reduce the heat to low and whisk as it simmers for about 3 minutes, or until it reaches your desired thickness. If it thickens too much, whisk in water, 1 tablespoon at a time, as needed.
5. Add the lemon juice, salt, and black pepper and whisk to combine.
6. Divide the cooked pasta between 4 plates, top with the sauce, and garnish with fresh herbs (if using).
7. Store leftovers in an airtight container in the refrigerator for up to 1 day.

EXTRA PROTEIN VARIATION

Top the pasta with 8 ounces chopped cooked chicken, vegan chicken, or dairy-free Italian sausage (chicken, pork, or vegan) before topping with the sauce.

PASTA PRIMAVERA

MAKES 4 TO 6 SERVINGS

The sauce on this pasta is made with a roux for a lighter cream sauce than Alfredo. The recipe is a perfect entrée for highlighting fresh summer produce, yet it still acts as warm comfort food on chilly winter nights.

12 ounces uncooked linguine or pasta of choice (gluten free, if needed)
1 pound fresh vegetables (zucchini, summer squash, red bell pepper, carrots, broccoli, etc.), sliced or broken into florets
2 teaspoons grapeseed or olive oil
¼ cup minced yellow onion (about ⅓ small onion)
2 or 3 garlic cloves, minced (1 to 1½ teaspoons)
1 teaspoon dried oregano *or* 1 tablespoon minced fresh oregano
½ teaspoon dried thyme *or* 1½ teaspoons minced fresh thyme
¼ cup white wine
¼ cup dairy-free buttery spread (can substitute olive oil)
¼ cup all-purpose flour, whole wheat flour, or all-purpose gluten-free flour blend
2 cups warm unsweetened plain dairy-free milk beverage (do not use one with added protein)
¾ teaspoon salt, or to taste
¼ to ½ teaspoon white pepper or freshly ground black pepper, to taste

1. Cook the pasta according to the package directions while preparing the rest of the recipe.
2. Steam the vegetables until tender, about 5 to 8 minutes.
3. Heat the oil in a large saucepan over medium-low heat. Add the onion and sauté for 3 minutes, or until translucent.
4. Add the garlic, oregano, and thyme and sauté for 1 minute.
5. Stir in the wine and buttery spread. Cook until the buttery spread has melted and the ingredients are well combined, about 1 minute.
6. Add the flour while continuously whisking to form a smooth paste. Cook while whisking the paste for about 2 minutes. It should smell nutty and take on a golden hue.
7. Slowly pour in the milk beverage while whisking. Whisk and cook until the sauce is smooth and reaches your desired thickness, about 5 minutes.
8. Add the salt and pepper and stir to combine.
9. Put the cooked pasta in a large bowl. Add the vegetables and sauce and gently toss to coat.
10. Store leftovers in an airtight container in the refrigerator for up to 1 day.

EXTRA PROTEIN VARIATION

Add 8 to 12 ounces chopped cooked white fish, trout, salmon, chicken, or tempeh, or one 15-ounce can drained and rinsed chickpeas with the vegetables and sauce.

CREAMED SPINACH PASTA

MAKES 4 SERVINGS

Once I discovered that pine nuts could be magically transformed into a rich cream with the simple whiz of a blender, it seemed only fitting that they should act as a base for a basil-spiked sauce. This sauce has a slightly rich, almost buttery feel on its own and can be used without the spinach if you decide to go another flavor route.

> 8 ounces uncooked angel hair pasta or pasta of choice (gluten free, if needed)
> ½ cup pine nuts, plus extra for garnish
> 1 cup water, plus additional as needed
> 1½ tablespoons cornstarch (can substitute arrowroot starch)
> ¾ to 1 teaspoon salt, or to taste
> ¼ teaspoon garlic powder
> 2 to 4 tablespoons chopped fresh basil
> White pepper or freshly ground black pepper, to taste
> 5 to 6 ounces baby spinach leaves
> PINE NUT PARMA SPRINKLES (page 202), for garnish (optional)

1. Cook the pasta according to the package directions while preparing the rest of the recipe.
2. Put the pine nuts in your spice grinder or food processor. Process into a clumpy powder or paste, about 1 minute.
3. Put the pine nut paste, water, cornstarch, ¾ teaspoon salt, and garlic powder in your blender. Blend until smooth and creamy, about 1 minute.
4. Pour the nut cream through a fine-mesh sieve (to catch any remaining nut bits) into a medium saucepan over medium-low heat. Cook, whisking often, until the sauce thickens to your desired consistency, about 3 minutes. If it thickens too much, whisk in a little more water.
5. Stir in the basil and cook for 1 minute.
6. Whisk in the pepper and more salt, if desired.
7. Drain the pasta, but do not rinse it. Return the pasta to its pan, off the heat, and stir the spinach leaves into the hot noodles. Cover the pan and let the spinach steam for a few minutes.
8. Add the sauce to your pasta and spinach and stir to evenly coat.
9. Serve the pasta topped with extra pine nuts or Parma sprinkles, if desired.
10. This is best eaten immediately, but you can store leftovers in an airtight container in the refrigerator for up to 1 day.

....

EXTRA PROTEIN VARIATION

Add 8 to 12 ounces chopped cooked white fish, trout, salmon, chicken, or tempeh, or one 15-ounce can drained and rinsed chickpeas with the sauce.

....

HOMEMADE CHEEZE TORTELLINI

MAKES 30 TO 40 TORTELLINI (3 TO 4 SERVINGS)

Finding dairy-free cheese tortellini is no easy feat, so I decided to make my own! They're fun to assemble, and you can easily customize the cheesy filling. Thus far, we've enjoyed them filled with ALMOND RICOTTA (page 196), CASHEW CHEEZE WHEEL (page 198), and SEEDY CHEEZE (page 200). This tortellini works well in soups, and it pairs nicely with most sauces, including dairy-free pesto, marinara, light primavera (page 321), herb- or garlic-infused buttery spread, or olive oil with crushed red pepper and salt.

> 1 cup semolina flour or all-purpose flour
> ⅓ cup white whole wheat flour (can substitute all-purpose flour if using semolina)
> ⅜ teaspoon salt
> Up to ½ cup water
> ¾ cup dairy-free soft cheese (see headnote)

1. In a medium bowl, whisk together the flours and salt. Slowly whisk in the water, bringing the dough together with your hands when it gets too thick to stir. Add the water as needed to get cohesive dough that is just barely sticky and still workable.

2. Turn out the dough onto a floured work surface. Knead it for 5 minutes, or until fairly smooth and elastic. Let the dough rest for 5 minutes.

3. Place a small bowl of water next to your work surface. Flour the work surface and your rolling pin.

4. Divide the dough in half. Cover one half with a tea towel and place the other half on your floured work surface.

5. Roll the dough as thin as you can muster, ideally about ¹⁄₁₆ inch.

6. Cut the dough with a 2¾-inch biscuit cutter or a wide glass. Pull up the scraps and combine them with the covered dough.

7. Drop 1 teaspoon of the dairy-free soft cheese into the middle of a tortellini. Tap your finger in the water and wet the outer edge of the tortellini. Fold it in half, pressing the area around the filling first to seal, and then pressing your way outward to fully seal the half moon. You will quickly see if you've overfilled the tortellini. If some squirts out, just make sure to reseal the tortellini before proceeding. Take the two ends of the half moon, bring them together, and pinch to seal. Dust the tortellini with flour to prevent sticking. Repeat with the remaining dough circles and cheese.

8. Repeat steps 5 to 7 with the second ball of dough and scraps.

9. Take any scraps, reroll, and repeat steps 5 to 7.

10. To cook the tortellini, bring a large pot of water to a boil. Gently drop the tortellini in the boiling water and boil for 6 to 12 minutes (size, thickness, and altitude will affect the cooking time), or until tender to the bite. Remove with a slotted spoon and add to soups or sauces.

11. Store cooked leftovers in an airtight container in the refrigerator for up to 1 day.

FREEZING TIPS: This tortellini freezes well when frozen prior to cooking. As you make them, space them out on baking sheets that will fit in your freezer. Place the baking sheet(s) in your freezer for 2 hours. Place the frozen tortellini in airtight freezer bags and return them to your freezer. When ready to eat, pop your desired amount of frozen tortellini in boiling water and cook as instructed above. They may take a few more minutes to cook.

SPAGHETTI X'S & O'S

MAKES 4 SERVINGS

O-shaped pasta, otherwise known as anelletti, isn't always easy to find in stores. But alphabet pasta, wheat or gluten free, makes an equally delicious and even more fun stand-in. This saucy pasta tastes fresher than the canned version but uses many of the same ingredients, including carrots! They add natural sweetness and a little more body to the finish.

> 1 (15-ounce) can tomato sauce
> ⅓ cup chopped soft-cooked carrots (see Cooked Carrots Tip on page 283)
> 1½ tablespoons nutritional yeast flakes
> 1 tablespoon grapeseed, olive, or rice bran oil
> 1 teaspoon onion powder
> ¼ teaspoon garlic powder
> ¼ teaspoon paprika
> ¼ teaspoon + ⅜ teaspoon salt, divided
> 1 cup unsweetened plain dairy-free milk beverage (do not use one with added protein)
> 8 ounces alphabet, ring, or other fun shaped pasta (gluten free, if needed, but not a quinoa-based variety)
> Black pepper, to taste (optional)

1. Put the tomato sauce, cooked carrots, nutritional yeast, oil, onion powder, garlic powder, paprika, and ¼ teaspoon salt in your blender. Blend until smooth, about 1 minute.

2. Pour the tomato sauce mixture into a large saucepan. Add the milk beverage to your blender and briefly blend, to catch any remaining sauce in your blender. Pour the tomato–milk beverage mixture into the saucepan and stir to combine.

3. Place the saucepan over medium heat and bring the sauce to a low boil. Reduce the heat to medium-low and let simmer for about 10 minutes, while you prepare the pasta.

4. Cook the pasta according to the package directions for al dente. Drain but do not rinse the cooked pasta.

5. Add the cooked pasta to your sauce and stir to combine. Cook, while stirring, for 2 to 3 minutes.

6. Season with the remaining ⅜ teaspoon salt, or to taste, and black pepper (if using).

7. Store leftovers in an airtight container in the refrigerator for up to 1 day.

SHELLS 'N' BUTTERNUT BAKE

MAKES 4 SERVINGS

You could say that the key ingredients in this creamy pasta dish are butternut squash and cashews. But it wasn't until I discovered the perfect seasoning blend from Jenn at **VeggieInspired.com** that this recipe was perfected. Jenn swears it is the touch of nutmeg that puts it over the top, but I think it's her combination of Dijon mustard, paprika, and turmeric that gives it just the right flavor. The cheesiness isn't identical to mac and cheese, but I promise that it's delicious in its own right.

12 ounces uncooked small pasta shells (gluten free, if needed) (can substitute elbows, farfalle, or fusilli shapes)

⅓ cup raw cashews

1¼ cups mashed cooked butternut squash (see How to Roast Squash below)

¾ to 1 cup water

1 tablespoon lemon juice

1¼ teaspoons + ⅛ teaspoon salt, divided

1 teaspoon Dijon mustard

¼ teaspoon onion powder

¼ teaspoon garlic powder

¼ teaspoon black pepper

⅛ teaspoon smoked paprika

⅛ teaspoon ground turmeric

⅛ teaspoon ground nutmeg

½ cup bread crumbs (gluten free, if needed)

1 tablespoon olive oil

1 garlic clove, minced (about ½ teaspoon) (can substitute ⅛ teaspoon garlic powder)

1. Cook the pasta according to the package directions for al dente while preparing the rest of the recipe.

2. Preheat your oven to 350°F.

3. Put the cashews in your spice grinder or food processor. Process until powdered, about 1 minute.

4. Put the cashew powder, butternut squash, ¾ cup water, lemon juice, 1¼ teaspoons salt, mustard, onion powder, garlic powder, pepper, smoked paprika, turmeric, and nutmeg in your blender. Blend until smooth and creamy, about 2 minutes. Blend in ¼ cup more water for saucier pasta, if desired.

5. Drain and rinse the cooked pasta and return it to the pan. Add the butternut sauce and stir to evenly coat.

6. Transfer the pasta and sauce to a medium casserole dish and level it out.

7. In a small bowl, whisk together the bread crumbs, oil, garlic, and remaining ⅛ teaspoon salt until the oil is evenly distributed. Sprinkle the crumb mixture evenly over the casserole.

8. Bake for 20 to 30 minutes, or until the crumbs are browned.

9. Store leftovers in an airtight container in the refrigerator for up to 1 day.

HOW TO ROAST SQUASH: *Cut a butternut squash in half lengthwise and scrape out the seeds and stringy bits from each half. Place the halves cut side down in a greased baking dish. Bake at 350°F for about 1 hour, or until the flesh is quite tender. Let cool, facedown, for 15 to 20 minutes. Scrape out the flesh and use it as mashed butternut squash.*

EXTRA PROTEIN VARIATION

Add 8 ounces chopped cooked chicken or dairy-free Italian sausage (chicken, pork, or vegan), or one 15-ounce can drained and rinsed chickpeas with the sauce. Leftover cooked and crumbled bacon or chopped ham (regular or vegan) also go well.

BRAZILIAN-STYLE STROGANOFF

MAKES 6 TO 8 SERVINGS

The Brazilian version of stroganoff typically includes tomato sauce, onions or mushrooms, and heavy whipping cream. Instead of dairy cream, I use the luxurious taste and texture of raw cashews to create my version of this rich and comforting dish. Traditional Brazilian stroganoff is served over rice, but we like it over noodles, too.

1 pound dry egg noodles or fusilli (gluten free, if needed) *or* 1½ cups uncooked rice
2 tablespoons grapeseed or olive oil
1 pound cremini or button mushrooms, thinly sliced
1 pound lean ground beef or vegan ground round
2 or 3 garlic cloves, minced (about 1 to 1½ teaspoons)
1 teaspoon + 1 teaspoon salt, or to taste, divided
¼ to ½ teaspoon black pepper, to taste
1 (14-ounce) can unsalted crushed tomatoes
1 teaspoon dried oregano
⅔ cup raw cashews
1 cup water, plus additional as needed
1 teaspoon lemon juice
⅓ cup chopped fresh flat-leaf parsley, for garnish (optional)

1. Cook the pasta or rice according to the package directions while preparing the rest of the recipe.

2. Heat the oil in a large skillet over medium heat. Add the mushrooms and cook for 5 minutes, stirring occasionally.

3. Add the beef or vegan "meat," garlic, 1 teaspoon salt, and pepper (use ½ teaspoon for more of a peppery kick). Cook while breaking the meat up, until cooked through, about 5 minutes. Drain off any excess liquid.

4. Stir in the tomatoes and oregano. Reduce the heat to low and simmer for 5 minutes.

5. Put the cashews in your spice grinder or food processor. Process until powdered, about 1 minute.

6. Put the cashew powder, water, and lemon juice in your blender. Blend until smooth and creamy, about 1 minute.

7. Pour the nut cream through a fine-mesh sieve (to catch any remaining cashew bits) into the tomato sauce. Stir in the remaining 1 teaspoon salt.

8. Let the sauce simmer for about 3 minutes, or until thickened to your desired consistency. If it thickens too much, stir in a little more water.

9. Plate the pasta or rice and top it with the sauce. Sprinkle each serving with chopped parsley, if desired.

10. Store leftovers in an airtight container in the refrigerator for up to 1 day.

ONION VARIATION

Omit the mushrooms. Quarter and thinly slice 1 large or 2 medium yellow onions. Sauté the onions in the olive oil over medium heat for 10 minutes. Proceed with the recipe as written.

SESAME SOBA NOODLES WITH KALE

MAKES 4 TO 6 SERVINGS

This flavorful noodle dish is an easy way to get nutrient-rich kale into your diet. You can replace the kale with Swiss chard, but it doesn't provide as much usable calcium as kale.

12 ounces udon, soba, or spaghetti noodles (gluten free, if needed)
1 large bunch kale (1 to 1½ pounds)
2 tablespoons white or black sesame seeds
1 tablespoon avocado, peanut, or other high-heat oil (see page 148)
1 tablespoon minced fresh ginger
1 tablespoon + 2 tablespoons soy sauce (can substitute gluten-free tamari or soy-free coconut aminos), divided
Water, as needed
2 tablespoons sesame oil
1 green onion, thinly sliced, for garnish (optional)

1. Cook the pasta according to the package directions while preparing the rest of the recipe.
2. Cut the thick stems away from the kale leaves and slice the leaves into strips.
3. Put the sesame seeds in a large skillet over medium heat. Stir the sesame seeds until they darken slightly and become fragrant, about 3 minutes. Remove the seeds to a small bowl.
4. Add the oil to your skillet. Add the ginger and sauté for 1 minute.
5. Turn the heat up to medium-high. Add the kale and 1 tablespoon soy sauce. Stir-fry the greens until they are wilted but still slightly crunchy, about 3 minutes. As the kale cooks, you can add water, 1 tablespoon at a time, but only if needed. If you end up with excess liquid once the kale is cooked, drain it.
6. Add the cooked pasta, remaining 2 tablespoons soy sauce, sesame oil, and toasted sesame seeds to the kale and toss to combine.
7. Serve topped with green onion, if desired.
8. Store leftovers in an airtight container in the refrigerator for up to 1 day.

EXTRA PROTEIN VARIATION

Add 8 to 12 ounces chopped cooked chicken, pork, or tempeh, or baked tofu, or one 15-ounce can drained and rinsed chickpeas with the pasta.

CHINESE FIVE-SPICE NOODLES

MAKES 4 SERVINGS

This dish has subtle flavor and gentle warm heat that is comforting on both warm and cool days.

    8 ounces dry rice noodles/sticks (similar to linguine in width)
    ½ cup orange juice
    2 tablespoons soy sauce (can substitute gluten-free tamari or soy-free coconut
        aminos), plus additional for serving
    2 teaspoons agave nectar or honey
    1 teaspoon grated orange zest
    1 teaspoon Chinese five-spice powder
    ¼ teaspoon crushed red pepper
    ¼ teaspoon salt
    1 tablespoon olive or peanut oil
    1 medium to large yellow onion, cut into thin wedges (about 2 cups)
    1 cup thinly sliced or shredded carrot (about 1 medium carrot)
    12 ounces portobello, cremini, or button mushrooms, thickly sliced
    2 or 3 garlic cloves, minced (about 1 to 1½ teaspoons)
    8 ounces small broccoli florets (about 4 cups)

1. Cook the rice noodles according to the package directions for al dente while preparing the rest of the recipe.
2. In a small bowl, whisk together the orange juice, soy sauce, sweetener, zest, five-spice powder, crushed red pepper, and salt.
3. Heat the oil in a large skillet over medium heat. Add the onion and carrot and sauté until just beginning to soften, about 4 minutes.
4. Add the mushrooms and garlic and sauté for 1 minute.
5. Add the broccoli, cover, and cook for 2 to 4 minutes, or until the broccoli is crisp-tender.
6. Drain but do not rinse the cooked noodles. Add the cooked noodles and orange sauce to the vegetables. Cook while stirring the ingredients to coat for about 2 minutes.
7. Plate the noodles and serve with extra soy sauce, if desired.
8. Store leftovers in an airtight container in the refrigerator for up to 1 day.

....

EXTRA PROTEIN VARIATION

Add 8 ounces chopped cooked chicken or pork or baked tofu with the noodles.

....

LASAGNA BÉCHAMEL

MAKES 8 SERVINGS

This recipe was shared with me by my friend Cybele Pascal, author of *The Whole Foods Allergy Cookbook* and founder of **CybelesFreeToEat.com**. She created this dish to use up fresh tomatoes from her neighbor and quickly discovered that it's better than the high-fat, dairy-filled versions of days past.

8 ounces dry lasagna noodles (gluten free, if needed)
1 medium eggplant, peeled and sliced into ¼-inch rounds
¼ cup + 3 tablespoons olive oil, divided
¼ cup + 2 tablespoons rice flour or oat flour (can substitute all-purpose flour)
2 cups hot unsweetened plain dairy-free milk beverage
Pinch ground nutmeg
1 bay leaf
Salt, to taste
Freshly ground black pepper, to taste
2 large portobello mushrooms, sliced into ¼-inch strips
12 shiitake or button mushrooms, sliced
3 ripe medium tomatoes, seeded and sliced into thin rounds
4 cups dairy-free red sauce (store-bought or PANTRY MARINARA on page 330)
20 basil leaves
½ cup bread crumbs (gluten free, if needed) or cornflake crumbs

1. Preheat your oven to 350°F.
2. Cook the pasta according to the package directions while preparing the rest of the recipe.
3. Lay the sliced eggplant on a plate and heat in your microwave on high for 2 minutes, or until just tender.
4. Heat the ¼ cup oil in a saucepan over medium heat. Add the flour and cook for 2 minutes, whisking continuously. Slowly pour in the milk beverage, while whisking until smooth. Add the nutmeg and bay leaf.
5. Bring the sauce to a low boil. Reduce the heat to low and simmer for 10 minutes, whisking often.
6. Remove the sauce from the heat. Discard the bay leaf and whisk in the salt and pepper.
7. Drizzle 1 tablespoon oil in the bottom of a 9 × 13-inch baking dish. Cover the bottom of the pan with half of the eggplant slices. Cover the eggplant with half of both types of mushrooms, followed by half of the sliced tomatoes. Cover the vegetables with 1½ cups red sauce and top with 10 basil leaves. Drizzle with half of the cream sauce. Cover with a layer of half of the lasagna noodles. Drizzle 1 tablespoon oil over the noodles. Layer with the remaining vegetables, another 1½ cups red sauce, the remaining 10 basil leaves, and remaining cream sauce. Top with the remaining lasagna noodles and spread the remaining 1 cup red sauce on to cover the noodles. Sprinkle the crumbs over the top and drizzle with the remaining 1 tablespoon oil.
8. Bake, uncovered, for 1 hour. Let cool completely. Refrigerate overnight, if time permits, before serving. Cut the lasagna while cool. Serve chilled or reheat individual portions, if desired.
9. Cover and store leftovers in an airtight container in the refrigerator for up to 2 days.

VERY VEGGIE LASAGNA

MAKES 8 SERVINGS

It was my personal mission to pack as many vegetables as possible into a single pan of lasagna, while still eliciting a seal of approval from my husband. This recipe easily passes the test, though he still prefers his veggie lasagna with some added ground beef.

PANTRY MARINARA

2 tablespoons grapeseed or olive oil
1 cup diced yellow onion (1 small to medium onion)
2 to 4 garlic cloves, minced (1 to 2 teaspoons)
1 teaspoon dried thyme *or* 1 tablespoon fresh minced thyme
1 teaspoon dried oregano *or* 1 tablespoon fresh minced oregano
Pinch crushed red pepper
2 (14-ounce) cans unsalted diced tomatoes (can substitute 2 pounds fresh tomatoes, diced)
1 cup vegetable broth
2 tablespoons tomato paste
1 tablespoon balsamic vinegar
2 teaspoons agave nectar, honey, or cane sugar
½ teaspoon salt

VEGGIE LASAGNA

12 dry lasagna noodles (gluten free, if needed)
1 batch TOFU RICOTTA (page 197) or COTTAGE-STYLE CHEEZE (page 201), *or* 1½ batches ALMOND RICOTTA (page 196), *or* 2 batches RICH & NUTTY RICOTTA (page 198)
2 cups baby spinach, chopped
1 tablespoon olive oil
1 pound zucchini, diced
1 red or green bell pepper, cored and diced
8 ounces button or cremini mushrooms, diced
PINE NUT PARMA SPRINKLES (page 202) or SUNFLOWER GRATED PARMA (page 202), for garnish (optional)
Chopped olives, for garnish (optional)

1. **To make the pantry marinara,** heat the oil in a large skillet over medium-low heat. Add the onion and sauté until soft and translucent, about 5 to 7 minutes.

2. Add the garlic, thyme, oregano, and crushed red pepper and sauté for 3 minutes.

3. Add the tomatoes, broth, tomato paste, vinegar, sweetener, and salt and stir to combine. Let the sauce simmer, uncovered, for 30 to 40 minutes, stirring occasionally. Let cool for 10 minutes.

4. Transfer the sauce to your blender (in batches, if needed) and pulse several times until somewhat smooth, but still a little chunky (see page 289 for tips).

5. **To make the lasagna,** cook the noodles according to the package directions while preparing the rest of the recipe.

6. Preheat your oven to 350°F.

7. In a medium bowl, stir together the dairy-free ricotta or cottage-style cheese and chopped spinach.

8. Heat the oil in a large skillet over medium-low heat. Add the zucchini and bell pepper and sauté until lightly softened, about 5 minutes.

9. Add the mushrooms and sauté until tender, about 5 minutes. Drain any excess liquid.

10. Set aside 1 cup marinara, and stir the rest into the vegetables. Simmer the marinara with the vegetables for 5 to 10 minutes.

11. Cover the bottom of a 9 × 13-inch baking dish with the reserved 1 cup marinara. Add a layer of 3 lasagna noodles. Cover the noodles with half of the spinach-ricotta mixture, then another layer of 3 noodles. Cover with half of the vegetable marinara, then another layer of 3 noodles. Cover with the remaining spinach-ricotta mixture, followed by the last layer of 3 noodles. Thoroughly cover the noodles with the remaining vegetable marinara.

12. Bake, uncovered, for 30 to 35 minutes, or until bubbly. Let cool for 10 minutes.

13. Serve topped with Parma and/or chopped olives, if desired.

14. Cover and store leftovers in an airtight container in the refrigerator for up to 2 days.

EXTRA PROTEIN VARIATION

Add 1 pound cooked lean ground beef, turkey, or vegan ground round to the vegetable marinara sauce before layering it in the lasagna.

CHAPTER 28

MORE MARVELOUS MAINS
Comforting Meal-Worthy Recipes

GOOD TO KNOW FOR THIS CHAPTER

DON'T LET THE INGREDIENT LISTS INTIMIDATE YOU. Some of these dishes may seem complicated due to the number of ingredients. But many of these are just spices and flavors that you probably purchase regularly. I rarely use premade spice blends since they can sometimes harbor dairy.

NATURAL CONVENIENCES ARE GREAT HELPERS. Make dinner easier with bagged baby spinach leaves, sliced mushrooms, jarred minced or crushed garlic and ginger, or other pre-prepped single ingredients. In many cases, they aren't even more expensive than their "as is" counterparts.

EVEN SIMPLE INGREDIENTS CAN VARY. I bet you didn't know that select brands of corn tortillas are much higher in calcium than others. The same goes for refried beans and tofu. Check the nutrition facts on different brands if minerals are a high priority in your diet.

CAULI-RICE ISN'T ALL OR NOTHING. For some extra vegetables, you can substitute cauliflower "rice" for the grain in many of these recipes. However, it doesn't have to be a straight swap. I often stir one part "riced" and cooked cauliflower in with one part cooked rice. My husband doesn't usually even know the vegetable is in there with this method. For cauliflower "rice" cooking methods, see my cookbook *Eat Dairy Free*.

NOT ALL CHILI POWDERS ARE CREATED EQUAL. Regular chili powder can vary from relatively mild to very hot. I typically use a medium-heat chili powder, unless otherwise noted. But you can use your heat of choice to spice a recipe up or down without losing flavor. Chipotle chili powder has a smokier flavor and is usually on the hot side.

PALEO EGGPLANT CANNELLONI WITH FRESH TOMATO-BASIL SAUCE

MAKES 3 TO 4 SERVINGS

My husband proclaimed this entrée to be "restaurant quality"! I was expecting it to taste good, but the luxurious results surprised us both. There is a little prep time involved, but the sauce and ricotta can be made in advance for a meal that comes together quickly. I like to serve it with a simple side dish, like steamed vegetables or a green salad.

> 1 medium eggplant (1¼ to 1½ pounds)
> ½ to ¾ teaspoon salt, plus additional for the eggplant
> 1 tablespoon olive oil, plus additional for the eggplant
> 2 garlic cloves, minced (about 1 teaspoon)
> 1 pound tomatoes, diced
> ⅛ to ¼ teaspoon black pepper
> ¼ cup chopped fresh basil
> 1 batch RICH & NUTTY RICOTTA (page 198)
> 2 cups baby spinach leaves, chopped (see Spinach Tip below)
> Sliced or chopped olives (black, kalamata, or green), for garnish (optional)

1. Cut the ends off the eggplant and optionally peel it. Cut the eggplant lengthwise into long, thin slices, roughly ⅛ to ¼ inch thick. Sprinkle one side of the slices with some salt and let them sit for 30 minutes, salt side up.

2. Heat the oil in a medium skillet over low heat. Add the garlic and sauté for 2 minutes.

3. Add the tomatoes, ½ teaspoon salt, and ⅛ teaspoon pepper. Let the sauce simmer for 20 to 30 minutes, or until the tomatoes have softened and released some juices.

4. Stir in the basil and simmer for 3 minutes. Season to taste with additional salt and pepper, if desired.

5. In a medium bowl, stir together the dairy-free ricotta and chopped spinach.

6. Preheat your oven on broil.

7. Wipe excess moisture and salt from the eggplant slices with a paper towel or clean tea towel. Lightly brush each side of the slices with oil, and place them on a baking sheet. Broil for 3 to 4 minutes per side, until softened and browned but not burned.

8. Turn off the broiler and preheat your oven to 400°F.

9. Spread half of the tomato sauce in the bottom of a 9 × 13-inch baking dish.

10. Scoop 1 to 2 tablespoons dairy-free ricotta onto one end of each eggplant slice. Roll the slices up, and place them, seam side down, in the sauce in your baking dish.

11. Spread the remaining tomato sauce over the eggplant rolls to coat.

12. Bake, uncovered, for 30 to 40 minutes, or until the eggplant rolls are quite tender.

13. Top each serving with sliced or chopped olives, if desired.

14. Cover and store leftovers in an airtight container in the refrigerator for up to 2 days.

SPINACH TIP: *When organic spinach is on sale, or if I have some baby spinach leaves on their last day, I freeze them in the bag. When it's time for this recipe, I roughly measure 2 cups, and then crumble the frozen leaves with my fingers.*

GUACAMOLE ENCHILADAS IN RED SAUCE

MAKES 4 SERVINGS

Enchiladas sans cheese? Yes, it's true! The richness of the filling more than compensates for the dairy in Americanized enchiladas. I often make this homemade red enchilada sauce because it's so easy and delicious. However, you can swap in a 15-ounce jar or can of your favorite dairy-free enchilada sauce, if preferred.

RED ENCHILADA SAUCE

3 tablespoons avocado, grapeseed, olive, or rice bran oil

3 tablespoons cornstarch (can substitute arrowroot starch)

2 tablespoons chili powder

1 teaspoon ground cumin

2 cups vegetable or chicken broth

½ cup tomato sauce

2 teaspoons cane sugar, agave nectar, or honey

1 teaspoon dried oregano

½ teaspoon salt

GUACAMOLE ENCHILADAS

2 very ripe medium avocados, pitted and peeled

1 to 1½ tablespoons lime juice, to taste

½ cup SILKEN SOUR CREAM (page 189), SOUR CASHEW CREAM (page 189),
   SOUR COCONUT CREAM (page 190), or store-bought dairy-free sour cream alternative,
   plus extra for serving

3 green onions, thinly sliced

¼ cup fresh flat-leaf parsley or cilantro, minced

1 small jalapeño pepper, seeded and minced

1 garlic clove, minced (about ½ teaspoon)

½ teaspoon ground cumin

¼ teaspoon salt

1 cup raw cashews, finely chopped

1 cup cooked chopped chicken, vegan chicken, or tempeh

10 to 12 corn or white flour tortillas (6- or 8-inch)

1. **To make the enchilada sauce**, heat the oil in a medium saucepan over medium heat. Add the starch and whisk while cooking for 1 minute.

2. Add the chili powder and cumin and whisk while cooking for 1 minute.

3. Gradually pour in the broth while whisking to eliminate any lumps. Add the tomato sauce, sugar, oregano, and salt and whisk to combine. Reduce the heat to medium-low and cook for 5 to 10 minutes, whisking occasionally, until the sauce thickens a little. It will thicken more when baking your enchiladas.

4. **To make the enchiladas**, preheat your oven to 350°F.

5. Put the avocado flesh and lime juice in a medium bowl, and mash until relatively smooth. Add the dairy-free sour cream alternative, green onions, parsley or cilantro, jalapeño, garlic, cumin, and salt and stir to thoroughly combine. Fold in the cashews and chicken or tempeh.

6. Pour a shallow layer of enchilada sauce (just enough to cover) in a 9 × 13-inch baking dish.

7. Lay a tortilla in the enchilada sauce in the baking dish, and place some of the avocado-cashew mixture along one side of the tortilla. Roll it up and place the enchilada to one side of the baking dish. Repeat with the remaining tortillas and avocado-cashew mixture.

8. Pour the enchilada sauce over the enchiladas to evenly coat. If using the homemade sauce, there will likely be extra. Store leftovers in an airtight container for up to 3 days, or freeze to use later.

9. Cover the baking dish with aluminum foil and bake for 30 minutes.

10. Serve each enchilada topped with a dollop of dairy-free sour cream alternative.

11. Cover leftover enchiladas and store them in the refrigerator for up to 1 day.

MUSHROOM & SAGE STUFFED BELL PEPPERS

MAKES 6 SERVINGS

This "meaty" vegetarian dish is wonderful with thick bell peppers. They're complemented by the hearty herbed filling, which has a delicious stuffing flavor vibe.

¾ cup dry brown lentils
1½ cups dry long-grain or jasmine brown rice
4 cups mushroom broth (can substitute vegetable broth)
½ cup water
1 tablespoon + 6 teaspoons olive oil, divided
½ teaspoon garlic powder
1 teaspoon salt
8 ounces cremini or button mushrooms, chopped
1 to 2 cups packed baby spinach leaves (optional)
1 teaspoon dried sage
Freshly ground black pepper, to taste
6 medium to large bell peppers (any color), tops and seeds removed
Garlic- or jalapeño-stuffed green olives, chopped (optional)

1. Rinse the lentils in a fine-mesh sieve until the water runs clear. Remove any stones.

2. Put the lentils, rice, broth, water, 1 tablespoon oil, garlic powder, and salt in a medium saucepan over medium heat. Bring the mixture to a boil. Cover and reduce the heat to low. Simmer for 40 to 45 minutes, or until the liquid is absorbed.

3. Remove the pan from the heat, and let sit for 5 to 10 minutes.

4. Preheat your oven to 350°F.

5. Stir the chopped mushrooms, spinach (if using), sage, and black pepper into the cooked rice mixture.

6. Stuff the bell peppers with the rice mixture, packing it in as needed.

7. Place the bell peppers in a large baking dish. Drizzle 1 teaspoon oil over each pepper.

8. Bake for 30 to 40 minutes, or until the peppers are soft.

9. Serve each pepper topped with chopped green olives, if desired.

10. Store leftovers in an airtight container in the refrigerator for up to 2 days.

RUSTIC ROASTED EGGPLANT PUTTANESCA

MAKES 6 SERVINGS

Rather than trying to mimic eggplant Parmesan, I opted for an equally satisfying sauce concept. I also roast the tomatoes, which adds so much depth of flavor that anchovies aren't missed in this puttanesca-style sauce.

  2 pounds cherry, grape, or sugar plum tomatoes
  4 or 5 garlic cloves, peeled
  1½ tablespoons + 2 tablespoons olive oil, divided
  ½ teaspoon + ½ teaspoon salt, divided, plus additional to taste
  ½ cup regular or vegan mayonnaise
  3 tablespoons water
  2½ cups panko or dry bread crumbs (gluten free, if needed)
  2 (1-pound) eggplants, optionally peeled, and sliced into ½-inch-thick rounds
  ½ cup chopped flat-leaf parsley, plus additional for garnish
  ½ cup pitted chopped kalamata olives, plus additional whole pitted olives for garnish
  ¼ cup capers
  2 teaspoons dried oregano
  ¼ teaspoon crushed red pepper

1. Preheat your oven to 375° F.
2. Place the tomatoes and garlic on a baking sheet with high sides. Drizzle with the 1½ tablespoons olive oil, sprinkle with ½ teaspoon salt, and stir to evenly coat.
3. Bake for 30 to 40 minutes, or until the tomatoes are quite soft, bursting, and starting to brown. Let cool for 10 minutes. Leave the oven on.
4. Grease or line 2 baking sheets with parchment paper or silicone baking mats.
5. In a shallow bowl, whisk together the mayonnaise and water.
6. In another shallow bowl, stir together the panko and remaining ½ teaspoon salt.
7. One at a time, dip the eggplant slices in the mayo mixture to coat both sides and then dredge in the crumbs, pressing the crumbs on, as needed. Place the coated slices in a single layer on your prepared baking sheets.
8. Bake for 15 minutes. Carefully flip each slice and bake for 15 more minutes.
9. Transfer the cooled tomatoes, with juices, and garlic to your blender. Pulse several times, until mostly pureed but still slightly chunky.
10. Heat the remaining 2 tablespoons oil in a large skillet over medium-low heat. Add the parsley, chopped olives, capers, oregano, and crushed red pepper and sauté for 3 minutes.
11. Add the tomato-garlic sauce and simmer for 5 to 10 minutes, or until it reaches your desired thickness. Season the sauce with additional salt, if desired.
12. Plate the eggplant slices and top with the sauce. Garnish with parsley and whole olives.
13. Store leftover sauce and eggplant slices in separate airtight containers in the refrigerator for up to 2 days.

EXTRA PROTEIN VARIATION

For a heartier finish, you can stir 1 to 2 cups chopped cooked chicken, vegan chicken, or chickpeas in with the sauce.

DECONSTRUCTED FALAFEL BOWLS WITH TAHINI SAUCE

MAKES 4 SERVINGS

These savory bowls are rich in plant-based protein, fiber, and minerals from the quinoa, beans, and tahini sauce. The recipe is spiked with fresh falafel flavors for a unique but fulfilling anytime dish.

1 cup dry quinoa
⅓ cup water, plus additional as needed
⅓ cup tahini
1 tablespoon lemon juice, or to taste
⅜ teaspoon + ½ teaspoon + ⅛ teaspoon salt, divided, or to taste
⅛ teaspoon garlic powder (see Garlic Note below)
¼ cup olive oil
1 cup diced yellow onion (1 small to medium onion)
1 garlic clove, minced (about ½ teaspoon) (optional)
1½ teaspoons ground cumin
½ teaspoon ground coriander
Pinch cayenne pepper
1 (15-ounce) can chickpeas/garbanzo beans, drained and rinsed
¼ teaspoon black pepper, to taste
Optional vegetable extras: 1 diced medium cucumber, 1 diced cluster tomato,
    1 shredded raw carrot, ½ cup diced cooked carrot, ½ cup diced red bell pepper, or
    ⅓ cup diced roasted red bell pepper
¼ cup minced fresh flat-leaf parsley

1. Bring a pot of water to a boil like you would for pasta. Thoroughly rinse the quinoa in a fine-mesh sieve. Add the quinoa to the water, stir, and boil for 15 to 18 minutes, or until the grains are tender and have rings around them. Drain and return the quinoa to the pot, off the heat. Cover and let sit for 5 to 10 minutes.

2. Put the water, tahini, lemon juice, ⅜ teaspoon salt, and garlic powder in your blender. Blend until smooth and creamy, about 30 seconds. Thin with more water for a drizzly consistency, if desired.

3. Heat the oil in a large skillet over medium-low heat. Add the onion and sauté until translucent, about 3 minutes.

4. Add the garlic (if using), cumin, coriander, and cayenne pepper and sauté for 30 seconds.

5. Stir in the cooked quinoa, garbanzo beans, ½ teaspoon salt, and black pepper and sauté for 1 minute.

6. Remove the skillet from the heat and stir in any vegetable extras. Season with the remaining ⅛ teaspoon salt.

7. Divide the quinoa mixture between 4 bowls. Dollop or drizzle each serving with tahini sauce and sprinkle with parsley.

8. Store leftover quinoa mixture and sauce in separate airtight containers in the refrigerator for up to 2 days.

GARLIC NOTE: Raw garlic doesn't go over well in our home, so I use garlic powder in the tahini sauce. But if you prefer the authentic edge of raw garlic you can substitute 1 garlic clove.

LENTIL CURRY IN A HURRY

MAKES 4 SERVINGS

This quick and easy dish has a mild, yet slightly spicy flavor that will please kids and spouses alike. My curry-hating husband devoured every last lentil, stating, "I guess I do like curry sometimes." For him, I use just 1½ teaspoons of curry powder, but feel free to use 2 teaspoons if you have a curry-loving household.

1 cup red lentils
2 teaspoons grapeseed, olive, or rice bran oil
½ cup chopped yellow onion (½ small to medium onion)
2 cups water
1½ to 2 teaspoons curry powder, to taste
1 teaspoon chili powder
½ teaspoon ground mustard powder
½ cup full-fat or lite coconut milk
½ teaspoon salt
4 cups cooked white or brown rice

1. Rinse the lentils in a fine-mesh sieve until the water runs clear. Remove any stones.
2. Heat the oil in a medium saucepan over medium heat. Add the onion and sauté until tender and translucent, about 3 to 5 minutes.
3. Add the water, lentils, curry powder, chili powder, and mustard and stir to combine. Bring the mixture to a low boil. Cover, reduce the heat to medium-low, and cook for 10 to 15 minutes, or until the lentils are tender.
4. Stir in the coconut milk and salt. Simmer, uncovered, for 3 to 5 minutes.
5. Divide the rice between 4 plates and top with the lentil curry.
6. Store leftover lentils and rice in separate airtight containers in the refrigerator for up to 2 days.

ADD-IN IDEAS

FRUIT: Dice 1 medium tomato or mash 1 small banana and stir it in with the coconut milk.

VEGETABLES: Stir 2 cups chopped spinach, kale, or lightly steamed cauliflower or broccoli in with the coconut milk.

TOFU SAAG PANEER

MAKES 3 TO 4 SERVINGS

Sarah Hatfield, my associate editor, is my Indian food expert since she and her husband enjoy it as often as possible. When I asked her if she thought a dairy-free paneer was possible, she said it already exists—it's called tofu! There are some tofu saag paneer recipes out there, but most are still surprisingly rich in dairy. Sarah went the extra mile, making this popular Indian dish completely dairy free and family-friendly.

6 cups + 1 cup water, divided
2 teaspoons + 1 teaspoon salt, divided, plus additional if needed
1 (14-ounce) package firm tofu, drained and diced into ½-inch cubes
5 to 6 ounces baby spinach leaves
1 medium yellow onion, roughly chopped
3 garlic cloves, smashed
1-inch piece fresh ginger, peeled
½ jalapeño pepper, seeded (optional)
2 tablespoons coconut oil (can substitute your favorite cooking oil)
1½ teaspoons ground cumin
1 teaspoon garam masala
½ teaspoon curry powder
⅛ teaspoon ground nutmeg
⅛ teaspoon cayenne pepper (optional)
1½ cups full-fat coconut milk
1 tablespoon lemon juice
2 cups cooked white or brown rice

1. Pour the 6 cups water into a large pot over medium-high heat. Bring it to a boil. Reduce the heat to low and add the 2 teaspoons salt. Add the tofu, turn off the heat, and let sit for 5 minutes.
2. Gently drain the tofu.
3. Steam the spinach until wilted, about 2 minutes. Let it cool for 3 minutes, then press out any excess water. Chop the spinach.
4. Put the onion, garlic, ginger, and jalapeño in your food processor. Process until minced. If you don't have a food processor, mince these ingredients with a knife.
5. Heat the oil in a large skillet over medium heat. Add the onion mixture and sauté for 5 minutes.
6. Stir in the remaining 1 cup water, remaining 1 teaspoon salt, cumin, garam masala, curry powder, nutmeg, and cayenne (if using). Simmer for 5 minutes.
7. Transfer the mixture to your blender or food processor. Add the spinach and blend until smooth, about 1 minute (see page 289 for tips).
8. Pour the spinach mixture back into your skillet. Add the coconut milk, lemon juice, and tofu and simmer for 5 minutes. Season with more salt, to taste, if desired.
9. Divide the rice between 3 to 4 plates. Top with the tofu paneer to serve.
10. Store leftover saag paneer and rice in separate airtight containers in the refrigerator for up to 1 day.

POWER STIR-FRY

MAKES 4 SERVINGS

I managed to pack numerous protein- and mineral-rich ingredients into this rich, delicious, and fulfilling stir-fry. It's got a slight Thai peanut influence, but with more flavor depth from the almond butter and molasses.

1 pound firm or extra firm tofu

1 tablespoon + 2 tablespoons + 2 tablespoons soy sauce (can substitute gluten-free tamari), divided

½ cup creamy almond butter (can substitute sunflower seed butter for nut free)

½ cup hot water, plus additional as needed

¼ cup apple cider vinegar or rice vinegar

2 tablespoons blackstrap molasses (can substitute honey or maple syrup)

¼ to ½ teaspoon crushed red pepper

2 tablespoons olive, peanut, or rice bran oil

1 medium to large yellow onion, cut into ¾-inch wedges (about 2 cups)

4 garlic cloves, minced (about 2 teaspoons)

1 tablespoon minced fresh ginger

12 ounces broccoli florets

1 red bell pepper, cored and cut into ¾-inch wedges

3 to 4 cups cooked quinoa or brown rice

½ cup sliced almonds, for garnish (optional)

1 small lime, cut into 4 wedges, for serving

1. Drain and lightly press the tofu, using a tea towel or paper towels, to remove any excess water. Cut it into ½-inch cubes.

2. Put the tofu in a medium bowl. Add the 1 tablespoon soy sauce and stir to combine. Let sit for 10 to 15 minutes.

3. In a medium bowl, whisk together the almond butter, hot water, vinegar, 2 tablespoons soy sauce, molasses, and crushed red pepper.

4. Heat the oil in a large skillet over medium heat. Add the onion and sauté for 2 minutes.

5. Add the garlic and ginger and sauté for 1 minute.

6. Add the broccoli, bell pepper, and remaining 2 tablespoons soy sauce. Sauté until the vegetables are crisp-tender, about 4 to 5 minutes.

7. Add the tofu and sauté for 2 minutes, or until heated through.

8. Remove the skillet from the heat and stir in the almond butter sauce. If it thickens too much, thin with additional water, 1 tablespoon at a time, until it reaches your desired consistency.

9. Divide the cooked quinoa or rice between 4 plates and top with the tofu mixture. Garnish with sliced almonds, if desired. Serve with lime wedges for seasoning to taste.

10. Store leftover stir-fry and rice in separate airtight containers in the refrigerator for up to 1 day.

HAWAIIAN TERIYAKI BOWLS

MAKES 4 SERVINGS

One of my favorite meals is the humble rice bowl. This simple, everyday version infuses homemade teriyaki sauce with the sweet, citrusy flavors of pineapple.

- 1 (14-ounce) can crushed or chunk pineapple in juice (do not drain)
- ½ cup + 2 tablespoons soy sauce (can substitute gluten-free tamari or soy-free coconut aminos)
- 2 tablespoons mirin or white wine (see Wine Note below)
- 1 to 2 teaspoons sesame oil
- ½ cup lightly packed brown sugar (can substitute coconut sugar)
- 2 teaspoons cornstarch (can substitute arrowroot starch)
- ½ teaspoon crushed red pepper (optional)
- ½ teaspoon garlic powder *or* 4 garlic cloves, smashed
- ¼ teaspoon ground ginger *or* 1 tablespoon chopped fresh ginger
- 4 cups cooked brown or white rice
- 2 pounds steamed vegetables (broccoli, cauliflower, carrots, snow peas, etc.)

1. Put the pineapple with juice, soy sauce, mirin or wine, sesame oil, brown sugar, starch, crushed red pepper (if using), garlic, and ginger in your blender. Blend until relatively smooth, about 1 minute.
2. Pour the sauce into a medium saucepan over medium-low heat. Cook, whisking occasionally, for 10 minutes, or until it thickens to your desired consistency.
3. Divide the rice between 4 bowls, top with the steamed vegetables, and ladle some sauce over the vegetables.
4. Store leftover vegetables and rice in separate airtight containers in the refrigerator for up to 1 day. Store leftover sauce in an airtight container in the refrigerator for up to 3 days.

WINE NOTE: Mirin is a Japanese rice wine that contains a good dose of sweetness. I have used both mirin and white wine in this recipe with good success. The white wine is just a bit less sweet.

....

EXTRA PROTEIN VARIATION

This simple dish also goes well with 1 pound chopped cooked chicken, salmon, trout, baked tofu, or tempeh.

....

GRILLED CHEEZE SANDWICHES

MAKES 2 SANDWICHES

With a jar of powdered cheeze mix at the ready, these comforting sandwiches take mere minutes to whip up! The instant cheesy sauce quickly thickens into a melty, slightly stretchy cheese consistency.

½ cup POWDERED CHEEZE MIX (page 207)
½ cup water
1 teaspoon lemon juice
Regular or vegan mayonnaise or dairy-free buttery spread, for spreading
4 slices bread (gluten free, if needed)

1. Put the cheeze mix and water in your blender. Blend until smooth, about 1 minute.
2. Pour the mixture into a small saucepan over medium heat and bring it to a low boil. Reduce the heat to low, and cook, while whisking, for about 2 minutes. It should become very thick.
3. Remove the pan from the heat and whisk in the lemon juice.
4. Spread a thin layer of the mayonnaise or buttery spread on 1 side of each bread slice.
5. Flip 2 of the slices over and top them with the cheesy mixture.
6. Top the cheesy slices with the other 2 slices, mayo/buttery side out.
7. Preheat a skillet over medium-low heat. Add the sandwiches and grill for about 2 to 3 minutes per side, or until browned to your liking. Enjoy immediately.

GREAT FILLING IDEAS: Sandwich one or more of these in your grilled cheeze for a tasty flavor twist: roasted red bell peppers, vegan or turkey deli meat, sliced beefsteak or heirloom tomatoes, sliced dill pickles, green chiles or sliced hot peppers, fresh herbs, sliced avocado, caramelized onions, bacon (vegan, turkey, or pork), or dairy-free pesto.

BUILD YOUR OWN TACO BAR

MAKES 4 TO 6 SERVINGS

Taco night has been a fun and easy dinner in our home for many years. My homemade seasoning is quick to whip up, without fear of fillers or allergens, and the choice of toppings can be whatever you have on hand.

1 tablespoon chili powder
1½ teaspoons ground cumin
1 teaspoon salt
½ teaspoon paprika
½ teaspoon black pepper (optional)
¼ teaspoon garlic powder
¼ teaspoon onion powder
¼ teaspoon dried oregano
⅛ to ¼ teaspoon crushed red pepper

1 tablespoon avocado, grapeseed, olive, or rice bran oil
1 pound lean ground beef, ground turkey, chopped chicken, or vegan ground round
   (see Vegan Protein Note below)
8 to 12 corn tortillas
Toppings of choice (see Dairy-Free Taco Bar Toppings below)

1. In a small bowl, whisk together the chili powder, cumin, salt, paprika, black pepper
   (if using), garlic powder, onion powder, oregano, and crushed red pepper.
2. Heat the oil in a medium skillet over medium heat. Add the meat or vegan ground round
   and cook while breaking it up, until cooked through, about 5 minutes. Add the seasoning
   and sauté for 2 to 3 minutes.
3. Transfer the cooked meat to a serving bowl.
4. Dampen 2 paper towels, and place 4 tortillas between them. Microwave the tortillas for
   30 to 60 seconds, or until warm and pliable. Repeat with the remaining tortillas. Keep
   the tortillas covered when serving.
5. Put several taco bar toppings in individual bowls and let everyone build their own!
6. Cover leftovers and store them in their individual bowls in the refrigerator for up to 1 day.

*VEGAN PROTEIN NOTE: Beyond straight meat alternatives, you can use about
2½ cups cooked beans (or one 16-ounce can if using refried beans) or chopped tempeh for the
protein. Heat any of these options with the spice blend above for a few minutes.*

DAIRY-FREE TACO BAR TOPPINGS

Avocado, diced
Banana peppers, stemmed
Caramelized onions
Corn
Fresh cilantro
Guacamole (see Easy Guacamole Recipe below)
Hot sauce
Jalapeño peppers, sliced or seeded and diced
Lettuce or cabbage, shredded
Lime wedges
Olives (black or green), sliced
Onions, diced
Pico de gallo
Salsa
Tomatoes, chopped

EASY GUACAMOLE RECIPE

In a medium bowl, mash together the flesh of 3 ripe avocados, juice of 1 lime (about
2 tablespoons), and ½ to 1 teaspoon salt (to taste). Stir in ½ cup diced red onion, up to
¼ cup chopped fresh cilantro, 1 diced small tomato, and 1 teaspoon minced garlic.
Optionally stir in ½ teaspoon ground cumin, a pinch cayenne pepper, or 1 seeded,
minced jalapeño pepper.

SWEET POTATO & BLACK BEAN TAQUITOS

MAKES 8 TAQUITOS

These crispy bites are secretly nutritious. The beans and tortillas are calcium rich
(check the label of the latter as brands differ), while the sweet potatoes add more fiber and
micronutrients. I keep the filling relatively mild, because we like to enjoy them with salsa or
hot sauce and guacamole. But you can double the diced green chiles or increase the
chili powder if a spicier filling is desired.

> 2 cups peeled and diced sweet potatoes (about 10 ounces)
> ¾ cup cooked black beans
> 1 teaspoon + 1 teaspoon lime juice, divided
> ⅛ teaspoon + ½ teaspoon salt, divided
> ½ teaspoon chili powder
> ¼ teaspoon ground cumin
> ¼ teaspoon smoked paprika
> ⅛ teaspoon black pepper
> 1 tablespoon canned roasted diced green chiles
> 8 corn tortillas
> Oil or oil spray, as needed
> 8 toothpicks, soaked in water
> Guacamole, salsa, hot sauce, and/or dairy-free sour cream, for serving

1. Steam the sweet potatoes until quite tender, about 10 to 12 minutes.
2. Preheat your oven to 400°F.
3. In a small bowl, stir together the beans, 1 teaspoon lime juice, and ⅛ teaspoon salt.
4. In another small bowl, whisk together the remaining ½ teaspoon salt, chili powder, cumin, paprika, and black pepper.
5. Put the cooked sweet potatoes in a medium bowl. Add the spice mix, remaining 1 teaspoon lime juice, and green chiles. Mash the potatoes and seasonings together with a fork or potato masher until relatively mashed but a bit chunky. Stir in the beans.
6. Dampen 2 paper towels, and place 4 tortillas between them. Microwave the tortillas for 30 to 60 seconds, or until warm and pliable.
7. Brush or spray one side of a tortilla with oil. Flip and spoon about 3 tablespoons of the sweet potato mixture across the bottom quarter of the tortilla. Roll it up as tightly as possible, place on a baking sheet, and put a water-soaked toothpick through the center to help hold it closed. Repeat with the remaining 3 warmed tortillas.
8. Repeat steps 6 and 7 with the remaining 4 tortillas.
9. Bake for 15 to 20 minutes, or until the tortillas are crisp.
10. Serve with guacamole, salsa, hot sauce, and/or dairy-free sour cream for dipping.
11. Store leftovers in an airtight container in the refrigerator for up to 2 days.

....

PROTEIN VARIATION

I like to use black beans in this recipe because they provide fiber and minerals like calcium, too. But you can swap in ¾ cup seasoned ground beef or vegan ground round.

....

VEGGIE TOSTADAS WITH AVOCADO CREMA

MAKES 8 TOSTADAS

The vegetable-bean blend for this flavorful mini-meal can be made in advance to quickly enjoy a tostada or two when cravings strike. We keep the seasoning relatively mild and sprinkle on hot sauce for personalized heat.

¾ cup mashed avocado (about 2 medium ripe avocados)
⅓ cup coconut cream
1 tablespoon fresh lime juice
¼ teaspoon + ½ teaspoon salt, divided
1½ teaspoons chili powder
¾ teaspoon ground cumin
½ teaspoon smoked paprika
¼ teaspoon ground coriander
⅛ teaspoon black pepper
1½ teaspoons grapeseed, rice bran, avocado, or olive oil
1 medium zucchini (about 8 ounces), cut into ½-inch chunks
½ cup diced bell pepper (any color)
¼ cup minced poblano pepper
¾ cup cooked black beans
½ cup corn kernels (fresh or frozen and thawed)
8 tostadas (store-bought or see How to Make Tostadas below)
Sliced olives, for garnish (optional)
Hot sauce, for serving (optional)

1. Put the avocado, coconut cream, lime juice, and ¼ teaspoon salt in a medium bowl. Mash with a fork or blend with a hand mixer to thoroughly combine.

2. In a small bowl, whisk together the chili powder, cumin, paprika, remaining ½ teaspoon salt, coriander, and black pepper.

3. Heat the oil in a medium skillet over medium heat. Add the zucchini, bell pepper, and poblano pepper and sauté for 5 minutes, or until the vegetables begin to look tender.

4. Add the beans, corn, and spice mix and sauté for 1 to 2 minutes, or until everything is well combined and heated through.

5. Spread the avocado crema on the tostadas and top with the bean and vegetable mixture, pressing it into the spread. Sprinkle with sliced olives and serve with hot sauce (if using).

6. These are best eaten immediately, but the leftover components can be stored in separate airtight containers in the refrigerator for up to 1 day.

HOW TO MAKE TOSTADAS: Brush 8 corn tortillas lightly with oil on both sides. Place the tortillas in a single layer on a baking sheet and bake at 400°F for 6 minutes. Flip and bake for 4 to 7 more minutes, or until crisped up to your liking.

EXTRA PROTEIN VARIATION

Add ½ pound seasoned and cooked ground turkey, beef, or vegan ground round with your toppings. You can alternatively use a taco-seasoned protein from the recipe on page 342.

CHAPTER 29

WARM SIDES
Greens to Grains Recipes

GOOD TO KNOW FOR THIS CHAPTER

I FOCUS ON VERSATILITY. The sides in this chapter are intended as basics that you can easily whip up and pair with most main dishes.

SIDES CAN BE THE BASE OF A GREAT MEAL. I've included "Make It a Meal" options for several of these recipes to turn them into a light but fulfilling lunch or dinner without the need for another entrée recipe.

THE INGREDIENTS ARE OPTIMIZED FOR EASE, COST, AND NUTRITION. Space is limited in books, so I chose to stick with ingredients that you can find in almost any grocer for a fair price year-round, and that offer the most dairy-free nutrition bang for your buck. Yes, your local stores have bok choy, too!

BRING ON THE BOK CHOY

MAKES 3 TO 4 SERVINGS

This calcium-rich side dish uses the tang of lemon rather than the sodium of soy for a flavor that is sweet, sour, and spicy all in one. Consequently, the flavor pairs well with most main dishes. And this dish is very quick to make. Just make sure all of your ingredients are prepared, measured, and next to the stove before beginning.

2 tablespoons avocado, rice bran, or other high-heat oil (see page 148)
1 medium yellow onion, quartered and thinly sliced (about 1½ cups)
4 garlic cloves, minced (about 2 teaspoons)
1 tablespoon grated fresh ginger
½ teaspoon salt
⅛ to ¼ teaspoon crushed red pepper, to taste
1½ pounds bok choy or baby bok choy, coarsely chopped (about 7 cups)
½ pound broccoli florets (about 3 cups)
2 tablespoons lemon juice
2 teaspoons honey, agave nectar, or cane sugar

1. Heat the oil in a large skillet or wok over medium-high heat. Add the onion, garlic, ginger, salt, and crushed red pepper and stir-fry for 2 minutes.
2. Add the bok choy and broccoli and stir-fry for 2 minutes.
3. Add the lemon juice and sweetener and stir-fry for 2 to 3 minutes, or until the broccoli and bok choy are crisp-tender.
4. Store leftovers in an airtight container in the refrigerator for up to 2 days.

MAKE IT A MEAL: *Stir-fry ¾ to 1 pound lightly salted chopped chicken, tempeh, or tofu in 1 to 2 tablespoons high-heat oil over medium-high heat until lightly browned and cooked through. Add it to the stir-fry during the last minute of cooking.*

KALE & SWEET ONION SAUTÉ

MAKES 4 SERVINGS

Kale may look like just another leafy green, but it's a member of the hearty cruciferous family. So unlike spinach, it's not only loaded with minerals such as calcium, but it also holds its structure quite well when cooked. This easy, nutrient-packed side was inspired by a wonderful Bobby Flay recipe.

> 1½ tablespoons avocado, rice bran, or other high-heat oil (see page 148)
> ½ medium to large sweet onion, sliced (about 1 cup)
> 1 garlic clove, minced (about ½ teaspoon) (optional)
> 10 to 12 ounces coarsely chopped kale (leaves and stems)
> ½ cup vegetable or chicken broth
> 2 tablespoons red wine vinegar (can substitute balsamic vinegar)
> ⅛ teaspoon salt, or to taste
> Freshly ground black pepper, to taste (optional)

1. Heat the oil in a large pot or skillet (with a lid) over medium heat. Add the onion and sauté until lightly browned, about 5 to 7 minutes.
2. Add the garlic (if using) and sauté for 30 seconds.
3. Raise the heat to medium-high and stir in the kale and broth. Cover, reduce the heat to medium-low, and cook for 5 minutes, or until the stems are somewhat tender.
4. Uncover and increase the heat to medium. Add the vinegar and sauté until any excess liquid has evaporated.
5. Season the vegetables with salt and pepper (if using).
6. Store leftovers in an airtight container in the refrigerator for up to 2 days.

BROCCOLI DIJON

MAKES 4 TO 6 SERVINGS

This recipe incorporates one of my favorite seasonings, Dijon mustard. Studies have shown that mustard helps increase the absorption of broccoli micronutrients. But Dijon can be quite pungent, so I've added an optional sweetener. It helps temper the flavor but doesn't actually make the sauce sweet. We enjoy this recipe both with and without the added sweetener, but the version without is slightly thicker and clings a little more to the florets.

> 1 pound broccoli florets (about 6 cups)
> ¼ cup buttery spread or BAKEABLE BUTTER (page 192), melted
> 2 tablespoons Dijon mustard
> 1 tablespoon lemon juice
> 1 tablespoon honey or agave nectar (optional)

1. Steam the broccoli florets for 5 to 10 minutes, or until they reach your desired tenderness.
2. Put the florets in a colander and shake to remove any excess water, and then transfer them to a large bowl.

3. In a small bowl, whisk together the melted buttery spread, mustard, lemon juice, and sweetener (if using).

4. Pour the sauce over the broccoli and toss to coat.

5. Plate the broccoli and drizzle on any remaining sauce from the bowl.

6. Store leftovers in an airtight container in the refrigerator for up to 2 days.

CREAMY CAULIFLOWER GRATIN

MAKES 6 SERVINGS

This fulfilling side dish gets its gratin name from the bread crumb topping, but no cheese is required. It's a flavorful way to get my resident cauliflower-hater to polish off his entire meal. I originally created it for my column in *Allergic Living* magazine. But my friend Alexa Croft, who photographed it for the magazine, insisted that it must be in this cookbook, too! For a more colorful side, use orange, purple, or green cauliflower, or a combination of all three.

¼ cup dairy-free buttery spread or BAKEABLE BUTTER (page 192)
1 large yellow onion, chopped (about 2½ cups)
¼ cup all-purpose flour or sweet white rice flour (for gluten free)
¼ cup regular or vegan mayonnaise
1¾ to 2 cups chicken or vegetable broth
¾ teaspoon salt, or to taste
⅛ teaspoon white pepper
Pinch ground nutmeg
1½ pounds cauliflower, chopped into small ¾-inch florets (about 7 cups)
½ to 1 cup panko bread crumbs (gluten free, if needed)

1. Preheat your oven to 350°F.

2. Melt the buttery spread in a large skillet over medium heat. Add the onion and sauté for 3 minutes or until it just starts to soften.

3. Reduce the heat to medium-low and add the flour. Cook, while stirring, for 2 minutes. Stir in the mayonnaise. Gradually whisk in the broth, as needed, until smooth. Cook for 3 minutes, or until a slightly thick sauce forms.

4. Remove the skillet from the heat and whisk in the salt, white pepper, and nutmeg. Add the cauliflower florets and toss to coat.

5. Pour the cauliflower with sauce into an 8 × 8-inch or 9 × 9-inch baking dish, and shake or press with a spoon to level out. Evenly sprinkle your desired amount of bread crumbs over the cauliflower.

6. Bake for 50 minutes, or until the cauliflower is tender and the crumbs are golden brown.

7. Let cool for 5 minutes before serving.

8. Cover and store leftovers in the refrigerator for up to 2 days.

MASHED POTATOES & MISO-MUSHROOM GRAVY

MAKES 4 SERVINGS

This comforting dish is satisfying on its own, but it also pairs well with most home-style mains. I tested olive oil, coconut oil, buttery spread, and even mayonnaise in these mashed potatoes, but coconut oil and buttery spread were the clear winners. For the gravy, the outcome depends heavily on the broth that you use, so be sure to use one that you like.

MASHED POTATOES
2 pounds yellow potatoes, cut into 1-inch cubes
¼ cup dairy-free buttery spread or coconut oil
¾ to 1 teaspoon salt, or to taste
Freshly ground black pepper, to taste
Up to ¼ cup unsweetened plain dairy-free milk beverage (can substitute broth)

MUSHROOM GRAVY
¼ cup olive oil
4 ounces mushrooms, halved and sliced (about 1 cup)
¼ cup diced yellow or sweet onion (about ⅓ small onion)
¼ cup whole wheat or all-purpose flour (can substitute sweet white rice flour or a gluten-free all-purpose flour blend)
½ teaspoon dried thyme
1½ to 2½ cups mushroom or vegetable broth
1½ teaspoons white miso (gluten free or soy free, if needed)
⅛ to ¼ teaspoon salt, or to taste
⅛ teaspoon black pepper

1. **To make the potatoes**, put the potatoes in a large pot and cover them with water. Cover the pot and bring the water to a boil. Cook for 20 minutes, or until the potatoes are very tender. Drain well and return the potatoes to the pot (off the heat) to help any remaining water evaporate.

2. Add the buttery spread or oil to the potatoes and mash. Add the salt and pepper and mash to combine. Add the milk beverage, if needed, to get your desired consistency. For a coarser mash, use a fork. For a light and fluffy whipped consistency, use a handheld mixer.

3. **To make the gravy**, heat the oil in a large saucepan or skillet with high sides over medium heat. Add the mushrooms and onion and cook for 5 minutes, stirring occasionally, or until the vegetables begin to brown.

4. Add the flour and thyme, and cook, while whisking or stirring, for 3 minutes. The flour should take on a golden hue.

5. Slowly whisk in 1½ cups of the broth or stock. Cook, while whisking, for about 5 minutes. Whisk in more broth or stock, as needed, to get the gravy consistency you desire.

6. Remove the gravy from the heat and whisk in the miso, salt, and pepper.

7. Serve the gravy as is, strain it through a fine-mesh sieve for a creamy finish, or transfer it to your blender and blend in the mushrooms and onions.

8. Divide the potatoes between 4 plates or bowls, and top with the gravy, to serve.

9. Store leftover gravy and potatoes in separate airtight container in the refrigerator for up to 2 days.

MAKE IT A MEAL: *Lightly season and cook ¾ pound ground beef, turkey, or vegan ground round in 1½ teaspoons olive oil over medium heat, until cooked through. Stir it into the gravy before serving.*

ROASTED GARLIC VARIATION

Preheat your oven to 400°F. Slice the top off 1 head of garlic to expose the cloves. Brush the top with olive oil and wrap the garlic head in aluminum foil. Roast for 45 to 60 minutes, or until the tops of the cloves are golden brown and the individual cloves appear to have separated from the side walls of the head. Allow the garlic to cool, and then squeeze the bottom of the head to pop the garlic cloves out. Lightly mash the cloves and add them to the potatoes along with the buttery spread or oil.

LEFTOVER MASHED POTATO CAKES VARIATION

Make small patties out of the leftover potatoes and dust them with flour (gluten free, if needed) or panko crumbs. Heat 2 to 4 tablespoons of high-heat oil (see page 148) in a skillet over medium-high heat. Fry the potato patties until browned, about 2 to 3 minutes per side. For cakes that hold together better, blend 1 egg or egg white into the leftover mashed potatoes before forming the patties.

ANYTIME OVEN-ROASTED POTATOES

MAKES 4 TO 6 SERVINGS

This recipe is a simple crowd-pleaser—and a great alternative to the milk-rich side dishes at potlucks and family dinners. In fact, my grandma requested that I bring a big batch to her birthday.

2 pounds yellow potatoes, cut into ¾-inch cubes
2 tablespoons grapeseed or olive oil
2 large garlic cloves, minced (about 1 teaspoon)
½ teaspoon dried basil
½ teaspoon dried oregano
½ teaspoon dried parsley
½ teaspoon dried thyme
½ teaspoon dried dill
½ teaspoon salt
¼ to ½ teaspoon crushed red pepper

1. Preheat your oven to 450°F and grease or line a baking sheet with parchment paper or a silicone baking mat.

2. Put the potatoes on your prepared baking sheet. Drizzle on the oil and sprinkle the garlic over the potatoes. Toss to coat.

3. Put the basil, oregano, parsley, thyme, dill, salt, and crushed red pepper in a small dish or spice grinder. Stir to combine or process for 10 seconds in the spice grinder for finer herbs.

4. Sprinkle the herb blend over the potatoes and toss to evenly coat. Spread the potatoes out into a single layer so the pieces aren't touching one another.

5. Roast for 15 minutes. Stir the potatoes, spread them back into a single layer, and roast for 10 to 20 minutes, or until evenly browned.

6. Store leftovers in an airtight container in the refrigerator for up to 2 days.

MAKE IT A MEAL: Add 1 pound sliced cooked dairy-free chicken sausage or vegan sausage to the baking sheet in a single layer during the last 10 minutes of roasting.

SEASONED OVEN FRIES

MAKES 3 TO 4 SERVINGS

One evening I got a hankering for seasoned French fries, but you can't always trust the restaurant versions to be dairy free. So I decided to bake up my own with a nice blend of everyday spices. If you live in a dry climate, these fries will crisp up fairly well, but it's hard to get a crisp exterior in more humid climates without a deep fryer. Either way, these are delicious and definitely satisfy French fry cravings.

> 1 pound russet potatoes, Yukon gold potatoes, or sweet potatoes, optionally peeled
> 2 teaspoons avocado, peanut, or rice bran oil
> ½ teaspoon paprika
> ½ teaspoon mild chili powder (can substitute a medium or spicy chili powder)
> ½ teaspoon garlic powder
> ½ teaspoon onion powder
> ½ teaspoon salt
> ⅛ teaspoon crushed red pepper

1. Preheat your oven to 425°F and grease a baking sheet or line it with parchment paper.
2. Slice the potatoes into ¼-inch rounds or French fries and put them in a large bowl. Drizzle on the oil and toss to combine.
3. In a small bowl, whisk together the paprika, chili powder, garlic powder, onion powder, salt, and crushed red pepper.
4. Sprinkle the seasoning blend over the potatoes and toss to evenly coat.
5. Transfer the potato slices to your prepared baking sheet. Spread the potatoes out into a single layer so the pieces aren't touching one another.
6. Bake for 15 minutes. Flip the fries and bake for 15 to 25 minutes, or until tender but golden.
7. Store leftovers in an airtight container in the refrigerator for up to 2 days.

ROASTED SWEET POTATO & GREENS SALAD

MAKES 4 TO 6 SERVINGS

This satisfying salad is heartier than your average iceberg bowl. In addition to the warm roasted sweet potatoes and rich, flavorful dressing, it's topped with roasted chickpeas. They add healthy crunch to salads, and can even stand in as a unique, protein-rich alternative to croutons.

- 1½ pounds sweet potatoes, peeled and cut into ½-inch chunks
- 1½ tablespoons + 1 teaspoon grapeseed, olive, or rice bran oil, divided
- ½ teaspoon + ⅛ teaspoon salt, divided
- ⅛ teaspoon black pepper
- 1 (15-ounce) can chickpeas/garbanzo beans *or* 1½ cups cooked chickpeas/garbanzo beans, drained, rinsed, and patted dry
- 8 to 10 cups baby spinach or seasonal greens of your choice (12 to 16 ounces)
- 1 batch BALSAMIC TAHINI DRESSING (page 288)
- Dried cranberries, for garnish (optional)
- Freshly ground black pepper, to taste (optional)

1. Preheat your oven to 450°F and grease 2 baking sheets or line them with parchment paper.
2. Put the sweet potatoes on your prepared baking sheet. Drizzle with the 1½ tablespoons oil and sprinkle with the ½ teaspoon salt and pepper. Toss to evenly coat. Spread the potatoes into a single layer so the pieces aren't touching one another.
3. Put the chickpeas on the other prepared baking sheet. Drizzle with the remaining 1 teaspoon oil and sprinkle with the remaining ⅛ teaspoon salt. Toss to evenly coat. Spread the chickpeas out on the baking sheet.
4. Roast the sweet potatoes and chickpeas for 15 minutes. Stir and spread them back into a single layer. Roast for 10 to 20 minutes, or until the sweet potatoes are lightly browned and the chickpeas are crispy. Let cool completely.
5. Divide the spinach or greens between 4 to 6 plates or bowls. Top each salad with some roasted sweet potatoes, crispy chickpeas, and dressing. Sprinkle each salad with dried cranberries (if using) or freshly ground black pepper (if using).
6. Store leftover sweet potatoes in an airtight container in the refrigerator for up to 1 day, and leftover chickpeas for up to 3 days.

MAKE IT A MEAL: *Double the roasted chickpeas by increasing the chickpeas to 2 cans or 3 cups, the oil to 2 teaspoons, and the salt to ¼ teaspoon. Or top the salads with 2 cups cooked and lightly seasoned chopped chicken or vegan chicken.*

....

SUMMER VARIATION

Substitute sliced cucumbers and shredded carrots for the roasted sweet potatoes.

....

BLACKSTRAP BARBECUE BEANS

MAKES 6 SERVINGS

Some brands of baked beans are high in calcium, but making them at home guarantees a plant-based, mineral-rich side. This easy stovetop recipe uses a good dose of blackstrap molasses and is also lower in sugars than most baked beans. But if you prefer a sweeter finish, just double the brown sugar.

1 tablespoon oil
½ cup diced yellow onion (½ small to medium onion)
1 garlic clove, minced (about ½ teaspoon)
1 (8-ounce) can tomato sauce
1 cup water
2 tablespoons packed brown sugar (can substitute coconut sugar)
2 tablespoons blackstrap molasses
2 tablespoons apple cider vinegar
1 teaspoon Worcestershire sauce (vegan, if needed)
½ teaspoon ground mustard powder
¼ teaspoon chipotle chile powder
¼ teaspoon liquid smoke
3 (15-ounce) cans beans (any combination of pinto, white, Great Northern, or navy beans), drained and rinsed
½ teaspoon salt, or to taste

1. Heat the oil in a large pot over medium-low heat. Add the onion and sauté for 5 minutes, or until translucent. Add the garlic and sauté for 1 minute.

2. Add the tomato sauce, water, brown sugar, molasses, vinegar, Worcestershire, mustard, chile powder, and liquid smoke and stir to combine. Stir in the beans.

3. Increase the heat to medium and bring the mixture to a low boil. Reduce the heat to low and simmer, uncovered, for 1 hour. Stir every 10 minutes, and add more water, as needed, if it thickens too much.

4. Stir in the salt and serve warm.

MAKE IT A MEAL: Serve the beans over cooked rice (¾ cup per serving) and top with steamed carrots or roasted sweet potatoes.

SPANISH-STYLE BARLEY

MAKES 4 TO 6 SERVINGS

I love this recipe for its ease of preparation, its unique texture, and the ability to adjust the heat and taste based on our latest favorite salsa. Cooked barley has some heft to it, with a rustic yet slightly creamy consistency and a tender but firm bite.

2 tablespoons grapeseed or olive oil
1 cup quick-cooking or regular pearl barley, rinsed
1 cup chopped yellow onion (1 small to medium onion)
2 garlic cloves, minced (about 1 teaspoon)
3 cups vegetable or chicken broth
1 cup salsa
½ teaspoon salt, or to taste
Freshly ground black pepper, to taste
1 (2¼-ounce) can sliced olives

1. Preheat your oven to 350°F.
2. Heat the oil in a large skillet over medium heat. Add the barley, onion, and garlic and sauté for 5 to 7 minutes, or until the onion begins to soften and the barley is lightly toasted.
3. Transfer the barley mixture to a medium Dutch oven or baking dish with a lid. Add the broth, salsa, salt, and pepper and stir to combine.
4. Cover and bake for 60 minutes if using quick-cooking barley, 90 minutes if using regular pearl barley.
5. If some liquid still remains, uncover the barley and bake for 10 to 15 more minutes, or until the remaining liquid cooks off.
6. Stir in the sliced olives.
7. Store leftovers in an airtight container in the refrigerator for up to 1 day.

MAKE IT A MEAL: Stir 6 cups chopped kale leaves or 1 cup cooked corn kernels into the barley during the last 10 minutes of cooking. Then stir one 15-ounce can of drained and rinsed pinto or black beans and/or 2 cups of cooked diced chicken into the cooked barley.

CREAMY POBLANO BAKED RISOTTO

MAKES 4 SERVINGS

This creamy risotto is so surprisingly easy to make, and the results are practically foolproof. The mild flavors of the poblano, lime juice, and corn complement one another perfectly, for a subtle yet alluring flavor that's far more versatile than you might think.

1 tablespoon avocado oil or olive oil
¼ cup diced yellow onion (about ⅓ small onion)
¼ cup diced poblano pepper (about 1 small pepper)
1 cup Arborio rice

1½ cups low-sodium chicken or vegetable broth or stock
1¼ cups full-fat coconut milk
1 tablespoon lime juice
½ teaspoon + ¼ to ½ teaspoon salt, divided
¼ teaspoon black pepper
½ cup cooked corn kernels

1. Heat the oil in a Dutch oven or oven-safe pot with a lid (9 to 10 inches wide works well) over medium-low heat. Add the onion and poblano pepper and sauté for 2 to 3 minutes, or until just beginning to soften. Add the rice and sauté for 3 to 4 minutes, or until very lightly toasted.

2. Add the broth or stock, coconut milk, lime juice, ½ teaspoon salt, and black pepper and stir to combine.

3. Cover and cook for 35 minutes (up to 40 minutes above 4,000 feet), or until the rice is tender but still a little al dente. It should look just a little bit soupy on the surface.

4. Add the corn and stir to combine. Add the remaining ¼ to ½ teaspoon salt, to taste.

5. This dish is best eaten immediately, but leftovers can be stored in an airtight container in the refrigerator for up to 1 day.

MAKE IT A MEAL: Add 1 pound sliced sautéed zucchini and 1 pound cooked chopped seasoned chicken, vegan or regular chorizo, vegan or regular dairy-free jalapeño sausage, or one 15-ounce can drained and rinsed black beans to the cooked risotto.

MULTI-GRAIN PILAF

MAKES 6 SERVINGS

This is a tasty, no-fuss alternative to plain old rice that offers a good dose of protein and fiber. Use it as a side dish or base for your favorite meal bowl. Feel free to mix and match the grains based on your preferences and what you have on hand.

½ cup millet
½ cup quinoa
½ cup brown rice
1 tablespoon coconut oil (can substitute olive oil or dairy-free buttery spread)
½ to 1 teaspoon salt
2¾ cups boiling water
¼ to ⅓ cup chopped fresh herbs (optional)

1. Preheat your oven to 375°F.
2. Rinse the millet, quinoa, and brown rice in a fine-mesh sieve.
3. Put the rinsed grains, oil, and salt in a medium Dutch oven or baking dish with a lid. Pour the boiling water over the grains and stir to combine.
4. Cover and bake for 1 hour. Let cool for 15 minutes.
5. Carefully remove the lid and fluff the grains with a fork. Stir in the fresh herbs (if using).
6. Store leftovers in an airtight container in the refrigerator for up to 1 day, or freeze to enjoy later.

CHAPTER 30

THE COOKIE JAR

Classic, Bar & Bakery Special Recipes

GOOD TO KNOW FOR THIS CHAPTER

CANE SUGAR IS PLAIN OLD WHITE GRANULATED SUGAR. At the store, you will see white sugar labeled most often as cane sugar, which is why I chose this wording. However, you can use sugar labeled as "white," "evaporated cane juice," or "beet" sugar instead.

MOST SUGAR IS VEGAN. Some brands of cane sugar are processed with bone char, but not as many as you might think. I used a certified vegan sugar for testing all the recipes in this book, and organic sugar is vegan, by their standards.

YOU CAN USE MY HOMEMADE BUTTERY SPREAD. If you have an issue with store-bought dairy-free buttery spread, you can swap in my BAKEABLE BUTTER (page 192) for the baked good recipes in this book. In most cases, it will produce very similar—and sometimes better!—results.

COOKIES CAN BE TEMPERAMENTAL AT HIGHER ALTITUDES. If you live above 4,000 feet, you might find that cookies, especially vegan ones, can come out greasy and flat. I have tested the recipes in this book at high altitude (4,500 feet specifically), and included adjustments, if needed. But before you bake, take note if the dough seems overly greasy. If it does, add more flour until it is just lightly greasy. If it's too dry and not sweet enough, add a little liquid sweetener, like agave nectar or maple syrup. If it's just a little too dry, splash in a little dairy-free milk beverage to get the right consistency.

NEVER ENOUGH CHOCOLATE CHIP COOKIES

MAKES 36 TO 48 COOKIES

Since finding a suitable non-hydrogenated margarine was difficult in my early dairy-free years, and living without home-baked cookies was not an option, I decided to venture into baking with oil. The results were surprisingly successful, and these cookies have become a staple at parties and in our home over the years. In fact, I have to act quickly when I take them out of the oven, before hungry hands attempt to tear the hot cookies right off the sheet!

2½ cups all-purpose flour or whole wheat pastry flour
1 teaspoon baking soda
½ teaspoon salt
1 cup firmly packed brown sugar
½ cup cane sugar
½ cup grapeseed, extra-light olive, rice bran, or melted coconut oil
1 to 2 tablespoons plain or unsweetened plain dairy-free milk beverage
1 teaspoon vanilla extract
2 large eggs (see Vegan Option below for egg free)
1 cup dairy-free semi-sweet chocolate chips

1. Preheat your oven to 375°F and line baking sheets with parchment paper or silicone baking mats.
2. In a medium bowl, whisk together the flour, baking soda, and salt.
3. Put the brown sugar, cane sugar, oil, milk beverage (1 tablespoon for puffier cookies, 2 tablespoons for flatter, chewier cookies), and vanilla in a large mixing bowl. Beat with a hand mixer until creamy.
4. Add the eggs to the mixing bowl and beat with a hand mixer until smooth. Gradually stir or beat in the flour mixture until fully incorporated. Fold in the chocolate chips.
5. Drop the dough by the large teaspoonful onto your prepared baking sheets about 2 inches apart.
6. Bake for 10 to 12 minutes, or until the cookies just begin to take on a light-brown hue.
7. Let cool on the baking sheets for 2 minutes before removing the cookies to a wire rack to cool completely.
8. Store in an airtight container at room temperature for up to 1 week, or put the cookies in plastic freezer bags and freeze to enjoy later.

VEGAN OPTION

Substitute a scant ½ cup (about 7 tablespoons) plain or unsweetened dairy-free yogurt plus 2 tablespoons ground flaxseed for the eggs.

COFFEEHOUSE COOKIES

MAKES 12 COOKIES

This fun java-inspired recipe was created by my good friend Hannah Kaminsky of BittersweetBlog.com. Hannah is a popular vegan cookbook author and a daily coffee connoisseur who isn't shy with caffeine infusions. But use caution when selecting your chocolate-covered ingredient; some brands do contain dairy. See GoDairyFree.org/gdf-ingredients for some dairy-free options.

1 cup all-purpose flour
1 teaspoon instant coffee powder
1 teaspoon baking powder
½ teaspoon baking soda
¼ teaspoon cream of tartar
¼ teaspoon salt
½ cup dark chocolate–covered espresso beans
¼ cup firmly packed dark brown sugar
¼ cup grapeseed, rice bran, or other neutral-tasting oil (see page 146)
¼ cup agave nectar or corn syrup
2 teaspoons vanilla extract

1. Preheat your oven to 350°F and line a baking sheet with parchment paper or a silicone baking mat.
2. In a large bowl, whisk together the flour, coffee powder, baking powder, baking soda, cream of tartar, and salt. Stir in the espresso beans.
3. Put the brown sugar, oil, liquid sweetener, and vanilla in a medium mixing bowl. Beat with a hand mixer until emulsified.
4. Pour the wet mixture into the dry ingredients and gently stir to combine.
5. Scoop relatively large balls of dough (slightly smaller than golf balls), roll them lightly into balls, and lightly flatten them onto your prepared baking sheet about 2 inches apart.
6. Bake for 8 to 12 minutes, or until slightly golden around the edges.
7. Let cool on the baking sheet for 15 minutes before removing the cookies to a wire rack to cool completely.
8. Store in an airtight container at room temperature for up to 1 week, or put the cookies in plastic freezer bags and freeze to enjoy later.

SOFT AND CHEWY OATMEAL COOKIES

MAKES 60 COOKIES

These cookies come out crispy on the outside but wonderfully soft and doughy on the inside. They may look a bit puffy when they emerge from the oven but will settle a bit as they cool.

 2 cups all-purpose flour or whole wheat pastry flour (increase to 2¼ cups above 4,000 feet)
 3 cups quick oats
 1 teaspoon ground cinnamon
 1 teaspoon baking soda
 ½ teaspoon salt
 1 cup dairy-free buttery spread or BAKEABLE BUTTER (page 192), softened (reduce to ¾ cup above 4,000 feet)
 1 cup firmly packed brown sugar
 ½ cup cane sugar
 6 tablespoons unsweetened applesauce (increase to ½ cup above 4,000 feet)
 2 tablespoons molasses
 1 teaspoon vanilla extract
 1 cup raisins or dried cranberries

1. Preheat your oven to 375°F and line baking sheets with parchment paper or silicone baking mats.

2. In a large bowl, whisk together the flour, oats, cinnamon, baking soda, and salt.

3. Put the buttery spread, brown sugar, and cane sugar in a large mixing bowl. Beat with a hand mixer until creamy. Add the applesauce, molasses, and vanilla and beat until creamy.

4. Gradually stir the dry mixture into the wet mixture until fully incorporated. Fold in the raisins or dried cranberries.

5. Shape the dough into walnut-size balls and place them on your prepared baking sheets about 2 inches apart.

6. Bake for 8 to 10 minutes (10 to 12 minutes above 4,000 feet) for soft and chewy cookies, or up to 12 minutes (14 minutes above 4,000 feet) for crispy cookies.

7. Let cool on the baking sheets for 3 minutes before removing the cookies to a wire rack to cool completely.

8. Store in an airtight container at room temperature for up to 1 week, or put the cookies in plastic freezer bags and freeze to enjoy later.

MAPLE PUMPKIN SPICE COOKIES

MAKES 30 TO 36 COOKIES

These wonderfully soft pumpkin cookies came onto my radar from a food allergy mom friend named Barb. I made a few tweaks for flavor, texture, and versatility and a new cookie addiction was born!

2 cups all-purpose flour
1 teaspoon baking powder
1 teaspoon baking soda
½ teaspoon salt
½ teaspoon + 1 teaspoon ground cinnamon, divided
¼ teaspoon ground nutmeg (can substitute more ground cinnamon)
1 cup pumpkin puree
1 cup + 2 teaspoons cane sugar, divided
½ cup organic palm shortening (can substitute melted coconut oil for chewier cookies)
2 tablespoons maple syrup
1 teaspoon vanilla extract

1. Preheat your oven to 350°F and line baking sheets with parchment paper or silicone baking mats.
2. In a medium bowl, whisk together the flour, baking powder, baking soda, salt, ½ teaspoon cinnamon, and nutmeg.
3. Add the pumpkin puree, 1 cup sugar, shortening, maple syrup, and vanilla to a large mixing bowl. Beat with a hand mixer until light and fluffy.
4. Gradually stir the flour mixture into the wet mixture. The dough will be rather sticky. If needed, chill the dough for 1 hour to make it a bit more manageable.
5. Drop the dough by the heaping tablespoonful onto baking sheets about 2 inches apart.
6. In a small bowl, whisk together the remaining 2 teaspoons sugar and remaining 1 teaspoon cinnamon. Evenly sprinkle the mixture on the cookie dough tops.
7. Bake for 10 to 14 minutes, or until the tops take on a golden hue.
8. Let cool on the baking sheets for 3 minutes before removing the cookies to a wire rack to cool completely.
9. Store in an airtight container at room temperature for up to 1 week, or put the cookies in plastic freezer bags and freeze to enjoy later.

FUDGE BROWNIE COOKIES

MAKES 24 COOKIES

These chocolaty cookies were the surprising result of several failed vegan brownie attempts. Naturally tender, chewy, and delicious with no need for eggs at all, these cookies were devoured at a dinner party in mere minutes. Of course, I didn't mention the secret ingredient . . .

1 cup all-purpose flour or whole wheat pastry flour
¼ cup cocoa powder
½ teaspoon baking soda
¼ teaspoon salt
1 cup cane sugar
6 tablespoons grapeseed, olive, rice bran, or melted coconut oil (reduce to ¼ cup above 4,000 feet)
6 tablespoons mashed ripe avocado (about 1 medium avocado)
1½ teaspoons vanilla extract
½ cup dairy-free semi-sweet chocolate chips

1. Preheat your oven to 375°F and line baking sheets with parchment paper or silicone baking mats.
2. In a medium bowl, whisk together the flour, cocoa powder, baking soda, and salt.
3. Put the sugar, oil, avocado, and vanilla in a medium mixing bowl. Beat with a hand mixer until combined and relatively creamy.
4. Gradually stir the flour mixture into the wet mixture. Fold in the chocolate chips. The dough will be rather stiff, so you may need to press some of the chocolate chips in when shaping.
5. Shape the dough into walnut-size balls and flatten them slightly onto your prepared baking sheets about 2 inches apart.
6. Bake for 10 to 12 minutes, or until the cookies appear baked on the outside but are soft in the center. Do not overbake them. The cookies will fall a bit as they cool.
7. Let cool on the baking sheets for 3 minutes before removing the cookies to a wire rack to cool completely.
8. Store in an airtight container at room temperature for up to 1 week, or put the cookies in plastic freezer bags and freeze to enjoy later.

GLUTEN-FREE OPTION

Substitute 1 cup oat flour (certified gluten free, if needed) for the flour and reduce the oil to ¼ cup.

GIRL SCOUT CARAMEL DELIGHT COOKIES

MAKES 24 COOKIES

Over the years, Girl Scout cookie producers have been adding more dairy-free options. But the ever-popular Caramel deLites (otherwise known as Samoas) are still loaded with milky ingredients. So I decided to make my own. They're a little more work than your average cookie, but very rewarding.

> ½ cup dairy-free buttery spread or BAKEABLE BUTTER (page 192)
> ¼ cup cane sugar
> 1 tablespoon unsweetened plain dairy-free milk beverage
> ½ teaspoon + ½ teaspoon vanilla extract, divided
> 1 to 1¼ cups all-purpose flour (up to 1½ cups above 4,000 feet)
> ⅛ teaspoon baking powder
> ⅛ teaspoon + ¼ teaspoon salt, divided
> 1 cup full-fat coconut milk
> ⅔ cup firmly packed brown sugar
> 1¼ to 1½ cups unsweetened shredded coconut
> 1 cup dairy-free semi-sweet chocolate chips
> 1 tablespoon coconut oil, buttery spread, or organic palm shortening

1. Preheat your oven to 350°F and line baking sheets with parchment paper or silicone baking mats.

2. Put the buttery spread, cane sugar, milk beverage, and ½ teaspoon vanilla in a medium mixing bowl. Beat with a hand mixer until creamy.

3. Add the 1 cup flour, baking powder, and ⅛ teaspoon salt to the wet ingredients and beat until well combined. Stir in up to ¼ cup of additional flour (up to ½ cup above 4,000 feet) to keep the dough from sticking to your hands.

4. Turn out the dough onto a lightly floured surface. Roll out or pat the dough until it is ⅛ to ¼ inch thick. Cut the dough with a 2¼-inch cookie or biscuit cutter. Carefully transfer the cut dough rounds to your prepared baking sheets.

5. Bake for 10 to 12 minutes (up to 16 minutes above 4,000 feet), or until the cookies just begin to brown around the edges. Let cool on the baking sheets while you prepare the caramel topping.

6. Put the coconut milk, brown sugar, and remaining ¼ teaspoon salt in a small saucepan over medium heat. Whisk to combine and bring the mixture to a low boil. Reduce the heat to medium-low, cover, and simmer for 10 minutes.

7. Uncover and continue to simmer the sauce, stirring occasionally, for 20 to 25 minutes, or until it looks like a somewhat thick caramel sauce. It will thicken more as it cools.

8. Remove the caramel mixture from the heat and stir in the remaining ½ teaspoon vanilla and the coconut. Use the maximum amount of coconut for a very thick topping.

9. Top each shortbread cookie with the caramel-coconut mixture and press it down lightly with damp hands to evenly cover.

10. Melt the chocolate chips with the oil, buttery spread, or shortening (see page 417 for How to Melt Chocolate).

11. Dip the shortbread bases in the chocolate and place them, chocolate side down, on parchment paper or a silicone baking mat to firm up. Drizzle the remaining chocolate over the tops.

12. Let the cookies sit until the chocolate is set. To speed up the process, you can place them in the refrigerator for 30 minutes.

13. Store in an airtight container at room temperature for up to 1 week, or put the cookies in plastic freezer bags and freeze to enjoy later.

RAW COOKIE DOUGH BITES

MAKES 25 TO 30 BITES

First raw eggs were the enemy. Then we found out that uncooked flour can be equally hazardous. Fortunately, all is not lost for cookie dough fans. These healthier bites offer a sweet hit that isn't overly sugary, and they are meant to be enjoyed without baking.

1½ cups raw cashews
½ cup coconut sugar (can substitute another granulated sugar)
⅓ cup flax seeds
¼ teaspoon ground cinnamon
¼ teaspoon salt
¼ cup melted coconut oil
¼ cup honey or agave nectar
¾ teaspoon pure vanilla flavoring or extract
½ cup dairy-free mini chocolate chips or add-ins of choice (optional)

1. Put the cashews, sugar, flax seeds, cinnamon, and salt in your food processor. Process until finely ground, about 1 minute.

2. Add the coconut oil, honey or agave nectar, and vanilla and process until a thick, smooth dough forms, about 2 minutes.

3. Transfer the dough to a bowl and stir in the chocolate chips or other add-ins (if using).

4. Enjoy as cookie dough or a sweet spread, or scoop the dough by the level tablespoonful and roll it into balls. Place the dough balls on plates lined with wax paper or parchment paper and lightly flatten them into thick cookie shapes.

5. Place the plates in the refrigerator and chill for 1 hour, or until the cookie dough bites have set up.

6. Store in an airtight container in the refrigerator for up to 3 weeks, or put the dough bites in plastic freezer bags and freeze to enjoy later.

NO FOOD PROCESSOR? *Put the cashews, sugar, flax seeds, cinnamon, and salt in your spice grinder and process until finely ground, about 30 seconds. You may need to do this in 3 or 4 batches, depending on the size of your grinder. Scrape the meal into a medium bowl and stir in the coconut oil, honey, and vanilla until thoroughly combined and smooth. Continue with the recipe starting at step 3.*

SALTY VARIATION

For salted cookie dough bites, increase the salt to ½ teaspoon and optionally sprinkle a few crystals of coarse sea salt atop each bite.

ENCHANTED BARS

MAKES 36 BARS

Made famous by a well-known sweetened condensed milk brand, magic cookie bars have a rich history that dates back to the 1800s. I've conjured up a dairy-free version that is reminiscent of those classic treats, but unique enough to deserve a charming new name.

2 to 2½ cups graham cracker or cookie crumbs (gluten free, if needed)
½ cup dairy-free buttery spread, melted (can substitute ¼ cup coconut oil +
    1 tablespoon grapeseed, rice bran, or other neutral-tasting oil)
¼ teaspoon ground cinnamon
Pinch salt
2 cups dairy-free semi-sweet mini chocolate chips
1⅓ cups unsweetened coconut flakes (can substitute sweetened shredded coconut
    for sweeter bars)
1 cup chopped walnuts, pecans, or cashews, optionally roasted and salted
    (omit for nut free)
1 batch EVERYDAY SWEETENED CONDENSED COCONUT MILK (page 191) or
    INSTANT SWEETENED CONDENSED MYLK (page 192)

1. Preheat your oven to 350°F and line a 9 × 13-inch baking dish with parchment paper.
2. Put 2 cups cracker or cookie crumbs in a medium bowl. Add the buttery spread, cinnamon, and salt and stir to evenly coat. If the mixture is a little too wet and greasy, add up to ½ cup more crumbs to get a moist, somewhat cohesive crumb mixture.
3. Firmly press the crumb mixture evenly into your prepared pan.
4. Put the chocolate chips, coconut, and nuts in your now-empty bowl. Drizzle on the sweetened condensed coconut milk and stir to evenly distribute and coat the ingredients.
5. Scrape the mixture onto the crust and gently spread it into an even layer.
6. Bake for 25 minutes, or until lightly browned around the edges.
7. Let cool completely, and optionally refrigerate, before lifting the parchment paper from the baking dish and placing the bars on a cutting board. Cut into small bars; they are very rich.
8. Store in an airtight container at room temperature or in the refrigerator for up to 3 days. Individual bars can be wrapped in plastic wrap and frozen to enjoy later.

CHIA BERRY CRUMB BARS

MAKES 9 TO 12 BARS

Classic crumb bars are loaded with butter and copious amounts of sugar. This delicious version is made dairy free with coconut oil, although you can substitute dairy-free buttery spread in a pinch. They're also more wholesome with chia seeds, less sugar, and the option for whole-grain flour.

> 1 cup all-purpose flour, whole wheat flour, or oat flour (certified gluten free, if needed)
> ½ cup packed brown sugar or coconut sugar
> ¼ teaspoon baking soda
> ¼ teaspoon salt
> 6 tablespoons coconut oil
> 2 tablespoons honey (can substitute agave nectar for vegan)
> 1 batch ROCKIN' RASPBERRY CHIA JAM (page 284)

1. Preheat your oven to 350°F and grease and flour an 8 × 8-inch baking dish.
2. Put the flour, sugar, baking soda, and salt in a large bowl and whisk to combine. Add the oil and honey and whisk until coarse crumbs form.
3. Press 2 cups of the crumb mixture firmly and evenly into the bottom of your prepared pan. Evenly spread on the chia jam to about ¼ inch from the edge. Evenly sprinkle the chia jam with the remaining streusel mixture and lightly press it down.
4. Bake for 20 to 25 minutes, or until golden.
5. Let cool completely before cutting into bars.
6. Cover and store at room temperature for up to 1 day or in the refrigerator for up to 3 days. Individual bars can be wrapped in plastic wrap and frozen to enjoy later.

O'HENRY BARS

MAKES 40 BARS

Sarah Hatfield, my associate editor, shared this updated version of her dairy-free recipe for homemade peanut butter Oh Henry! bars. They are a family favorite and impossible to resist!

    1 cup firmly packed brown sugar
    ⅔ cup dairy-free buttery spread or BAKEABLE BUTTER (page 192)
    4 cups rolled or quick oats (certified gluten free, if needed)
    ½ cup honey (can substitute corn syrup or agave nectar for vegan)
    1 tablespoon vanilla extract
    1 cup dairy-free semi-sweet chocolate chips
    ⅔ cup chunky peanut butter (can substitute sunflower seed butter for peanut free)

1. Preheat your oven to 350°F and grease a jelly roll pan or cookie sheet with high sides or line it with parchment paper.
2. Put the brown sugar and buttery spread in a large mixing bowl. Beat with a hand mixer until creamy. Add the oats, honey, and vanilla and stir to combine.
3. Pat the oat mixture firmly into your prepared pan.
4. Bake for 15 minutes, or until the center is just barely firm. Let cool completely.
5. Melt the chocolate chips with the peanut butter (see page 417 for How to Melt Chocolate).
6. Evenly spread the chocolate mixture on top of the oatmeal layer.
7. Let cool to room temperature and then refrigerate for 15 minutes before cutting into bars.
8. Cover and store at room temperature or in the refrigerator for up to 3 days. Individual bars can be wrapped in plastic wrap and frozen to enjoy later.

FABULOUS FUDGE BROWNIES

MAKES 9 TO 12 BROWNIES

This dessert is a house favorite, whether served alone or à la mode. I prefer the brownies cooled so that the chocolate chips re-solidify, but my husband likes them warm and gooey.

    ¾ cup baking flour of choice (see Flour Note following)
    ¼ cup cocoa powder
    ¼ teaspoon salt
    1 cup cane sugar
    2 large eggs (see Vegan Dark Chocolate Brownie Option following for egg free)
    ¼ cup grapeseed, olive, rice bran, or melted coconut oil
    1½ teaspoons vanilla extract
    ½ cup unsweetened shredded coconut (optional)
    ⅓ to ½ cup dairy-free semi-sweet or dark chocolate chips
    ¼ cup chopped walnuts (optional)

1. Preheat your oven to 350°F and grease an 8 × 8-inch baking dish.
2. In a medium bowl, whisk together the flour, cocoa powder, and salt.
3. Put the sugar, eggs, oil, and vanilla in a medium mixing bowl. Whisk or beat with a hand mixer until creamy.
4. Gradually stir the flour mixture into the wet mixture. Fold in the coconut (if using).
5. Scrape the batter into your prepared dish and level it out. Sprinkle the chocolate chips and nuts (if using) evenly over the brownie batter.
6. Bake for 25 to 35 minutes, or until a toothpick inserted into the center of the brownies comes out clean and the brownies are relatively firm to the touch.
7. Let cool for at least 10 minutes before cutting. They will set up more as they cool.
8. Cover and store at room temperature or in the refrigerator for up to 3 days. Individual brownies can be wrapped in plastic wrap and frozen to enjoy later.

FLOUR NOTE: All-purpose, whole wheat, spelt, and other wheat flours produce great results in this recipe. For gluten-free brownie lovers, I have successfully made this recipe with various types of grain-based gluten-free flours (like rice, millet, and sorghum) and all-purpose gluten-free flour blends. However, I would avoid using single grain-free flours, like coconut, almond, and chickpea/garbanzo bean. These might produce dry or overly dense results.

VEGAN DARK CHOCOLATE BROWNIE OPTION

Eggs are an integral component in brownies, which is why I couldn't suggest a simple swap. For the vegan version, increase the cocoa powder to ½ cup and add 1 tablespoon ground flaxseed and ¼ teaspoon baking soda to the dry ingredients. In the wet ingredients, increase the oil to 5 tablespoons (use 3 tablespoons oil plus 2 tablespoons water above 4,000 feet), decrease the sugar to ⅓ cup, and add ⅓ cup maple syrup or your liquid sweetener of choice. Prepare and bake as instructed above.

PEANUT BUTTER BROWNIE VARIATION

Add 2 heaping tablespoons peanut butter or sunflower seed butter to the wet mixture. You can still use or omit the coconut or walnuts—it's delicious each way!

LEMON STREUSEL SQUARES

MAKES 16 BARS

A while back, I came across an intriguing recipe on the Internet for lemon streusel bars. While I do enjoy lemon bars, the concept of a brown sugar streusel sounded so much better. However, the recipe called for sweetened condensed milk. After some experimentation, I created a delicious sweetened condensed coconut milk, which works perfectly in this recipe.

1 batch RICH SWEETENED CONDENSED COCONUT MILK (page 190)
⅓ to ½ cup fresh-squeezed lemon juice (about 2 lemons; see Lemon Note below)
2 teaspoons grated lemon zest
¾ cup dairy-free buttery spread or organic palm shortening, softened
1 cup firmly packed brown sugar
2 cups all-purpose flour or whole wheat pastry flour
1½ cups rolled oats
¼ teaspoon salt

1. Preheat your oven to 350°F and grease an 8 × 8-inch, 9 × 9-inch, or 7 × 11-inch baking dish.
2. In a medium bowl, whisk together the sweetened condensed coconut milk, lemon juice, and lemon zest.
3. Put the buttery spread or shortening and brown sugar in a large mixing bowl. Beat with a hand mixer until creamy. Add the flour, oats, and salt and whisk until coarse crumbs form.
4. Set aside 2 cups of the streusel mixture and press the remaining streusel into the bottom of your prepared baking dish.
5. Spread the lemon-coconut filling over the streusel crust. Sprinkle the filling with the reserved 2 cups streusel. Gently pat the streusel into the filling.
6. Bake for 30 to 35 minutes (or 35 to 45 minutes if using an 8 × 8-inch dish), or until the streusel is lightly golden and slightly firm to the touch.
7. Let cool completely before cutting into fourths each way.
8. Cover and store at room temperature or in the refrigerator for up to 3 days. Individual lemon squares can be wrapped in plastic wrap and frozen to enjoy later.

LEMON NOTE: My lemon-loving in-laws said, "Bring on the lemon!" They loved the bars with a full ½ cup of lemon juice, proclaiming that even more would be good. My husband and my grandmother, however, like lemon in moderation. They preferred the bars with ⅓ cup lemon juice, which had a little less bite. I liked both. You choose which version works best for you.

LEMON STREUSEL TARTLETS VARIATION

Pat the streusel base into 16 muffin cups lined with cupcake liners. Divide the filling evenly between the muffin cups, and top each with the remaining streusel. Pat the streusel gently into the filling. Bake for 20 to 25 minutes, or until the tops are golden and they appear set. Allow the tartlets to cool in the cups for at least 10 minutes before serving.

CHAPTER 31

TAKE THE CAKE

All-Occasion Cake and Frosting Recipes

GOOD TO KNOW FOR THIS CHAPTER

CAKES CAN BE TOO BOISTEROUS AT HIGH ALTITUDE. If you live above 4,000 feet, cake recipes often require minor modifications for best results. I've tested the following recipes at 4,500 feet and included high altitude adjustments, if needed. Most of the time, a simple leavener reduction does the trick. I usually reduce both the baking soda and the baking powder by 25 to 50 percent (the latter at 5,000 feet or above). In some cases where both baking soda and baking powder are required, I might just omit the baking powder.

YOU CAN SOLVE SUNKEN CUPCAKES. At high altitudes, sunken cupcakes usually indicate too much leavener. If they are just lightly indented, reduce the leavener by 25 percent on the next batch, but if they are completely caved in, reduce the leavener by 50 percent. At low altitudes, overly moist cupcakes or not enough leavener is more often the cause. Add a little more flour in your next batch or increase the baking powder by ⅛ to ½ teaspoon. If you aren't vegan or allergic to eggs, and the recipe doesn't include eggs, it can help to add 1 or 2 eggs (no other adjustments needed) with the wet ingredients. Eggs help in both rising and fortifying the cake structure. As for the failed batch, fill the indent with frosting, jam, or another filling, and enjoy!

MAKE THEM SPECIAL WITH TOPPINGS. This is a mix-and-match style chapter with all the basic cake and frosting needs, plus a couple of fun extras. You can garnish them for various occasions with natural sprinkles, dairy-free cookie or graham crumbles, whole or half dairy-free cookies, fresh berries, dairy-free chocolate chips, melted and molded dairy-free chocolate (recipes starting on page 419), or favorite candies.

BAKING WITH BOX CAKE MIXES

Birthday cakes are a big deal in the dairy-free world, especially when dealing with milk-allergic or intolerant little ones. While I always prefer a cake baked from scratch, you still have some options when it comes to cake mixes. These can be especially helpful for someone who isn't dairy free but is baking for a party with dairy-free or vegan guests.

START WITH

1 box dairy-free cake mix (see Choosing Your Cake Mix below)

WHISK IN ONE OF THE FOLLOWING

BOX INGREDIENTS: Some cake mixes are dairy free from start to finish. They merely call for eggs, oil, and water. Vegan cake mixes, which don't call for eggs, are also available.

MODIFIED BOX INGREDIENTS: If the cake mix calls for milk, substitute an equal amount of your favorite plain or unsweetened plain milk beverage. If the cake mix calls for butter, substitute an equal amount of dairy-free buttery sticks (if creaming) or neutral-tasting oil (if melted; see page 146). If you want to replace the eggs, visit **GoDairyFree.org/egg-subs** for options.

PUMPKIN PUREE: Use one 15-ounce can pumpkin puree in place of the eggs, oil, and water. The results will be a little more dense and moist, but are loved by many. This is a great option for white, chocolate, carrot, or spice cake mixes.

SODA: Use one 12-ounce can plain seltzer water or flavored soda in place of the oil, water, and even the eggs for a vegan cake. Just be sure to choose a variety that goes well with the flavor of your cake. The results will be quite moist, but many people like this version better than using the box ingredients.

CHOOSING YOUR CAKE MIX: *Surprisingly, dozens of brands and flavors are dairy free, and there are even vegan and allergy-friendly options available. The mainstream brands work best with the options above, and many are kosher pareve. However, some of the smaller brands include their own options for special diet baking. I've listed a bunch at* **GoDairyFree.org/cake**.

BANANA CRUMB COFFEE CAKE

MAKES 9 TO 12 SERVINGS

According to my husband, this cake could be sold at Starbucks. The first time I made it, the two of us polished off the entire pan within 24 hours. Since our waistlines don't need quite that much cake, I now make sure to bake it when there are more mouths around to feed. Nonetheless, if you are making this for a get-together or a bigger household, you can double the entire recipe and bake it in a 9 × 13-inch pan.

CRUMB TOPPING
⅓ cup chopped pecans or walnuts (can substitute quick oats or rolled oats for nut free)
¼ cup firmly packed brown sugar
2 to 3 tablespoons all-purpose flour or whole wheat pastry flour
½ teaspoon ground cinnamon
2 tablespoons cold dairy-free buttery spread or coconut oil

BANANA CAKE
1½ cups all-purpose flour (can substitute part whole wheat pastry flour)
1 teaspoon baking powder
½ teaspoon baking soda (reduce to ¼ teaspoon above 4,000 feet)
½ teaspoon ground cinnamon
¼ teaspoon ground nutmeg
¼ teaspoon salt (⅜ teaspoon if using oil)
1 cup ripe mashed banana (2 to 3 bananas)
¼ cup coconut oil or dairy-free buttery spread, softened or melted
    (can substitute your favorite baking oil)
¼ cup firmly packed brown sugar
¼ cup cane sugar
3 tablespoons maple syrup
1 tablespoon ground flaxseed

1. Preheat your oven to 350°F and grease an 8 × 8-inch baking dish.
2. **To make the crumb topping**, put the nuts, brown sugar, 2 tablespoons flour, and cinnamon in a medium bowl and whisk to combine. Add the buttery spread or oil and whisk until coarse crumbs form. If the mixture is too wet, whisk in 1 more tablespoon flour.
3. **To make the banana cake**, put the flour, baking powder, baking soda, cinnamon, nutmeg, and salt in a medium bowl and whisk to combine.
4. Put the banana, oil or buttery spread, brown sugar, cane sugar, maple syrup, and flaxseed in a large mixing bowl. Beat with a hand mixer until relatively smooth and creamy.
5. Add the dry mixture to the wet mixture and stir to combine. Do not overmix; some small lumps are okay.
6. Scrape the batter into your prepared baking dish and level it out. Evenly sprinkle the crumb topping on the batter.
7. Bake for 30 to 40 minutes, or until a toothpick inserted into the center of the cake comes out clean.
8. Cover and store at room temperature for up to 2 days. Individual slices can be wrapped in plastic wrap and frozen to enjoy later.

SWEET APPLE SNACKIN' CAKE

MAKES 9 TO 12 SERVINGS

I typically use Granny Smith or Golden Delicious apples in this wonderfully moist and tender cake. They stay a bit firm when baked and offer a nice contrast to the sweetness.

    1⅔ cups all-purpose flour or whole wheat pastry flour
    1 teaspoon baking soda (reduce to ½ teaspoon above 4,000 feet)
    1 teaspoon ground cinnamon
    ⅛ teaspoon ground nutmeg
    ¼ teaspoon salt
    ¾ cup unsweetened applesauce
    ½ cup dairy-free buttery spread or organic palm shortening, softened
        (can substitute your favorite baking oil)
    ½ cup firmly packed brown sugar
    ½ cup cane sugar (reduce by 1 tablespoon above 4,000 feet)
    1 tablespoon white vinegar or apple cider vinegar
    1 or 2 apples, peeled, cored, and cut into ¼-inch-thick slices or chunks

1. Preheat your oven to 350°F and grease an 8 × 8-inch baking dish.
2. Place the flour, baking soda, cinnamon, nutmeg, and salt in a medium bowl and whisk to combine.
3. Add the applesauce, buttery spread or shortening, brown sugar, cane sugar, and vinegar to a large mixing bowl. Beat with a hand mixer until relatively creamy.
4. Add the dry mixture to the wet mixture and stir to combine. Do not overmix; some small lumps are okay. The batter will be quite thick.
5. Layer the apple chunks or slices in the bottom of your prepared baking dish.
6. Scrape the batter over the top of the apples and level it out.
7. Bake for 25 to 35 minutes (30 to 40 minutes above 4,000 feet), or until the cake is firm to the touch and a toothpick inserted into the center of the cake comes out clean. Let cool for 10 minutes in the pan.
8. Run a knife around the edge of the cake to loosen. Invert the cake onto a plate or cutting board to release it before slicing.
9. Cover and store at room temperature for up to 1 day, or in the refrigerator for up to 3 days. Individual slices can be wrapped in plastic wrap and frozen to enjoy later.

YELLOW BIRTHDAY CAKE

MAKES TWO 9-INCH CAKE LAYERS (10 TO 12 SERVINGS)

There is something so rewarding about baking a birthday cake from scratch. This versatile cake can be dressed up any way you like it, and was even the base recipe I adapted to create my PINEAPPLE UPSIDE-DOWN CAKE recipe (page 376).

    2¾ cups all-purpose flour
    1½ teaspoons baking powder (reduce to 1 teaspoon above 4,000 feet)

½ teaspoon baking soda

½ teaspoon salt

4 large eggs, separated

¾ cup dairy-free buttery spread, softened (can substitute a neutral-tasting oil, see page 146)

2 cups cane sugar (reduce to 1¾ cups above 4,000 feet)

1 tablespoon white vinegar or apple cider vinegar

2 teaspoons vanilla extract

1 cup + 3 tablespoons dairy-free milk beverage

1 batch frosting recipe of choice (recipes beginning on page 384) (optional)

1. Preheat your oven to 350°F and grease and flour a 9 × 13-inch baking dish or two 9-inch round cake pans.

2. In a large bowl, whisk together the flour, baking powder, baking soda, and salt.

3. Put the egg whites in a medium mixing bowl. Beat with your hand mixer until the whites fluff up and are stiff but not dry.

4. Put the buttery spread and sugar in a large mixing bowl. Beat with your hand mixer until creamy. Add the egg yolks, vinegar, and vanilla and beat for 2 minutes, or until the mixture looks light and fluffy.

5. Add about one-third of the flour mixture to the wet mixture in your large mixing bowl, followed by about one-third of the milk beverage, and beat just to combine; do not overmix. Repeat two more times until the flour mixture and milk beverage are used up.

6. Gently fold the stiff egg whites into the batter.

7. Scrape the batter into your prepared pan(s) and even it out.

8. Bake for 35 minutes, or until a toothpick inserted into the center of the cake comes out clean.

9. Let cool for 15 minutes in the pan(s), before removing the cake(s) to a wire rack to cool completely before frosting.

10. Cover the unfrosted cake and store at room temperature for up to 2 days. Once frosted, it should be refrigerated for up to 3 days, or individual slices can be wrapped in plastic wrap and frozen to enjoy later.

VEGAN OPTION

The yellow color in this type of cake typically comes from egg yolks. But with a few changes, this dessert can be egg free. Omit the eggs. Increase the milk beverage to a scant 1¾ cups, the flour to 3 cups, the baking powder to 2 teaspoons (1¾ teaspoons above 4,000 feet), and the baking soda to 1 teaspoon (½ teaspoon above 4,000 feet). Add ½ teaspoon ground turmeric to the dry ingredients to achieve a notable yellow hue. Bake as directed above. The vegan option will also fit into 8-inch round pans, but with the smaller pans, the baking time should be reduced to 20 to 28 minutes.

CUPCAKE VARIATION

Line 24 muffin cups with cupcake liners. Divide the batter between the liners and bake at 350°F for 20 to 26 minutes, or until a toothpick inserted into the center of a cupcake comes out clean.

PINEAPPLE UPSIDE-DOWN CAKE

MAKES 18 TO 24 SERVINGS

The first time I baked this cake was for my Hawaiian food–loving friend, Barb. It has a moist crumb and perfectly gooey topping that's impossible to resist. I make it as one large cake, but you can divide the ingredients between two 9-inch round cake pans, if preferred.

6 tablespoons + ¾ cup dairy-free buttery spread, divided
½ cup firmly packed brown sugar
⅓ cup sweetened or unsweetened shredded coconut (optional)
1½ cups crushed pineapple, drained but juice reserved
2¾ cups all-purpose flour
1½ teaspoons baking powder (reduce to 1 teaspoon above 4,000 feet)
½ teaspoon baking soda
½ teaspoon salt
4 large eggs, separated
2 cups cane sugar (reduce to 1¾ cups above 4,000 feet)
2 teaspoons vanilla extract
1¼ cups pineapple juice

1. Preheat your oven to 350°F.
2. Melt the 6 tablespoons buttery spread and pour it into a 9 × 13-inch baking dish. Tilt the pan to evenly distribute the buttery spread. Evenly sprinkle on the brown sugar and coconut (if using). Spread the crushed pineapple evenly over the top.
3. In a large bowl, whisk together the flour, baking powder, baking soda, and salt.
4. Put the egg whites in a medium mixing bowl. Beat with your hand mixer until the whites fluff up and are stiff but not dry.
5. Put the remaining ¾ cup buttery spread and sugar in a large mixing bowl. Beat with your hand mixer until creamy. Add the egg yolks and vanilla and beat for 2 minutes, or until the mixture looks light and fluffy.
6. Add about one-third of the flour mixture to the wet mixture in your large mixing bowl, followed by about one-third of the pineapple juice, and beat just to combine; do not overmix. Repeat two more times until the flour mixture and juice are used up.
7. Gently fold the stiff egg whites into the batter.
8. Scrape the batter into your prepared pan and even it out.
9. Bake for 35 minutes, or until a toothpick inserted into the center of the cake comes out clean.
10. Run a knife around the edge of the cake to loosen. Invert the cake onto a serving platter or cutting board to release it before slicing.
11. Cover and store at room temperature for up to 1 day, or in the refrigerator for up to 3 days. Individual slices can be wrapped in plastic wrap and frozen to enjoy later.

> ### VEGAN OPTION
>
> Omit the eggs. Increase the pineapple juice to a scant 1¾ cups, the flour to 3 cups, the baking powder to 2 teaspoons (1¾ teaspoons above 4,000 feet), and the baking soda to 1 teaspoon (½ teaspoon above 4,000 feet). Bake as directed above.

SIMPLY WONDERFUL WHITE CAKE

MAKES 10 TO 12 SERVINGS

This classic cake is delightfully sweet, but not too sweet, allowing the frosting to take center stage. But if desired, you can increase the sugar to 1 cup. For a birthday cake, double the entire recipe and bake it in a 9 × 13-inch pan or two 8-inch round cake pans.

1½ cups all-purpose flour
1 teaspoon baking powder (reduce to ¾ teaspoon above 4,000 feet)
1 teaspoon baking soda (reduce to ½ teaspoon above 4,000 feet)
½ teaspoon salt
¾ cup cane sugar
¼ cup grapeseed, rice bran, or other neutral-tasting oil (see page 146)
1 tablespoon white vinegar
1 teaspoon vanilla extract
1 cup plain or vanilla dairy-free milk beverage
1 batch frosting recipe of choice (recipes beginning on page 384) (optional)

1. Preheat your oven to 350°F and grease an 8 × 8-inch baking dish.
2. In a medium bowl, whisk together the flour, baking powder, baking soda, and salt.
3. In a large mixing bowl, whisk together the sugar, oil, vinegar, and vanilla. Stir in the milk beverage. Add the flour mixture and stir until the batter is smooth.
4. Scrape the batter into your prepared baking dish and even it out.
5. Bake for 28 to 35 minutes, or until a toothpick inserted into the center of the cake comes out clean.
6. Let cool completely before frosting or slicing.
7. Cover the unfrosted cake and store at room temperature for up to 2 days. Once frosted, it should be refrigerated for up to 3 days, or individual slices can be wrapped in plastic wrap and frozen to enjoy later.

....

CUPCAKE VARIATION

Line 12 muffin cups with cupcake liners. Divide the batter between the liners and bake at 350°F for 18 to 22 minutes, or until a toothpick inserted into the center of a cupcake comes out clean.

....

CHOCOLATE WACKY CAKE

MAKES 10 TO 12 SERVINGS

Various versions of this naturally vegan war-era cake are prepared every day. Not only can it be prepared with inexpensive, common pantry items, but it is also an easy one to mix up by hand. For a birthday cake, double the entire recipe and bake it in a 9 × 13-inch pan or two 8-inch round cake pans.

1½ cups all-purpose flour
1 cup cane sugar
¼ cup cocoa powder
1 teaspoon baking soda (reduce to ½ teaspoon above 4,000 feet)
½ teaspoon salt
⅓ cup grapeseed, rice bran, or other neutral-tasting oil (see page 146)
1 tablespoon white vinegar
1 teaspoon vanilla extract
1 cup cold water or unsweetened plain or chocolate dairy-free milk beverage
1 batch frosting recipe of choice (recipes beginning on page 384) (optional)

1. Preheat your oven to 350°F and grease an 8 × 8-inch baking dish.
2. In a large bowl, whisk together the flour, sugar, cocoa powder, baking soda, and salt.
3. Make 3 small wells in the flour mixture. Pour the oil into one well, the vinegar into the second, and the vanilla into the third. Pour the cold water or milk beverage over everything and stir until a relatively smooth batter forms.
4. Scrape the batter into your prepared baking dish and even it out.
5. Bake for 30 to 35 minutes, or until a toothpick inserted into the center of the cake comes out clean.
6. Let cool completely before frosting or slicing.
7. Cover the unfrosted cake and store at room temperature for up to 2 days. Once frosted, it should be refrigerated for up to 3 days, or individual slices can be wrapped in plastic wrap and frozen to enjoy later.

CUPCAKE VARIATION

Line 12 muffin cups with cupcake liners. Divide the batter between the liners and bake at 350°F for 18 to 22 minutes, or until a toothpick inserted into the center of a cupcake comes out clean.

CARROT SPICE CUPCAKES

MAKES 16 CUPCAKES

I originally made these cupcakes for my column in *Allergic Living* magazine, so the recipe includes several special diet options. All are delicious, but the main recipe received rave reviews at a dinner party for fifteen where only the hostess was dairy free!

1½ cups all-purpose flour (see Gluten-Free Option below)
1½ teaspoons ground cinnamon
1 teaspoon baking powder
½ teaspoon baking soda
½ teaspoon ground nutmeg
¼ teaspoon ground ginger
¾ teaspoon salt
¾ cup firmly packed brown sugar
½ cup crushed pineapple with juice (do not drain)
½ cup grapeseed, rice bran, or melted coconut oil
2 large eggs (see Vegan Option below for egg free)
⅓ cup cane sugar
1¼ teaspoons vanilla extract
2 cups grated carrots
½ batch CREAM CHEEZE FROSTING (page 384)

1. Preheat your oven to 350°F and line 16 muffin cups with cupcake liners.
2. In a medium bowl, whisk together the flour, cinnamon, baking powder, baking soda, nutmeg, ginger, and salt.
3. Put the brown sugar, pineapple with juice, oil, eggs, cane sugar, and vanilla in a large mixing bowl. Beat with a hand mixer for 1 minute.
4. Add the dry mixture to the wet mixture and stir until the ingredients are just combined. Fold in the carrots.
5. Divide the batter between your prepared muffin cups. They should each be about two-thirds to three-fourths full.
6. Bake for 25 to 30 minutes, or until a toothpick inserted into the center of a cupcake comes out clean.
7. Remove the cupcakes to a wire rack to cool completely before frosting.
8. Store unfrosted cupcakes in an airtight container at room temperature for up to 1 day or in the refrigerator for up to 3 days. Once frosted, the cupcakes should be refrigerated or individually wrapped in plastic wrap and frozen to enjoy later.

GLUTEN-FREE OPTION

Substitute 1 cup brown rice flour (superfine if possible), ¼ cup tapioca starch, ¼ cup potato starch, and ¼ teaspoon xanthan gum for the all-purpose flour.

VEGAN OPTION

Omit the eggs and cane sugar. Add ¼ cup honey or agave nectar with the wet ingredients. Increase the baking soda to 1 teaspoon (½ teaspoon above 4,000 feet). This makes just 12 cupcakes.

ORANGE CHOCOLATE CHUNK CUPCAKES

MAKES 12 CUPCAKES

This is a special recipe that my friend Hannah Kaminsky shared with me specifically for this book. The cupcakes are naturally infused with orange, spiked with dark chocolate chunks, and garnished with a rich chocolate ganache.

1⅓ cups all-purpose flour
½ teaspoon baking powder (reduce to ¼ teaspoon above 4,000 feet)
½ teaspoon baking soda (reduce to ¼ teaspoon above 4,000 feet)
¼ teaspoon salt
3 ounces dairy-free dark chocolate, chopped
1 cup orange juice (fresh-squeezed if possible; about 4 oranges)
½ cup cane sugar
⅓ cup grapeseed, rice bran, or other neutral-tasting oil (see page 146)
1½ teaspoons grated orange zest
¼ teaspoon vanilla extract
1 batch DARK CHOCOLATE GANACHE FROSTING (page 387)

1. Preheat your oven to 350°F and line 12 muffin cups with cupcake liners.
2. In a large bowl, whisk together the flour, baking powder, baking soda, and salt. Stir in the chocolate chunks.
3. In a medium bowl, whisk together the orange juice, sugar, oil, zest, and vanilla.
4. Pour the wet mixture into the dry ingredients and stir just until combined.
5. Divide the batter between your prepared muffin cups.
6. Bake for 16 to 22 minutes (22 to 26 minutes above 4,000 feet), or until a toothpick inserted into the center of a cupcake comes out clean.
7. Remove the cupcakes to a wire rack to cool completely before frosting.
8. Store unfrosted cupcakes in an airtight container at room temperature for up to 2 days or in the refrigerator for up to 3 days. Once frosted, the cupcakes should be refrigerated or individually wrapped in plastic wrap and frozen to enjoy later.

CAKE VARIATION

Pour the batter into a lightly greased 8-inch round cake pan and bake for 20 to 25 minutes (25 to 30 minutes above 4,000 feet), or until a toothpick inserted into the center of the cake comes out clean. Double the recipe for a two-layer cake.

CHOCOLATE MUG CAKE

MAKES 1 SERVING

There's no need to ever feel left out. This recipe takes mere minutes for an instant personal cake that can be whipped up wherever a microwave exists. I've even included a single-serve frosting recipe for the literal icing on the cake!

CHOCOLATE MUG CAKE

3 tablespoons all-purpose flour

2 tablespoons cane sugar

1 tablespoon cocoa powder

⅛ teaspoon baking soda (reduce to ¹⁄₁₆ teaspoon above 4,000 feet)

Generous pinch salt

2 tablespoons water or unsweetened plain dairy-free milk beverage

1 tablespoon grapeseed, olive, or rice bran oil

½ teaspoon white vinegar or apple cider vinegar

⅛ teaspoon vanilla extract

1 tablespoon dairy-free mini chocolate chips (optional)

OPTIONAL CHOCOLATE FROSTING

2 tablespoons powdered confectioners' sugar

1½ teaspoons cocoa powder

1 teaspoon dairy-free buttery spread, softened

⅛ teaspoon vanilla extract or maple syrup

½ teaspoon water or unsweetened plain dairy-free milk beverage, as needed

1. **To make the mug cake**, put the flour, sugar, cocoa powder, baking soda, and salt in a microwave-safe mug or ramekin and whisk to combine. Add the water or milk beverage, oil, vinegar, and vanilla and whisk to combine. Stir in the chocolate chips (if using).

2. Microwave the cake on high for 60 to 90 seconds, or until puffed up and gently firm to the touch. The cook time can vary by microwave, humidity, and altitude; be careful not to overcook it.

3. **To make the frosting**, put the powdered sugar and cocoa powder in a small bowl and whisk to break up any clumps. Add the buttery spread and vanilla or maple syrup and whisk until smooth. If it is too thick, whisk in the water or milk beverage.

VANILLA MUG CAKE

MAKES 1 SERVING

Vanilla fans need a single-serve treat, too! This one has an optional dairy-free buttercream for a piece of birthday cake indulgence.

VANILLA MUG CAKE

3 tablespoons all-purpose flour
1½ tablespoons cane sugar
⅛ teaspoon baking powder
Generous pinch salt
2 tablespoons water or unsweetened plain dairy-free milk beverage
1 tablespoon grapeseed, rice bran, or other neutral-tasting oil (see page 146)
¼ teaspoon white vinegar
⅛ to ¼ teaspoon vanilla extract

OPTIONAL BUTTERCREAM

1 tablespoon dairy-free buttery spread, softened
½ teaspoon dairy-free milk beverage or water
⅛ teaspoon vanilla extract
3½ to 4 tablespoons powdered confectioners' sugar, or as needed

1. **To make the mug cake**, put the flour, sugar, baking powder, and salt in a microwave-safe mug or ramekin and whisk to combine. Add the water or milk beverage, oil, vinegar, and vanilla and whisk to combine.

2. Microwave the cake on high for 60 to 90 seconds, or until puffed up and gently firm to the touch. The cook time can vary by microwave, humidity, and altitude; be careful not to overcook it.

3. **To make the buttercream**, put the buttery spread, milk beverage or water, and vanilla in a small bowl and whisk to combine. Whisk in the powdered sugar until smooth and until your desired sweetness is reached.

MINI BERRY CHEEZECAKES

MAKES 12 MINI CHEEZECAKES

Most dairy-free cheesecake recipes are a little on the soft side. But these delicious, single-serve desserts are infused with blueberries or strawberries for fruity flavor that actually helps them set up to a wonderfully rich consistency.

1½ cups raw cashews
1 batch COOKIE CRUMB CRUST, Graham Cracker Variation (page 401)
⅔ cup coconut cream, melted
½ to 1 cup freeze-dried strawberries, blueberries, or raspberries, to taste
½ to ⅔ cup honey or agave nectar, to taste
¼ cup lemon juice
¼ cup coconut oil, melted
1 teaspoon pure vanilla flavoring or extract
¼ teaspoon salt
Fresh berries or berry sauce, to serve (optional)

1. Put the cashews in a container and cover with a few inches of water. Cover and place in the refrigerator to soak for 6 hours or overnight. Drain and rinse the cashews.

2. If not using silicone muffin cups, line 12 muffin cups with cupcake liners.

3. Divide the crumb crust mixture between the muffin cups and firmly press down to pack it in as a bottom crust.

4. Put the soaked cashews, melted coconut cream, freeze-dried berries, sweetener, lemon juice, melted oil, vanilla, and salt in your blender. Blend until smooth, about 3 minutes.

5. Scrape the mixture onto your prepared crusts and level it out by tapping the muffin cups on the counter.

6. Freeze for 2 hours, or until set.

7. Pop the cheezecakes out of the muffin cups. If using cupcake liners, peel them off before serving the cheezecakes topped with fresh berries or berry sauce, if desired. They will keep fairly well at room temperature for up to 2 hours, but are best served cold.

8. Store in an airtight container in the refrigerator for up to 1 week, or individually wrap and freeze the cheezecakes to enjoy later.

WHIPPED VANILLA ICING

MAKES 2 TO 2½ CUPS (ENOUGH TO FROST AN 8- OR 9-INCH DOUBLE-LAYER CAKE)

This deliciously addictive white icing is a cross between rich frosting and fluffy whipped cream.

> 1 cup cold plain or unsweetened plain dairy-free milk beverage
> ¼ cup all-purpose flour or white rice flour (for gluten free)
> 1 teaspoon vanilla extract
> ½ cup dairy-free buttery spread or sticks, softened
> ½ cup organic palm shortening
> 1 cup cane sugar

1. In a small saucepan, whisk together the cold milk beverage and flour until no lumps remain.
2. Place the pan over medium heat. Cook, while whisking, until it takes on a pudding-like texture, about 4 minutes.
3. Remove the pan from the heat and whisk in the vanilla.
4. Put the buttery spread or sticks, shortening, and sugar in a large mixing bowl. Beat with a hand mixer until quite creamy, about 3 minutes.
5. Add the pudding-like mixture to your mixing bowl. Beat until the icing is fluffy, about 3 minutes.
6. Store leftover frosting in an airtight container in the refrigerator for up to 1 week. Beat the chilled frosting with your hand mixer for 30 seconds to soften before using.

CREAM CHEEZE FROSTING

MAKES 2 TO 2½ CUPS (ENOUGH TO FROST AN 8- OR 9-INCH DOUBLE-LAYER CAKE)

Two cups of powdered confectioners' sugar is my standard quantity in this recipe. But I find that the versatility of cream cheese frosting lends itself well to numerous recipes where more or less sweetener may be desired. So I've included a wide sweetener range for you to customize it to taste.

> 8 ounces dairy-free cream cheese alternative
> ½ cup coconut cream
> 1 teaspoon pure vanilla flavoring or extract
> Generous pinch salt
> 1 to 4 cups powdered confectioners' sugar, to taste (see headnote)

1. Put the cream cheese alternative, coconut cream, vanilla, and salt in a medium mixing bowl. Beat with a hand mixer until light and creamy, about 2 minutes.
2. Sift in the powdered sugar, 1 cup at a time, and beat on low speed to incorporate it.
3. Store leftover frosting in an airtight container in the refrigerator for up to 1 week. Beat the chilled frosting with your hand mixer for 30 seconds to soften before using.

BUTTERCREAM FROSTING

MAKES APPROXIMATELY 3 CUPS (MORE THAN ENOUGH TO FROST AN 8- OR 9-INCH DOUBLE-LAYER CAKE)

This recipe is a simple dairy-free riff on classic buttercream, and my personal go-to recipe for frosting almost any type of cake.

1 cup dairy-free buttery sticks or spread, softened
1 teaspoon pure vanilla flavoring or extract
3½ to 4 cups powdered confectioners' sugar
1 to 4 tablespoons plain or unsweetened plain dairy-free milk beverage, as needed

1. Put the buttery spread or sticks in a large mixing bowl. Beat with a hand mixer until creamy, about 2 minutes. Add the vanilla and beat just until combined.
2. Sift in the powdered sugar, 1 cup at a time, and beat on low speed to incorporate it.
3. Turn the hand mixer up to medium or high speed and whip the frosting for 2 minutes. Beat in the milk beverage as needed to reach your desired consistency.
4. Store leftover frosting in an airtight container in the refrigerator for up to 1 week. Beat the chilled frosting with your hand mixer for 30 seconds to soften before using.

FROSTING VARIATIONS

DECORATOR'S BUTTERCREAM: Substitute ½ cup organic palm shortening for ½ cup of the buttery spread or sticks.

PURE WHITE FROSTING: Substitute 1 cup organic palm shortening for all of the buttery spread or sticks and add a generous pinch of salt with the vanilla. Optionally add ½ teaspoon almond extract with the vanilla extract.

PEANUT BUTTER FUDGE FROSTING

MAKES 1½ CUPS (ENOUGH TO FROST AN 8- OR 9-INCH CAKE LAYER)

This sweet, rich, and addictive frosting is from my associate editor, Sarah Hatfield, and her peanut butter–loving household of six.

> ½ cup creamy peanut butter (substitute sunflower seed butter for peanut free)
> ¼ cup dairy-free buttery spread or sticks
> ¼ cup plain dairy-free milk beverage
> 1 teaspoon pure vanilla flavoring or extract
> Pinch salt
> 2 cups powdered confectioners' sugar

1. Put the peanut butter, dairy-free buttery spread or sticks, milk beverage, vanilla, and salt in a large mixing bowl. Sift in the powdered sugar.

2. Beat with a hand mixer on medium speed just until smooth, about 1 minute. Do not overmix.

3. Store leftover frosting in an airtight container in the refrigerator for up to 1 week. Beat the chilled frosting with your hand mixer for 30 seconds to soften before using.

FUDGY CHOCOLATE FROSTING

MAKES 2½ CUPS (ENOUGH TO FROST AN 8- OR 9-INCH DOUBLE-LAYER CAKE)

This fudgy frosting made an entire two-tiered white birthday cake vanish in minutes!

> ½ cup dairy-free buttery spread or sticks
> 3 tablespoons agave nectar or honey
> 2 tablespoons unsweetened plain dairy-free milk beverage
> 1 teaspoon pure vanilla flavoring or extract
> 2½ cups powdered confectioners' sugar
> ½ cup cocoa powder

1. Put the dairy-free buttery spread or sticks, liquid sweetener, milk beverage, and vanilla in a large mixing bowl. Beat with a hand mixer until creamy, about 2 minutes.

2. Sift in the powdered sugar and cocoa. Beat on low speed until the ingredients are mostly incorporated.

3. Turn the hand mixer up to medium or high speed and whip the frosting until fluffy, about 2 minutes.

4. Store leftover frosting in an airtight container in the refrigerator for up to 1 week. Beat the chilled frosting with your hand mixer for 30 seconds to soften before using.

DARK CHOCOLATE GANACHE FROSTING

MAKES 2¼ CUPS (ENOUGH TO FROST 18 CUPCAKES OR THE OUTSIDE OF AN 8-INCH DOUBLE-LAYER CAKE)

Traditional ganache, like my recipe on page 423, is a simple blend of chocolate and cream. But this version has some extra ingredients to give it a sweet frosting finish. Nonetheless, it still retains amazing flavor depth and intense dark chocolate appeal.

> 6 ounces dark chocolate, chopped
> ¼ cup lite coconut milk
> ½ cup dairy-free buttery spread
> Pinch salt (optional)
> 1½ cups powdered confectioners' sugar

1. Melt the chocolate with the coconut milk (see page 417 for How to Melt Chocolate).
2. Pour the chocolate mixture into a medium mixing bowl and let cool to room temperature.
3. Add the buttery spread and salt. Sift in the powdered sugar. Beat with a hand mixer on low speed until the ingredients are mostly incorporated.
4. Turn the hand mixer up to medium or high speed and whip the frosting until fluffy, about 2 minutes.
5. Store leftover frosting in an airtight container in the refrigerator for up to 1 week. Beat the chilled frosting with your hand mixer for 30 seconds to soften before using.

BUTTERLESS SPICE FROSTING

MAKES 2 CUPS

This is a great make-ahead frosting. The spices meld and the consistency thickens as it chills overnight. Since it is made without shortening or margarine, this creamy topper is a little denser than your average fluffy frosting. So I prefer it atop cookies, cupcakes, or as a dessert-like spread on graham crackers.

 1 cup raw cashews
 ¼ cup plain or unsweetened plain dairy-free milk beverage, plus additional as needed
 4 teaspoons grapeseed, rice bran, or other neutral-tasting oil (see page 146)
 ¼ teaspoon pure vanilla flavoring or extract
 ¾ teaspoon ground cinnamon
 ¼ teaspoon ground nutmeg or allspice
 ¼ teaspoon ground ginger
 Pinch ground cloves
 Pinch salt
 2 cups powdered confectioners' sugar

1. Put the cashews in your spice grinder (in batches) or food processor. Process them until they pass the powder stage and begin to clump, about 2 minutes.

2. Put the cashew paste, milk beverage, oil, vanilla, cinnamon, nutmeg or allspice, ginger, cloves, and salt in a medium mixing bowl. Beat with a hand mixer until creamy, about 2 minutes.

3. Sift in the powdered sugar. Beat on low speed until it is mostly incorporated.

4. Turn the hand mixer up to medium or high speed and beat the frosting until creamy, about 2 minutes. If it is too thick, beat in more milk beverage, 1 tablespoon at a time, until it reaches your desired consistency.

5. Cover and place the frosting in the refrigerator for several hours or overnight. It will thicken a bit as it chills. If it is too thick, beat in more milk beverage, 1 tablespoon at a time, until it reaches your desired consistency.

6. Store leftover frosting in an airtight container in the refrigerator for up to 1 week.

CHAPTER 32

PUDDING, MOUSSE & PIE, OH MY!

Crusts to Crustless Recipes

GOOD TO KNOW FOR THIS CHAPTER

PREMADE CRUSTS ARE OFTEN DAIRY FREE. Bakeries tend to use butter in their crusts, but the premade graham, cookie, and traditional pie crusts sold in the baking aisle and freezer section at most major grocers are usually dairy free. Nevertheless, I've included basic, easy crust recipes that let you have more control over the exact ingredients.

SEVERAL INGREDIENTS HAVE NATURAL THICKENING POWER. This chapter includes coconut milk/cream, avocado, melted chocolate, tofu, chia seeds, and starch to give you examples of how different dairy-free ingredients work to create body and thickness without dairy.

IN SOME CASES, THE TYPE OF MILK BEVERAGE CAN MAKE A DIFFERENCE. In many recipes, I leave the type of milk beverage up to you. But in some recipes, a richer milk beverage, like coconut, produces a superior result. And in puddings and sauces, I often recommend against using a milk beverage with added protein. Some protein-infused milk beverages can clump or create a less-pleasing texture when thickened.

PUDDINGS CAN BE MADE INTO PIE FILLINGS. Use part or all lite or full-fat coconut milk in place of the milk beverage in the pudding recipes in this chapter for a thicker pie filling. The latter will produce the richest, firmest results.

ONE 10-OUNCE BAG OF CHOCOLATE CHIPS CONTAINS ABOUT 1½ CUPS. Many dairy-free brands are sold in 10-ounce bags, which is why you will see me use this quantity often. But if you need to convert, every 2 ounces of chocolate chips or chopped chocolate is roughly a scant ⅓ cup.

HOW TO MAKE INSTANT BOX PUDDING

Although this isn't a from-scratch recipe, it's a top request among readers. If you have ever tried preparing instant pudding by simply substituting dairy-free milk beverage, you've likely ended up with somewhat soupy pudding. Fortunately, I've discovered many ways to perfectly thicken that quick mix without a drop of dairy.

START WITH

1 (3.9-ounce) package dairy-free instant pudding mix (see Jell-O Pudding Note below)

WHISK IN ONE OF THE FOLLOWING

THICKENING CASHEW MILK: Put ¼ cup cashews in your spice grinder and process until powdered and beginning to clump, about 2 minutes. Put the cashew paste and 1 cup cold water in your blender. Blend until smooth and creamy, about 1 minute. Add another 1 cup cold water and blend to combine. Pour the fresh cashew milk beverage through a fine-mesh strainer into a glass measuring cup. Whisk 2 cups of this cashew milk beverage into your pudding mix. Cover and refrigerate. It will be soft set within 5 minutes, but you can chill it for longer for a firmer pudding.

LITE COCONUT MILK: Whisk 2 cups chilled lite coconut milk or ½ cup chilled full-fat coconut milk plus 1½ cups cold water into the pudding mix. Cover and refrigerate. It will be soft set within 5 minutes, but you can chill it for longer for a firmer pudding.

LESS UNSWEETENED MILK BEVERAGE: Whisk 1¼ to 1½ cups unsweetened dairy-free milk beverage into the pudding mix. Cover and refrigerate. It will be soft set within 5 minutes. This is a sweeter, more concentrated pudding, so using unsweetened milk beverage is essential.

MILK BEVERAGE + OIL: In a small saucepan, whisk together 1¾ cups + 2 tablespoons cold plain or unsweetened plain milk beverage and the pudding mix until smooth. Place the pan over low heat and warm for just 1 to 2 minutes, while whisking. Whisk in 1½ tablespoons coconut oil or organic palm oil until smooth. Let cool to room temperature, cover, and refrigerate. It will need 2 hours or more to set up.

JELL-O PUDDING NOTE: Most flavors of the popular Jell-O brand of instant pudding mixes are made without milk ingredients and are certified kosher pareve. However, a select few do contain dairy. Check the ingredient statement and contact the company to discuss cross-contamination potential if that is a concern for you.

INSTANT CREAMY MOUSSE VARIATION

Whisk 1 cup full-fat coconut milk or coconut cream and 1 cup cold water into the pudding mix and allow it to chill for 1 hour or more for a rich and luxurious treat.

PIE FILLING VARIATION

Pour one 14-ounce can or 11-ounce package full-fat coconut milk or coconut cream into a glass measuring cup. Add enough unsweetened plain dairy-free milk beverage to reach 2 cups. Whisk this into the pudding mix, pour it into your prepared pie crust, and even it out. Finish and chill the pie as directed by your recipe.

DOUBLE CHOCOLATE PUDDING

MAKES 6 SERVINGS

This sweet but rich chocolate pudding is a hit with kids and adults. But you can give it an even more grown-up flavor by using dark chocolate or increasing the chocolate chips to 1 cup.

3½ cups unsweetened plain dairy-free milk beverage (do not use one with added protein)
½ cup cane sugar (can substitute your sweetener of choice)
¼ cup cornstarch (can substitute arrowroot starch)
3 tablespoons cocoa powder
½ teaspoon salt
½ cup dairy-free semi-sweet chocolate chips
1½ teaspoons vanilla extract

1. Put the milk beverage, sugar, starch, cocoa powder, and salt in your blender. Blend until smooth, about 30 seconds.

2. Pour the mixture into a medium saucepan over medium heat. Bring it to a boil. Cook, while whisking, for 3 minutes.

3. Remove the pan from the heat and whisk in the chocolate chips and vanilla until smooth. Let cool to room temperature.

4. Serve the pudding warm or spoon it into a container, cover, and refrigerate to enjoy later. It will thicken more as it chills. If the pudding appears lumpy, whisk it until smooth.

5. Store in an airtight container in the refrigerator for up to 3 days.

BUTTAHSCOTCH PUDDING

MAKES 4 SERVINGS

This sweet treat is reminiscent of classic butterscotch pudding. It was created by my friend Hannah Kaminsky.

¼ cup dairy-free buttery spread
1 cup firmly packed dark brown sugar
¼ cup + 1¾ cups cold plain or unsweetened plain dairy-free milk beverage, divided (do not use one with added protein)
3 tablespoons cornstarch (can substitute arrowroot starch)
½ teaspoon salt
1 teaspoon vanilla extract

1. Melt the buttery spread in a medium saucepan over medium heat. Stir in the brown sugar and cook until it is dissolved, about 2 minutes.

2. In a small bowl, whisk together the ¼ cup milk beverage, starch, and salt until smooth.

3. Pour the cornstarch mixture into the saucepan, while whisking, until it is completely incorporated and smooth.

4. Add the remaining 1¾ cups milk beverage and whisk to combine. Once the mixture comes to a boil, cook while whisking for 1 minute. It should be relatively thick.

5. Remove the pan from the heat and whisk in the vanilla.

6. Pour the pudding into 4 individual serving dishes. Optionally place a piece of plastic wrap over the surface of each serving to prevent a skin from forming.

7. Place the pudding in your refrigerator and chill for 4 hours, or until set.

8. Cover and store leftovers in the refrigerator for up to 3 days.

VERSATILE VANILLA PUDDING

MAKES 4 SERVINGS

This easy pudding recipe performs best with a higher-fat milk beverage, like coconut, soy, or nut milk. But any milk beverage without added protein will do in a pinch.

⅓ cup cane sugar
3 tablespoons cornstarch (can substitute arrowroot starch)
¼ teaspoon salt
2 cups cold plain or unsweetened plain dairy-free milk beverage (do not use one with added protein)
1 tablespoon dairy-free buttery spread (optional)
1 teaspoon vanilla extract
Ground nutmeg, for garnish (optional)

1. In a medium saucepan, whisk together the sugar, starch, and salt. Slowly add the milk beverage while whisking, until smooth.

2. Place the pan over medium-low heat. Cook while whisking until the mixture thickens enough to coat the back of a metal spoon, about 5 to 10 minutes. If it begins to boil, reduce the heat to low.

3. Remove the pan from the heat and whisk in the buttery spread (if using) and vanilla.

4. Pour the pudding into 4 individual serving dishes, and sprinkle each with a pinch of nutmeg (if using). Optionally place a piece of plastic wrap over the surface of each serving to prevent a skin from forming.

5. Place the pudding in your refrigerator and chill for 2 hours, or until set.

6. Cover and store leftovers in the refrigerator for up to 3 days.

....

PUDDING VARIATIONS

INSTANT RICE PUDDING: After adding the vanilla, stir in 2 cups cooked brown or white rice. Optionally stir in ½ teaspoon ground cinnamon and/or ½ cup raisins. Chill as directed above.

BANANA PUDDING PARFAITS: Once the pudding has chilled and set, divide half of the pudding between 4 parfait glasses. Top the pudding with banana slices. Repeat the layers with the remaining half of the pudding and more banana slices. Garnish with vanilla wafer cookies.

CUSTARDY PUDDING: Lightly beat 1 or 2 egg yolks. Stir a small amount of the hot pudding into the egg yolks, and return it all to the pan. Cook and stir for 1 minute more before removing the pudding from the heat and stirring in the buttery spread and vanilla.

....

CREAMSICLE CHIA PUDDING

MAKES 2 SERVINGS

This sweet, bright chia pudding has an addictive orange-vanilla flavor and a unique consistency. It also packs in loads of bone-building nutrients: each serving includes roughly 10 percent of the RDA for calcium and magnesium, plus a hefty dose of fiber and omega-3 fatty acids. And it's just sweet enough for a treat, but healthy enough for a snack or light breakfast.

¾ cup fresh-squeezed orange, tangelo, or tangerine juice (about 2 oranges or tangelos or 3 tangerines)
¼ cup full-fat coconut milk or lite coconut milk
4 teaspoons honey or agave nectar, or to taste
½ teaspoon pure vanilla flavoring or extract
3 to 4 tablespoons white or black chia seeds (see Chia Seed Notes below)
¼ teaspoon grated orange, tangelo, or tangerine zest

1. In a medium bowl, whisk together the juice, coconut milk, sweetener, and vanilla. Add the chia seeds and zest and stir to combine.
2. Cover the bowl and refrigerate for 1 hour, or until thickened.
3. Cover and store leftovers in the refrigerator for up to 3 days.

CHIA SEED NOTES: If using full-fat coconut milk, start with 3 tablespoons chia seeds. You can add more after chilling if it's too thin for your tastes. White chia seeds are actually tan in color, but still let some of the orange color show through in this pudding. Black chia seeds will produce much darker results. But other than color, white and black chia seeds are nearly identical.

BLENDED VARIATION

For thicker instant pudding, put the juice, coconut milk, sweetener, vanilla, and chia seeds in your blender. Blend until relatively smooth. Pour the mixture into a bowl, stir in the zest, cover, and chill for about 10 minutes.

CHOCOLATE-COVERED BANANA MOUSSE

MAKES 6 SERVINGS

Venturing out on that "chocolate is healthy" limb, this quick and easy dessert does sway toward the nutritious side. Nonetheless, it still fulfills the need for a little indulgence. For an elegant presentation, layer it in parfait glasses with your favorite fresh berries.

1 (12-ounce) package firm silken tofu
2 very ripe medium bananas
8 ounces (about 1¼ cups) dairy-free semi-sweet chocolate chips or chopped
    dark chocolate
1 teaspoon pure vanilla flavoring or extract
⅛ teaspoon salt

1. Put the tofu and bananas in your blender or food processor. Process until smooth, about 1 minute.
2. Melt the chocolate (see page 417 for How to Melt Chocolate).
3. Add the melted chocolate, vanilla, and salt to the tofu-banana mixture in your blender or food processor. Blend until smooth and creamy, about 1 minute. Do not blend for too long, to avoid overheating the chocolate.
4. Scrape the mousse into 6 serving dishes. Cover and refrigerate for 1 hour, or until thickened.
5. Cover and store in the refrigerator for up to 1 day, or freeze the mousse for an ice cream–like treat later.

BANANA-FREE VARIATION

Soak 4 large pitted Medjool dates in ⅓ cup very hot or boiling water for 10 minutes. Use the dates with soaking water in place of the bananas.

DEATH BY CHOCOLATE MOUSSE

MAKES 6 SERVINGS

This easy mousse is delicious on its own, but it also makes a great pie filling. Pour it into a prepared pie crust and top it with COOL WHIPPED COCONUT CREAM (page 424) and shaved chocolate for a quick but impressive dessert!

> 1½ cups dairy-free semi-sweet or dark chocolate chips
> 1½ cups coconut cream
> 3 tablespoons powdered confectioners' sugar, or to taste
> 1½ teaspoons vanilla extract
> Generous pinch salt

1. Put the chocolate chips in a medium mixing bowl and put equal parts water and ice in a larger bowl to make an ice bath.

2. Heat the coconut cream in a small saucepan over medium heat until small bubbles begin to form around the edge.

3. Pour the hot coconut cream over the chocolate chips and let sit for 1 minute. Whisk until the chocolate is completely smooth. Add the sugar, vanilla, and salt and whisk until smooth. Let cool for 5 minutes.

4. Place the chocolate mixing bowl in the ice bath, but be careful not to let any drops of water get into the chocolate. Whisk or beat the chocolate with a hand mixer until the mousse begins to thicken and whip.

5. Scrape the mousse into 6 serving dishes, cover, and place them in your refrigerator to chill for 1 hour or more.

6. Cover and store in the refrigerator for up to 3 days, or freeze the mousse for an ice cream–like treat later.

....

LIGHTER VARIATION

Substitute lite coconut milk or unsweetened dairy-free milk beverage for the coconut cream, but reduce the amount to 1 cup.

....

KEY LIME MOUSSE PIE

MAKES 8 SERVINGS

This thick, creamy pie has a flavor that is reminiscent of Key lime pie, but with a much richer consistency. For single-serve presentation, layer graham cracker or vanilla wafer cookie crumbs with the pie filling and whipped coconut cream in clear glasses.

> 1 batch RICH SWEETENED CONDENSED COCONUT MILK (page 190)
> 1 large ripe avocado, pitted and peeled
> ¼ to ⅓ cup fresh-squeezed lime or Key lime juice (3 to 4 limes), to taste
> 1 batch COOKIE CRUMB CRUST (page 401) made with vanilla wafer cookies
> COOL WHIPPED COCONUT CREAM (page 424) (optional)

1. Put the sweetened condensed coconut milk, avocado, and lime juice in your blender. Blend until smooth and creamy, about 1 minute.
2. Pour the filling into your prepared pie crust and even it out.
3. Refrigerate for at least 2 hours, or until the filling is set.
4. Serve each slice topped with a dollop of whipped coconut cream (if using).
5. Cover and store leftovers in the refrigerator for up to 2 days. The filling may darken slightly.

CRAZY FOR COCONUT CREAM PIE

MAKES 8 SERVINGS

Cream pies have always been my dad's favorite dessert, so I made sure to run this recipe by him before including it in this book. Not only did it pass his test, but I think it also made me a cream pie fan! Unlike the typical processed filling, this one tastes fresh and rich, and is infused with pure coconut throughout.

1 (11-ounce) package or (14-ounce) can full-fat coconut milk
1¼ to 2 cups unsweetened coconut milk beverage
½ cup cane sugar
¼ cup cornstarch (can substitute arrowroot starch)
¼ teaspoon salt
1 tablespoon dairy-free buttery spread (can substitute coconut oil)
1½ teaspoons + 1 teaspoon vanilla extract, divided
1 cup + ⅓ cup unsweetened coconut flakes, divided
1 Easy Peasy Pie Crust (page 400) (can substitute a store-bought crust or
    gluten-free crust), baked and cooled
1 cup coconut cream
¼ cup powdered confectioners' sugar

1. Pour the coconut milk into a glass measuring cup and add enough coconut milk beverage to make 3 cups.

2. Pour the coconut milk mixture into a medium saucepan. Add the cane sugar, starch, and salt and whisk until smooth.

3. Place the pan over medium heat and bring the mixture to a boil. Cook, while whisking, for 3 minutes.

4. Remove the pan from the heat. Add the buttery spread and 1½ teaspoons vanilla and whisk to combine. Stir in the 1 cup coconut flakes. Let cool for 15 minutes.

5. Pour the coconut filling into your prepared pie crust and level it out. Let cool for 15 minutes.

6. Place the uncovered pie in the refrigerator to completely cool for about 30 minutes.

7. Put the remaining ⅓ cup coconut flakes in a pan over medium heat. Toast, stirring often, for 3 minutes, or until some of the flakes turn golden. Remove the flakes to a bowl to cool.

8. Put the coconut cream, powdered sugar, and remaining 1 teaspoon vanilla in a small mixing bowl. Beat with a hand mixer until creamy, about 1 minute. It may thin a bit, but should remain quite thick.

9. Once the pie is cool, spread the sweetened coconut cream on top and smooth it out. Sprinkle the toasted coconut flakes evenly on top of the coconut cream.

10. Lightly cover the pie with plastic wrap and refrigerate until set, about 4 hours.

11. Cover and store leftovers in the refrigerator for up to 3 days.

BANANA COCONUT CREAM PIE VARIATION

Use a deep-dish pie crust and layer banana slices (from 2 or 3 bananas) in the bottom of the pie crust just before adding the coconut filling.

MAPLE & BROWN SUGAR APPLE CRISP

MAKES 6 TO 8 SERVINGS

I think of apple crisp as a crustless Dutch apple pie, which is why I included it in this chapter. Using coconut oil in the butterless crisp topping adds richness and also makes for a wonderfully firm, crumbly top crust when chilled. Nonetheless, you can swap in melted buttery spread or your favorite neutral-tasting oil (see page 146) in a pinch.

1 cup + 1 tablespoon all-purpose flour, whole wheat pastry flour, or oat flour
   (for gluten free), divided
¾ cup quick oats (certified gluten free, if needed)
¾ cup + 2 tablespoons firmly packed brown sugar, divided
¾ teaspoon + ½ teaspoon ground cinnamon, divided
¼ teaspoon salt
⅛ teaspoon ground nutmeg
½ cup coconut oil, melted
2½ pounds baking apples (about 5 or 6 apples; see Sweetener Note below)
1 tablespoon lemon juice
2 tablespoons maple syrup
COOL WHIPPED COCONUT CREAM (page 424), SNICKERDOODLE CASHEW ICE CREAM
   (page 407), or PURELY VANILLA ICE CREAM (page 403), to serve (optional)

1. Preheat your oven to 350°F.
2. In a medium bowl, whisk together the 1 cup flour, oats, ¾ cup brown sugar, ¾ teaspoon cinnamon, salt, and nutmeg.
3. Add the oil and whisk or stir with a fork to combine. The mixture should look a little wet and clumpy, but still loose.
4. Peel and core the apples. Cut them into ¼-inch-thick slices and cut the slices in half.
5. Put the apple half slices in a large bowl. Add the remaining 2 tablespoons brown sugar, lemon juice, remaining 1 tablespoon flour, and remaining ½ teaspoon cinnamon. Toss to evenly coat the apples.
6. Transfer the apples to an 8 × 8-inch or 9 × 9-inch baking dish. Shake or gently tap the dish on the counter to pack them down a little and level them out.
7. Sprinkle the crumb mixture evenly over the apples. Evenly drizzle the maple syrup over the crumble.
8. Bake for 35 minutes, or until the apples are tender when poked with a toothpick. Let cool for 10 minutes.
9. Serve scoops of the warm crisp topped with whipped coconut cream or dairy-free ice cream, if desired.
10. Cover and store leftovers in the refrigerator for up to 3 days.

SWEETENER NOTE: If using Granny Smith apples, this crisp will have a sweet-tart finish. If you prefer a sweeter filling, either increase the brown sugar in the filling to ¼ cup or use a sweeter baking apple, like Golden Delicious, Braeburn, Fuji, or Jonagold.

EASY PEASY PIE CRUST

MAKES ONE 9-INCH PIE CRUST

This is my basic, go-to pie crust recipe for sweets and savories. To make both a top and a bottom crust, double the recipe.

1½ cups all-purpose flour or whole wheat pastry flour
½ to 1 tablespoon cane sugar (omit for a savory crust)
½ teaspoon salt
6 tablespoons grapeseed, rice bran, or other neutral-tasting oil (see page 146)
3 tablespoons cold water, plus additional as needed

1. In a medium bowl, whisk together the flour, sugar (if using), and salt.
2. Add the oil and water and stir until a dough forms, bringing it together with your hands when needed. If the dough is too dry, sprinkle in more water, as needed.
3. If not using immediately, tightly wrap the dough in plastic wrap and refrigerate for up to 2 days.
4. Press the dough into a 9-inch pie pan and crimp the edges as desired, or roll it out to make a crust. Use and bake the crust in your recipe as directed.

HOW TO BLIND BAKE: Blind baking is the term used for pre-baking a crust without the filling. For this recipe, blind baking works best with the Super-Flaky Coconut Oil Variation. Place a large square of parchment paper over the unbaked pie crust, lightly pressing it in against the edges and sides. Add pie weights, dried beans, dry rice, or other dry grains until the crust is two-thirds full. Place the crust in the refrigerator for 30 minutes. Bake for 20 minutes at 375°F. Remove the pie from the oven and lift out the parchment with the pie weights. Prick the bottom of the crust several times with a fork. Bake the crust for 15 to 20 more minutes, or until it is golden.

SUPER-FLAKY COCONUT OIL VARIATION

After step 1, whisk 6 tablespoons solid or semi-solid coconut oil into the dry mixture until coarse crumbs form. Add the cold water until it comes together into dough.

COOKIE CRUMB CRUST

MAKES ONE 9-INCH PIE CRUST

I've always been a sucker for crumb crusts, and they are so easy to make at home. I almost always use them unbaked, but I've included a baked version for those of you who prefer a toastier crust.

> 2 cups dairy-free crunchy cookie crumbs (see Cookie Notes below), plus additional as needed
> 2 tablespoons coconut oil, melted
> 2 tablespoons grapeseed, rice bran, or other neutral-tasting oil (see page 146), plus additional as needed

1. Put the cookie crumbs in a medium bowl. Drizzle in the two oils and stir to combine. The crumbs should come together into cohesive-looking clumps but shouldn't appear greasy. If too dry, add a little more neutral oil. If too greasy, add more crumbs.

2. Press the crumbs into an ungreased 8- or 9-inch pie pan or the bottom of a 9-inch springform pan.

3. Use in your recipe as directed.

COOKIE NOTES: Crumb crusts work best if the cookies are ground into very fine crumbs. For the most consistent results, process the cookies in a spice grinder, powerful blender, or food processor.

You can use chocolate, vanilla, graham, gingersnap, or your favorite crunchy cookies in this crust. Gluten-free cookies work well, too. It's also okay if they have chocolate chips in them.

....

CRUST VARIATIONS

GRAHAM CRACKER: Substitute graham cracker crumbs (regular, vegan, or gluten free) for the cookie crumbs. Many graham cracker crusts are sweetened, but I prefer mine without added sweetener. If you like a sweetened graham crust, add up to ¼ cup powdered confectioners' sugar.

BUTTERY: Substitute ¼ to ⅓ cup melted dairy-free buttery spread or BAKEABLE BUTTER (page 192) for all of the oil. The amount needed will vary a bit with the crumbs used.

BAKED: For a crispier crust, bake it for 5 to 10 minutes at 350°F.

....

CHAPTER 33

ICE CREAM SOCIAL

Assorted Scoops, Toppings & Frozen Treat Recipes

GOOD TO KNOW FOR THIS CHAPTER

PREP YOUR ICE CREAM MAKER. The biggest mistake when making homemade ice cream is neglecting to chill the insert ahead of time. For most ice cream makers, you need to place the bowl insert in the freezer at least 24 hours in advance. If you don't, the ice cream won't thicken. Check the manufacturer's instructions to confirm whether your machine must be prepped. It's also best to pre-chill the container that you'll be packing the finished ice cream into.

AN ICE CREAM MAKER ISN'T ESSENTIAL. Even inexpensive models (think $25) are extremely helpful. But if you don't have the space or budget, use one of these options:

Option 1—Freeze a shallow pan, like a 9 × 13-inch baking dish. Pour the ice cream mixture into the pan and freeze it until the edges start to freeze, about 30 to 45 minutes. Blend it with a hand mixer until creamy. Repeat this process 3 or 4 more times. Then cover and freeze until firm.

Option 2—Fill ice cube trays half full with the ice cream mixture. Freeze for about 1 hour, or until soft frozen. Blend the cubes in your food processor or blender (begin by pulsing) until creamy. If frozen solid, let the cubes defrost for 10 minutes before blending. Pack the soft serve into an airtight container and freeze for 3 hours or more.

YOU CAN BUILD YOUR OWN DAIRY-FREE ICE CREAM SUNDAE BAR. In addition to the sauces in this chapter, put out bowls of chopped allergy-friendly cookies, natural sprinkles, dairy-free chocolate chips, fresh berries, pitted or maraschino cherries, mini marshmallows (vegan, if desired), melted jam, chopped nuts, or favorite candies.

PURELY VANILLA ICE CREAM

MAKES ABOUT 1 QUART

I've tested countless pints of dairy-free vanilla ice cream over the years, but most taste more like coconut, soy, or cashew than vanilla. This version uses a simple emulsion of milk beverage and oil for a clean taste that's also adaptable to your special diet or food allergy needs. Enjoy it over slices of pie, cake, and crisp, or in a bowl with an easy homemade topping (recipes starting on page 414).

> 3 cups cold unsweetened plain or vanilla dairy-free milk beverage
>   (see Dairy-Free Milk Note below)
> ¾ cup cane sugar
> ½ cup non-GMO canola, rice bran, or other neutral-tasting oil (see page 146)
> 2 to 3 teaspoons vanilla paste or pure vanilla flavoring (can substitute vanilla extract
>   or the seeds from 1 whole vanilla bean), to taste
> Pinch salt
> ⅛ teaspoon xanthan gum or guar gum (see Gum Note below)

1. Put the milk beverage and sugar in your blender or food processor. Blend until the sugar dissolves, about 1 minute.
2. With the motor running, very slowly drizzle in the oil. Continue to blend until creamy and emulsified, about 1 minute.
3. Add the vanilla and salt and blend briefly to combine. Add the gum and blend for 1 minute. The mixture might appear a little gloppy at first, but it will settle.
4. Pour the mixture into a 4-cup or larger glass measuring cup and place it in the refrigerator to chill for at least 1 hour.
5. Whisk the mixture to smooth it out before churning. Churn the mixture in your prepared ice cream maker according to the manufacturer's directions.
6. Pack the soft ice cream into a freezer-safe container and freeze for at least 3 hours for hard-packed ice cream.

DAIRY-FREE MILK NOTE: *I find that pea protein milk yields the creamiest results and does the best job of letting the vanilla flavor shine through. Other milk beverages will work, but they tend to yield icier and less flavorful results. My second favorite option is lite coconut milk, but it does give a slight coconut vibe to the flavor. Two 14-ounce cans of lite coconut milk will yield about 3¼ cups.*

GUM NOTE: *Xanthan or guar gum helps bind the emulsion between the milk beverage and the oil so that your ice cream has a smoother, creamier finish with little to no ice crystals. It isn't absolutely essential (especially if you use lite coconut milk instead of milk beverage), but without it, the consistency will be more like a cross between ice milk and ice cream.*

CHOCOLATE PUDDIN' POP ICE CREAM

MAKES ABOUT 1 QUART

The richness of this chocoholic's dream is reminiscent of frozen pudding. I like the milky consistency best when packed and frozen for just a few hours, but you can also let it soften on the counter for 10 minutes if it has chilled for longer.

- ¼ cup + 1¼ cups plain dairy-free milk beverage, divided (do not use one with added protein)
- 4 teaspoons cornstarch, arrowroot starch, or tapioca starch
- 1½ cups full-fat coconut milk
- ⅔ cup cane sugar
- 2 tablespoons maple syrup or honey
- ¼ cup cocoa powder
- 3 ounces dairy-free semi-sweet chocolate chips or chopped chocolate (scant ½ cup)
- 2 teaspoons vanilla extract
- ¼ teaspoon salt

1. In a small bowl, whisk together the ¼ cup milk beverage and starch until smooth.
2. Put the remaining 1¼ cups milk beverage, coconut milk, sugar, and liquid sweetener in a medium saucepan. Sift in the cocoa powder and whisk to combine.
3. Place the pan over medium heat and whisk while bringing the mixture to a slow boil. Boil for 3 minutes, whisking occasionally.
4. Whisk the starch mixture again, and then whisk it into the mixture in your saucepan. Cook, while whisking, until thickened to a rich cream consistency, about 2 minutes.
5. Remove the pan from the heat. Add the chocolate, vanilla, and salt and whisk until smooth.
6. Pour the mixture into a 4-cup or larger glass measuring cup and let it cool to room temperature. Cover and refrigerate for at least 2 hours.
7. Churn the chilled mixture in your prepared ice cream maker according to the manufacturer's directions.
8. Pack the soft ice cream into a freezer-safe container and freeze for at least 3 hours for hard-packed ice cream.

FRESH STRAWBERRY ICE CREAM

MAKES ABOUT 1 QUART

This recipe contains just four ingredients, but the creamy texture and bright berry flavor prove that simplicity is bliss.

> 1 pound strawberries, hulled
> 1 (14-ounce) can full-fat coconut milk
> ⅔ cup cane sugar
> 1 tablespoon pure vanilla flavoring or extract

1. Put the strawberries, coconut milk, sugar, and vanilla in your blender. Blend until smooth and creamy, about 2 minutes.
2. Put the blender jar in the refrigerator and let the mixture cool for 1 hour or more.
3. Churn the chilled mixture in your prepared ice cream maker according to the manufacturer's directions.
4. Pack the soft ice cream into a freezer-safe container and freeze for at least 3 hours for hard-packed ice cream.

VERY CHERRY NICE CREAM

MAKES 2 SERVINGS

This healthy ice cream gets creamy sweetness from a base of fruit, but I like to add just a little cashew butter for an extra touch of nutrition—and luxury.

> 1 very ripe large banana, frozen and broken into chunks
> ⅔ cup frozen dark sweet cherries
> ½ to ⅔ cup 100% pure cherry juice (not tart)
> 2 tablespoons cashew butter (can substitute sunflower seed butter for nut free)
> ½ teaspoon pure vanilla flavoring or extract
> Generous pinch salt
> Sweetener, to taste (optional)
> Dairy-free mini chocolate chips or MAGICAL SHELL (page 414), to serve (optional)

1. Put the frozen banana, frozen cherries, ½ cup cherry juice, cashew butter, vanilla, and salt in your blender or food processor. Blend until smooth and creamy, about 1 minute. If it's too thick to blend, add a little more cherry juice, as needed, to get things moving.
2. Blend in sweetener, if desired.
3. Divide the soft serve between 2 dishes and serve immediately or pack it into a freezer-safe container and enjoy it later as a hard-packed ice cream. Serve topped with mini chocolate chips or magical shell topping, if desired.

PEANUT BUTTER PARAD-ICE CREAM

MAKES ABOUT 1½ QUARTS

This luxurious peanut butter ice cream has a double dose of indulgence with the addition of peanut butter chunks. If you want an even richer finish, substitute one 14-ounce can full-fat coconut milk for one can of the lite coconut milk.

PEANUT BUTTER ICE CREAM
2 (14-ounce) cans lite coconut milk
⅔ cup creamy peanut butter (can substitute sunflower seed butter for peanut free)
⅔ cup agave nectar, honey, maple syrup, brown sugar, or cane sugar, or to taste
2 teaspoons pure vanilla flavoring or extract
⅛ teaspoon salt (optional)

PEANUT BUTTER CHUNKS
3 tablespoons creamy peanut butter (can substitute sunflower seed butter for peanut free)
2 tablespoons agave nectar or honey
2 tablespoons coconut oil
¼ teaspoon pure vanilla flavoring or extract

1. **To make the peanut butter ice cream**, put the coconut milk, peanut butter, sweetener, vanilla, and salt (if using) in your blender. Blend until smooth and the sugar is dissolved, about 2 minutes.

2. Put the blender jar in the refrigerator and let the mixture cool for at least 1 hour.

3. **To make the peanut butter chunks**, put the peanut butter, sweetener, oil, and vanilla in a small saucepan over low heat. Heat, while whisking, until the mixture is smooth, about 2 minutes. Remove from the heat and let cool to room temperature.

4. Line a plate with a piece of wax paper or parchment paper. Pour the melted peanut butter chunk mixture onto the plate and spread it out with a silicone spatula, if needed, to about ¼-inch thickness.

5. Place the plate in the freezer for 15 minutes.

6. Cut the peanut butter chunk mixture into small pieces. Carefully break them up (they will be a little soft at room temperature) and return them to the freezer.

7. Churn the chilled mixture in your prepared ice cream maker according to the manufacturer's directions. When the ice cream is almost fully churned, add the frozen peanut butter chunks.

8. Pack the soft ice cream into a freezer-safe container and freeze for at least 3 hours for hard-packed ice cream.

SNICKERDOODLE CASHEW ICE CREAM

MAKES ABOUT 1 QUART

This premium dairy-free ice cream is insanely rich and creamy. Even when packed and fully frozen, it readily scoops. If you aren't in a cinnamon mood, feel free to omit the spice and just enjoy the vanilla and caramel notes as is.

1⅔ cups raw cashews
1 cup + ¾ cup unsweetened plain dairy-free milk beverage, divided
¾ cup firmly packed brown sugar (can substitute coconut sugar for less sweet)
3 tablespoons rice bran or other neutral-tasting oil (see page 146)
    (do not use coconut oil)
1½ teaspoons pure vanilla flavoring or paste (can substitute vanilla extract)
½ to 1 teaspoon ground cinnamon, to taste
⅜ teaspoon salt

1. Put the cashews in your spice grinder (in batches, if needed) or food processor. Process until powdered and beginning to clump, about 1 minute.
2. Put the 1 cup milk beverage and ground cashews in your blender. Blend until very smooth and creamy, about 2 minutes.
3. Add the remaining ¾ cup milk beverage, brown sugar, oil, vanilla, cinnamon, and salt. Blend until the sugar is dissolved, about 2 minutes.
4. Put the blender jar in the refrigerator and let the mixture cool and thicken for 2 hours or more.
5. Churn the chilled mixture in your prepared ice cream maker according to the manufacturer's directions.
6. Enjoy as soft serve or pack the soft ice cream into a freezer-safe container. Freeze for at least 3 hours for hard-packed ice cream.

TROPICAL COCONUT ICE DREAM

MAKES ABOUT 1½ PINTS

This ultra-premium ice cream is enriched with both full-fat coconut milk and cream of coconut, which is a sweetened coconut product often found near the alcohol in grocers. The recipe was created by my friend Hannah Kaminsky, who can't resist creating unique flavors. She pairs the coconut base with ginger and a twist of citrus for a Southeast Asian–style treat.

1 (14-ounce) can full-fat coconut milk
1 tablespoon cornstarch or arrowroot starch
1 (15-ounce) can cream of coconut
¼ cup cane sugar
½ teaspoon lemon or lime juice
2 teaspoons grated fresh ginger

1. Measure ¼ cup of the coconut milk and pour it into a small bowl. Add the starch and whisk until the starch is dissolved.

2. Put the remaining coconut milk, cream of coconut, sugar, lemon or lime juice, and ginger in a saucepan over medium heat. Bring the mixture to a boil.

3. Whisk the starch mixture again, and then whisk it into the mixture in your saucepan. Cook, while whisking, until slightly thickened, about 3 minutes. Remove the pan from the heat.

4. Pour the mixture into a 4-cup or larger glass measuring cup and let it cool to room temperature. Cover and refrigerate for at least 2 hours.

5. Churn the chilled mixture in your prepared ice cream maker according to the manufacturer's directions.

6. Enjoy as soft serve or pack the soft ice cream into a freezer-safe container. Freeze for at least 3 hours for hard-packed ice cream.

MINT STRACCIATELLA

MAKES 1½ PINTS

Stracciatella is a type of gelato with very fine chocolate flakes. The chocolate melts in your mouth for a more infused flavor experience than simply adding chocolate chips. The base of this ice cream gets a soft green hue from the avocados, which also help add body and richness.

> 1 (14-ounce) can regular coconut milk
> 1 cup plain or unsweetened plain dairy-free milk beverage
> ½ cup agave nectar or honey
> ¼ cup + 2 tablespoons cane sugar
> 2 small ripe avocados, pitted and peeled
> 1½ teaspoons peppermint extract, or to taste
> 1 teaspoon lemon juice
> ½ teaspoon pure vanilla flavoring or extract
> ⅛ teaspoon salt
> 4 ounces dairy-free semi-sweet chocolate chips or chopped dark chocolate

1. Put the coconut milk, milk beverage, liquid sweetener, sugar, avocado, peppermint, lemon juice, vanilla, and salt in your blender. Blend until smooth and creamy, about 2 minutes.

2. Place the blender jar in your refrigerator to chill for 1 hour or more.

3. Churn the chilled mixture in your prepared ice cream maker according to the manufacturer's directions.

4. While the ice cream is churning, melt the chocolate (see page 417 for How to Melt Chocolate). Let cool for 5 minutes.

5. Optionally drizzle the melted chocolate in a slow, thin stream into the ice cream maker when just a minute or two of churning remains. If doing this, skip step 7.

6. Pack the soft ice cream into a freezer-safe container.

7. If you skipped step 5, drizzle the melted chocolate over the packed ice cream. Freeze for 1 to 2 hours, or until mostly firm. Break the top chocolate layer up with a spoon into small pieces. Stir it into the ice cream.

8. Freeze the ice cream for at least 3 hours for hard-packed ice cream.

. . . .

MINT CHIP VARIATION

Do not melt the chocolate. Instead, add ⅓ cup dairy-free mini chocolate chips to the ice cream maker during the last few minutes of churning.

. . . .

DECADENT DARK CHOCOLATE SORBET

MAKES 1 PINT

Hannah Kaminsky insisted that I also share this sorbet recipe with you. She says you will be surprised at how rich it is, proclaiming it even more indulgent than full-fledged chocolate ice cream. Hannah uses Dutch-processed cocoa powder because it is less bitter. If you decide to swap in a natural cocoa powder, make sure it is a very mildly flavored one.

> ¼ cup + 1¾ cups warm water, divided
> 1 cup cane sugar
> 1 cup Dutch-processed cocoa powder
> 1 teaspoon vanilla extract
> ½ teaspoon salt

1. Put the ¼ cup water and sugar in a medium saucepan over medium heat. Let the sugar dissolve and come to a boil without stirring. Then cook, stirring occasionally, until the sugar becomes a golden caramel color, about 5 to 10 minutes.
2. Carefully whisk in the remaining 1¾ cups water. The caramel will seize up a bit; just continue to cook and whisk until the caramel is melted and smooth. Remove the pan from the heat.
3. Sift in the cocoa powder and whisk until smooth. Add the vanilla and salt and whisk to combine.
4. Pour the mixture into a 3-cup or larger glass measuring cup and let it cool to room temperature. Cover and refrigerate for at least 2 hours.
5. Churn the chilled mixture in your prepared ice cream maker according to the manufacturer's directions.
6. Pack the soft ice cream into a freezer-safe container. Freeze for at least 3 hours for hard-packed ice cream.

OATMEAL COOKIE ICE CREAM SANDWICHES

MAKES 10 ICE CREAM SANDWICHES

The tender cookies in this naturally gluten-free recipe were made specifically for freezing. Get creative with mixing and matching ice cream flavors and garnishes.

> 1 cup + 2 tablespoons rolled oats (certified gluten free, if needed)
> 1 tablespoon flax seeds
> 1 cup quick oats (certified gluten free, if needed)
> ½ teaspoon baking soda
> ¼ teaspoon salt
> ⅓ cup firmly packed brown sugar
> ¼ cup cane sugar
> ¼ cup grapeseed, rice bran, or other neutral-tasting oil (see page 146)

3 tablespoons plain or unsweetened plain dairy-free milk beverage
1 tablespoon maple syrup
½ teaspoon vanilla extract
2 pints dairy-free ice cream, your choice of flavors
Dairy-free mini chocolate chips or allergy-friendly sprinkles (optional)

1. Preheat your oven to 350°F and line 2 baking sheets with parchment paper or silicone baking mats.
2. Put the rolled oats and flax seeds in your spice grinder (in batches, if needed) or food processor. Process until powdered, about 1 minute.
3. In a medium bowl, stir together the oat-flax mixture, quick oats, baking soda, and salt.
4. Put the brown sugar, cane sugar, oil, milk beverage, maple syrup, and vanilla in a medium mixing bowl. Whisk or beat with a hand mixer until smooth, about 1 minute.
5. Add the oat mixture to the wet mixture and stir to combine.
6. Scoop the dough by the level tablespoon and place each mound a few inches apart on your prepared baking sheets. With the back of the tablespoon or damp hands, flatten the dough into uniform ¼-inch-high disks.
7. Bake for 10 to 12 minutes, or until just cooked with no shine remaining, but not yet golden.
8. Let cool on the baking sheets for 15 minutes before carefully removing the cookies to a wire rack to cool completely. They are fragile when warm, but will firm up.
9. Once the cookies have cooled to room temperature, remove the dairy-free ice cream from the freezer and place the cookies in your freezer to briefly chill while the ice cream softens enough to scoop, about 5 to 10 minutes.
10. Place 1 cookie, bottom side up, on a flat surface. Top with 1 or 2 scoops ice cream. Top with a second cookie, bottom side down, and gently press down to adhere and push the ice cream past the cookie edges. With a knife or spreader, smooth the ice cream to be flush with the cookie edges, adding more ice cream, if needed. Immediately place the cookie sandwich on parchment paper or a silicone baking mat in the freezer. Repeat with the remaining cookies and ice cream.
11. If using chocolate chips or sprinkles, spread the mini chocolate chips or sprinkles on a flat work surface. Roll each sandwich, like a wheel, in the garnish so it sticks to the ice cream. Place the sandwiches back in the freezer to firm up.
12. Once frozen solid, tightly wrap each ice cream sandwich in plastic wrap and store in the freezer.

CHOCOLATE-COATED VARIATION

Once the ice cream sandwiches are frozen solid, place a wire rack over parchment or wax paper. Melt 6 ounces dairy-free semi-sweet or dark chocolate chips with 4 teaspoons coconut oil or dairy-free buttery spread (see page 417 for How to Melt Chocolate). One at a time, remove each ice cream sandwich from the freezer, set it on the wire rack, and drizzle the melted chocolate over the top, swirling it out with the back of a spoon to drip down the cookie edges. As the chocolate sets up, return each sandwich to the freezer. Once solid, tightly wrap each ice cream sandwich in plastic wrap and store in the freezer.

MANGO-ORANGE SHERBET BARS

MAKES 12 BARS

If you're craving something cool and creamy but want to avoid churning ice cream, make these scrumptious sherbet bars! They're healthier than your average scoop, but packed with refreshing flavor.

> 2 cups pureed ripe mango (see Mango Note below)
> ¼ cup honey or agave nectar, or to taste
> 1 teaspoon fresh-squeezed lime juice
> 1 teaspoon pure vanilla flavoring or extract
> 1 cup orange juice (fresh squeezed if possible; about 3 oranges)
> ¾ cup full-fat coconut milk or coconut cream

1. Put the mango, sweetener, lime juice, and vanilla in your blender. Blend until smooth and the sweetener is dissolved, about 2 minutes.
2. Add the orange juice and coconut milk or cream and blend until creamy, about 1 minute.
3. Pour the mixture into ice-pop molds and freeze until set, about 4 hours. Alternatively, pour the mixture into 5-ounce paper cups, freeze for 1 hour (or until partially set), insert a wooden stick in each, and then freeze until set.

MANGO NOTE: You will need about 2 to 3 large mangoes, pitted and peeled, to get this amount of puree. Choose mangoes with low to no fibers, like Honey/Ataulfo, Keitt, or Kent. High-fiber mangoes leave little fibrous bits behind. Also, if your mangoes aren't sweet and ripe, increase the sweetener, to taste, and err on the sweet side. Desserts taste a little less sweet once frozen.

....

SHERBET VARIATIONS

SHERBET ICE CREAM: If you do have an ice cream maker, you can process this mixture in your ice cream maker for scoopable sherbet.

MANGO DREAMSICLES: For a creamier treat, omit the orange juice and double the coconut milk or cream. Increase the sweetener to ⅓ cup, or to taste.

....

PIÑA COLADA POPS

MAKES 8 TO 12 POPS

This is a fun and refreshing summer treat that plays off the coconut milk flavor rather than trying to mask it. And the touch of alcohol helps stave off ice crystals, because it doesn't freeze. Use just 1 tablespoon if you want the rum to remain undetected, or 2 tablespoons for a bigger hint of grown-up flavor.

> 1 (14-ounce) can full-fat coconut milk (can substitute lite coconut milk for icier pops)
> ⅔ cup crushed pineapple

⅓ cup agave nectar (can substitute simple syrup)

1 to 2 tablespoons rum, to taste (can omit for "virgin" pops)

1. Put the coconut milk, pineapple, and agave nectar in your blender. Blend for about 1 minute; some pineapple bits may remain, but it will be relatively smooth.

2. Add the rum and blend briefly to combine.

3. Pour the mixture into ice-pop molds and freeze until set, about 4 hours. Alternatively, pour the mixture into 5-ounce paper cups, freeze for 1 hour (or until partially set), insert a wooden stick in each, and then freeze until set.

FRUIT 'N' CREAM POPS

MAKES 4 TO 6 POPS

Watermelon and strawberry have evolved to be one of my favorite fruit combinations, and this is a cool way to enjoy them in the heat of summer. Feel free to reduce the sweetener in the watermelon-strawberry blend if your fruit is particularly ripe, but be aware that the end product will taste a little less sweet once frozen.

½ cup watermelon puree (about 4 ounces seedless watermelon flesh)

½ cup fresh or frozen sliced ripe strawberries

1 tablespoon + 1 tablespoon honey or agave nectar, divided

¼ teaspoon lime juice

½ cup coconut cream or full-fat coconut milk

¼ teaspoon pure vanilla flavoring or extract

1. Put the watermelon, strawberries, 1 tablespoon sweetener, and lime juice in your blender. Blend until smooth, about 1 minute. Pour the mixture into a glass measuring cup.

2. Rinse out your blender and add the coconut cream or milk, remaining 1 tablespoon sweetener, and vanilla. Blend until smooth, about 1 minute.

3. Pour the fruit blend into 4 to 6 ice-pop molds until they are roughly one-third full. Freeze the pops for 30 minutes.

4. Remove the pops from the freezer, and evenly divide the vanilla cream mixture between the pops to make the second layer. Freeze the pops for 30 minutes.

5. Remove the pops from the freezer, and pour the remaining fruit blend over the middle layer to make the third layer. Place the popsicle sticks into the pops and freeze for 1 to 2 hours, or until completely frozen.

CREAMY POP VARIATIONS

QUICK BLENDED POPS: Skip the layering. Instead, blend all the ingredients together. Fill the ice-pop molds and chill in the freezer for 2 hours or until they are frozen solid.

STRAWBERRY CREAM VARIATION: For a bigger fruit infusion, blend two ripe strawberries into the vanilla cream before pouring it into the molds.

CHOCOLATE MAGICAL SHELL

MAKES ¾ CUP

I love crackly chocolate atop ice cream, but the most popular brand does contain milk. So I created this simple dairy-free version.

> 1 cup dairy-free semi-sweet chocolate chips
> 1½ tablespoons coconut oil (can substitute organic palm oil for coconut free)
> 1½ teaspoons grapeseed, rice bran, or other neutral-tasting oil
> Pinch salt (optional)

1. Melt the chocolate (see page 417 for How to Melt Chocolate).
2. Add the two oils and whisk until smooth. It will be thin, for drizzling, but will set up on the ice cream. Whisk in the salt (if using).
3. Store in an airtight container at room temperature or in the refrigerator for up to 1 month. If it sets up, gently warm the sauce before using.

PEANUT BUTTER MAGICAL SHELL

MAKES GENEROUS ½ CUP

This rich topping is a little thicker than the chocolate version, but it still hardens for a delicious peanut buttery coating.

> ¼ cup creamy peanut butter (can substitute sunflower seed butter for peanut free)
> ¼ cup coconut oil, plus additional as needed
> ⅓ cup powdered confectioners' sugar
> ½ teaspoon vanilla extract

1. Put the peanut butter and coconut oil in a small saucepan over low heat. Cook, while whisking, until melted and smooth, about 2 minutes.
2. Remove the pan from the heat. Sift in the powdered sugar and add the vanilla. Whisk until smooth. If the mixture is too thick for drizzling, whisk in a little more coconut oil, 1 teaspoon at a time.
3. Let cool to room temperature before using.
4. Store in an airtight container at room temperature or in the refrigerator for up to 1 month. If it sets up, gently warm the sauce before using.

HOT FUDGE SAUCE

MAKES 1½ CUPS

This very rich dark chocolate sets up almost like fudge when chilled. But when warmed, it provides a thick cascade of luxury that you can enjoy atop ice cream or your favorite dessert.

> ¾ cup full-fat coconut milk or coconut cream
> ½ cup honey, agave nectar, or light corn syrup
> ½ cup + ½ cup chopped dairy-free dark chocolate, divided
> ⅓ cup firmly packed brown sugar
> ¼ cup cocoa powder
> ¼ teaspoon salt
> 2 tablespoons dairy-free buttery spread (can substitute coconut oil or your oil of choice)
> 1½ teaspoons vanilla extract

1. Put the coconut milk or cream, liquid sweetener, ½ cup chocolate, brown sugar, cocoa powder, and salt in a heavy saucepan over medium heat. Bring the mixture to a low boil, while whisking. Reduce the heat to low and cook for 4 minutes, whisking often.
2. Remove the pan from the heat and whisk in the remaining ½ cup chocolate, buttery spread, and vanilla until smooth. Let cool for 5 minutes before serving.
3. Store in an airtight container in the refrigerator for up to 1 week. If the sauce thickens too much as it chills, gently warm it before using.

SWEET & SILKY BUTTERSCOTCH SAUCE

MAKES 2 CUPS

This super sweet sauce adds that extra touch of indulgence to ice cream, apple crisp, or cake. It's adapted from a recipe I clipped from a magazine many years ago.

> 1 cup firmly packed brown sugar
> ⅔ cup agave nectar or light corn syrup
> ¼ cup dairy-free buttery spread
> ⅔ cup lite coconut milk
> 1 teaspoon pure vanilla flavoring or extract
> ⅛ teaspoon baking soda
> Scant ⅛ teaspoon salt

1. Put the sugar, liquid sweetener, and buttery spread in a medium saucepan over medium heat. Cook, while stirring, until the sugar has dissolved and the mixture comes to a full rolling boil. Allow it to boil, without stirring, for exactly 1 minute.
2. Remove the pan from the heat and let cool for 5 minutes.
3. Put the coconut milk, vanilla, baking soda, and salt in a glass measuring cup and whisk to combine.
4. Slowly pour the coconut milk mixture into the slightly cooled sauce, while whisking until smooth. Let cool for 5 minutes before serving.
5. Store in an airtight container in the refrigerator for up to 1 week. If it thickens too much as it chills, gently warm the sauce before using.

CHAPTER 34
SWEET EVERYTHINGS
Chocolates, Toppers &
Easy Treat Recipes

GOOD TO KNOW FOR THIS CHAPTER

DON'T BE TEMPTED TO USE VANILLA EXTRACT. In some recipes in this book, I specifically call for vanilla bean, vanilla powder, and/or pure vanilla flavoring. Don't be tempted to swap in a type of vanilla not called for. In some of the recipes that follow, alcohol (in regular vanilla extract) or liquid (in vanilla extract and flavoring) may produce less desirable results.

USE CAUTION WITH COCONUT MILK POWDER. Many brands contain a little bit of caseinate, which is milk protein. Some brands have emerged that are strictly dairy free, but be sure to scour the ingredients regardless of claims. I have seen a couple of brands mislabeled as vegan when they actually contained milk protein.

COCOA BUTTER AND CACAO BUTTER ARE THE SAME THING. Producers often use the term *cacao butter* to differentiate food-grade cocoa butter. But as long as it is labeled "food grade," cocoa or cacao butter will work in these recipes.

HOMEMADE CHOCOLATE DOESN'T WORK IN ALL BAKING NEEDS. Homemade chocolate is great for nibbling and no-bake applications. It can be melted and molded, stirred into granola bars, and tossed into trail mixes. However, it typically separates in baking, leaving behind odd greasy holes where the chocolate used to be. If you are melting and infusing the chocolate into your baked good, it may work well, but if you need those chunks to hold their shape, don't count on it.

THE REASON FOR THE BAKING ISSUES IS A LACK OF EMULSIFICATION. Homemade chocolate consists of a blend of cocoa butter, sugar, and solids (like cocoa powder). When baked, the cocoa butter liquefies and separates from the solids. Manufacturers either add lecithin (an emulsifier) or they "knead" the chocolate for up to 3 days using a process called conching to prevent separation.

BUT YOU CAN'T JUST ADD AN EMULSIFIER. Lecithin needs to be properly emulsified, and creating this emulsification at home without overheating the chocolate is tricky business. It's possible, but not an everyday kind of pursuit.

HOW TO MELT CHOCOLATE (5 METHODS)

Because we can't as easily buy dairy-free chocolate confections, melting your own chocolate for sweet recipes is often a part of dairy-free life. Not that I'm complaining. But there are various methods and important things to know for efficiency and to avoid wasting precious cacao. The transition from perfectly smooth melted chocolate to burned and practically useless chocolate can happen in mere seconds, especially when direct or high heat is used. Here is a rundown of the various techniques—and tips on how to master them.

Cheater Method: The Microwave

BEST FOR: Small batches, drizzling, speed and efficiency

HOW TO: Put the dairy-free chopped chocolate or chocolate chips in a microwave-safe bowl (with other ingredients, like oil, if the recipe calls for it). Microwave on high for 30 seconds, and then stir. Microwave on high for 30 more seconds, and stir vigorously. If the chocolate isn't completely melted, microwave on high for 15 more seconds, and stir vigorously. It should be fully melted and smooth, but do not overheat it—not even a little.

Traditional Method: Double Boiler

BEST FOR: Even heating, tempering (see Tempering on the next page), drizzling, preventing burned or degraded chocolate

HOW TO: Put water in the bottom of a double boiler so the top of the water is just below the upper pan. Put dairy-free chopped chocolate or chocolate chips in the upper pan, and then place the double boiler over low heat. Once the chocolate is partially melted, stir until it is fully melted. Remove from the heat to use. If drizzling, use a dry spoon or wipe any condensation from the bottom of the bowl before pouring.

My Favorite Method: CounterTop Double Boiler

BEST FOR: Even heating, tempering (see Tempering on the next page), drizzling, dipping, preventing burned or degraded chocolate

HOW TO: Put a few inches of very hot water (125°F to 160°F) in a pan on a work surface. Put a metal bowl in the water-filled pan so it is relatively secure and the bottom is touching the water. Add the dairy-free chopped chocolate or chocolate chips to the bowl. Once the chocolate is partially melted, stir until it is fully melted. The bowl can be removed from the heat, or left in the pan to keep the chocolate melted if dipping. The water will stay warm enough to keep it melted as you work. If drizzling, use a dry spoon or wipe any condensation from the bottom of the bowl before pouring.

Risky Method: StoveTop Style

BEST FOR: Recipes using dairy-free coconut cream or coconut milk

HOW TO: You can put dairy-free chopped chocolate or chocolate chips in a small saucepan over low heat and melt, while continuously stirring. This is a touchy method that often results in scorched chocolate. But if your recipe also calls for combining the melted chocolate with coconut milk or another very creamy dairy-free liquid, you can safely heat the two together in a saucepan over low heat, whisking often, until melted and smooth.

Semi-Pro Method: Tempering

BEST FOR: A glossier finish

HOW TO: Melt two-thirds of the dairy-free chocolate using one of the double boiler methods above. Clip on a candy thermometer. The chocolate should be hot, but you don't want it to exceed 120°F. Remove the pan or bowl of chocolate from the heat and gradually stir in the remaining third of the chocolate, letting it melt as you go. Let the chocolate cool at room temperature to about 82°F before using. This can take about 30 minutes. If it cools too much as you are dipping (appears matte and thickens), gently reheat it on the double boiler back to 80°F to 85°F.

Disaster-Prevention Tips

WHEN IS IT BURNED? Chocolate scorches when overheated, and becomes a bit darkened and slightly grainy in appearance. It is notably thicker than smooth melted chocolate, so you might think it isn't melted yet and be tempted to heat it longer. But this will only burn it more.

CAN BURNED CHOCOLATE BE SAVED? Sometimes it can. Immediately transfer the chocolate to a dry, cool bowl and whisk in some solid dairy-free chocolate chips. This might bring the chocolate temperature down quickly enough to recover it to a smooth consistency. If this doesn't work, spread the chocolate on parchment paper and refrigerate to set it up. Chop, and if it doesn't taste too scorched, use it in hearty recipes, like granola bars.

DON'T TOUCH THE WATER. Do not let any water (not even a drop) get into your melted dairy-free chocolate. This can cause it to seize.

CHOCOLATE-DIPPED COCONUT CRISPY CUPS

MAKES 8 TREATS

This riff on traditional rice crispy treats is butter free and lower in sugar, and it doubles as a special snack. These also stay crispy longer than most dairy-free recipes, since there is no water moisture from ingredients like margarine.

½ cup + 1 teaspoon coconut butter, softened, divided
¼ cup + 2 tablespoons honey or agave nectar
½ teaspoon pure vanilla flavoring or extract
Generous pinch salt
2 cups crispy brown rice cereal (certified gluten free, if needed)
½ to ¾ cup dairy-free semi-sweet or dark chocolate chips
¼ cup unsweetened shredded coconut, for decorating

1. Put the ½ cup coconut butter, sweetener, vanilla, and salt in a medium bowl and whisk to combine. Gently stir in the cereal until it is well coated.

2. Divide the crispy mixture between 8 silicone muffin cups or metal cups lined with cupcake liners. Firmly press the mixture into each cup using a piece of plastic wrap to prevent sticking. Refrigerate for 1 hour, or until firm.

3. Melt the chocolate chips with the remaining 1 teaspoon coconut butter (see page 417 for How to Melt Chocolate).

4. Pop the crispy treats out of their cups and dip the bottoms in the chocolate. Place them chocolate side up on a plate or in a container in a single layer. Use any remaining chocolate to smooth out and fill in the chocolate-dipped tops. Sprinkle with the coconut.

5. Refrigerate until set, about 10 minutes.

6. Store in an airtight container in the refrigerator for up to 1 week, or in the freezer to keep them firm and crispy.

IRRESISTIBLY EASY BUCKEYES

MAKES 24 TRUFFLES

Casually elegant, these glorified peanut butter cups earned me rave reviews at a close friend's wedding. For party favors, we wrapped a few little treats in tulle and placed one on each guest's plate. All night long, people I had never met approached me with recipe requests for "those incredible truffles." While I would love to gloat about my innovation and labor, the recipe is an embarrassingly easy riff on a classic that's named for its resemblance to the nut of the Ohio buckeye tree.

> ¾ cup creamy peanut butter (can substitute sunflower seed butter for peanut free)
> ¼ cup + ½ teaspoon dairy-free buttery spread or organic palm shortening, divided
> ½ teaspoon vanilla extract
> ¼ teaspoon salt (can omit if using salted peanut butter and buttery spread)
> 2 cups powdered confectioners' sugar
> 6 ounces semi-sweet or dark chocolate chips

1. Put the peanut butter, ¼ cup buttery spread or shortening, vanilla, and salt (if using) in a large mixing bowl. Sift in the powdered sugar. Beat with a hand mixer on low speed until smooth, about 2 minutes.
2. Pinch off pieces of the peanut butter mixture and roll them into 1-inch balls. Place them in a single layer on baking sheets lined with wax paper or parchment paper. Freeze until firm, about 15 to 20 minutes.
3. Melt the chocolate chips with the remaining ½ teaspoon buttery spread or shortening (see page 417 for How to Melt Chocolate).
4. One by one, dunk the chilled peanut butter balls about two-thirds of the way in the melted chocolate, and place them back on the baking sheets.
5. Refrigerate for 1 hour or freeze for 20 minutes, or until the chocolate is firm.
6. Store in an airtight container in the refrigerator for up to 2 weeks, or freeze to enjoy later.

ANYTIME TRUFFLES

MAKES 48 TRUFFLES

Luxurious truffles can be one of the simplest foods to prepare. Just make sure you use a good-quality dairy-free chocolate for the finest results.

> 1 pound dairy-free dark chocolate, coarsely chopped
> ¾ cup raw cashews
> ¾ cup water
> 2 tablespoons liqueur *or* 1 to 2 teaspoons flavor extract (optional)
> Cocoa powder, finely chopped nuts, powdered confectioners' sugar, or
> shredded coconut, for coating

1. Melt the chocolate (see page 417 for How to Melt Chocolate).
2. Put the cashews in your spice grinder (in batches) or food processor. Process until they pass the powder stage and begin to clump, about 2 minutes.

3. Put the cashew paste, water, and liqueur or extract (if using) in your blender. Blend until smooth and creamy, about 2 minutes.
4. Gently fold the cashew cream into the melted chocolate until smooth.
5. Cover and refrigerate for 4 hours, or until the chocolate is firm enough to scoop and handle. If it sets up too much, let it sit at room temperature for 10 minutes to soften.
6. Scoop 1-inch balls of the chocolate mixture and roll them in your choice of coating.
7. Store in an airtight container in the refrigerator for up to 1 week, or freeze to enjoy later.

NUT-FREE OPTION

Substitute 1 cup coconut cream for the cashews and water, and skip step 2.

CHOCOLATE-COATED VARIATION

Melt 10 ounces dairy-free dark or semi-sweet chocolate with 1 teaspoon oil. Dip the truffles in the chocolate to coat and place them on baking sheets lined with wax paper or parchment paper. Refrigerate for 1 hour, or until the chocolate is set.

FABULOUS FUDGE BITES

MAKES 16 TO 20 FUDGY BITES

I created this wonderfully easy recipe for So Delicious, to test out and highlight their rich "culinary" coconut milk (aka regular full-fat coconut milk in small aseptic packages). The recipe has since become a dairy-free staple in many homes.

⅓ cup full-fat coconut milk
4 teaspoons coconut oil
½ teaspoon vanilla extract *or* ¼ teaspoon peppermint, orange, or coffee extract
½ cup dairy-free semi-sweet chocolate chips or chopped dark chocolate
1½ cups powdered confectioners' sugar
¼ cup cocoa powder

1. Put the coconut milk and oil in a small saucepan over medium-low heat. Cook, whisking occasionally, until hot and just barely beginning to bubble. Remove the pan from the heat and stir in the vanilla.
2. Put the chocolate in a medium bowl and pour the hot coconut milk over the top. Let sit for 1 minute, and then whisk until smooth.
3. Sift the powdered sugar and cocoa into the chocolate mixture. Stir until thoroughly combined. The mixture will be quite thick.
4. Line 16 to 20 mini muffin cups with mini cupcake liners. Fill each liner about two-thirds to three-fourths full with the fudge mixture and level the chocolate out.
5. Refrigerate for 1 hour, or until firm.
6. Store in an airtight container in the refrigerator for up to 1 week, or freeze to enjoy later.

DULCE DE COCO

MAKES 1 CUP

Dulce de leche, or sweet milk, is a very thick, toffee-like caramel that's used as a spread, topping, or sweetener in many countries. This version uses coconut milk instead of dairy milk and was shared with us by the talented vegan cookbook author Hannah Kaminsky. I've used this recipe myself and can guarantee that the patience needed for preparation is greatly rewarded.

> 1 (14-ounce) can full-fat coconut milk
> 1 cup firmly packed dark brown sugar
> ¼ teaspoon salt
> ½ teaspoon vanilla extract

1. Put the coconut milk, sugar, and salt in a medium saucepan over medium-high heat. Bring the mixture to a boil, while whisking. Once boiling, reduce the heat to low, cover, and simmer for about 20 minutes.

2. Remove the lid and simmer, whisking occasionally, for 35 to 40 minutes, or until thickened.

3. Remove the pan from the heat and whisk in the vanilla. Let cool for at least 10 minutes before using. It will continue to thicken as it cools.

4. Store in an airtight container in the refrigerator for up to 1 week. If it thickens too much as it chills, gently warm the caramel mixture before using.

GOES-WITH-EVERYTHING CHOCOLATE GANACHE

MAKES 1½ CUPS

I'm not reinventing the wheel with this one. This is a tried and true, basic chocolate ganache recipe made dairy free. It can be used as a drizzle, pie or cake filling, or frosting!

> 10 ounces (about 1½ cups) dairy-free semi-sweet chocolate chips or chopped dark chocolate
> 1 cup full-fat coconut milk or cream
> ½ teaspoon vanilla extract
> Generous pinch salt

1. Put the chocolate in a medium bowl.
2. Put the coconut milk or cream in a small saucepan over medium heat. Cook, whisking often, until it just begins to boil. Remove the pan from the heat and whisk in the vanilla and salt.
3. Pour the hot coconut milk over the chocolate and let sit for 1 minute. Whisk until smooth.
4. For a pourable ganache, use it immediately.
5. For a filling or frosting, refrigerate the chocolate mixture for 10 minutes. Add equal parts water and ice to a larger bowl until about a quarter full. Place the chocolate bowl in the ice bath. Whip the ganache with a whisk or beat with a hand mixer until thick and fluffy, about 2 minutes.
6. Store leftover ganache in an airtight container in the refrigerator for up to 1 week. Beat the chilled ganache with your hand mixer for 30 seconds to soften before using.

COOL WHIPPED COCONUT CREAM

MAKES ABOUT 1 CUP

This whip is my go-to for a quick dollop or for making decadent recipes. But be sure to read my Whip Tips below before making your first batch.

>   1 cup coconut cream
>   2 to 4 tablespoons powdered confectioners' sugar, to taste
>   1 to 1½ teaspoons pure vanilla flavoring or extract, to taste
>   Pinch salt (optional)
>   Thickener (see Whip Tips below) (optional)

1. Chill a medium mixing bowl and a whisk or beaters in the freezer for 10 minutes.
2. Put the coconut cream in your chilled bowl and whisk or beat with a hand mixer until the mixture is smooth, creamy, and just slightly fluffy, about 1 minute.
3. Sift in the powdered sugar. Add the vanilla, salt (if using), and thickener (if using). Whisk or beat with a hand mixer on low speed to incorporate the ingredients.
4. Store in an airtight container in the refrigerator for up to 1 week. It will thicken more as it chills.

WHIP TIPS:

WHAT YOU SEE IS WHAT YOU GET. *Unlike dairy whipping cream, coconut cream doesn't thicken and become voluminous as it's whipped. So it's essential that you are using a thick coconut cream. Do not attempt to start this recipe with milk beverage or a runny coconut milk.*

THERE IS A SECRET INSTANT WHIP THICKENER. *For a whip that sets better and has more staying power at room temperature, modified starch works miracles. It's the magical ingredient in instant pudding. Use 2 teaspoons modified starch in this recipe. See* **GoDairyFree.org/gdf-ingredients** *for inexpensive options.*

MILKY POWDERS CAN ALSO HELP THICKEN. *Adding ¼ cup dairy-free milk powder or powdered cashews to this recipe will help thicken it further, but it won't be as fluffy and will slightly influence the consistency and taste. Soymilk powder works best, but coconut milk powder makes this a true coconut-flavored whip.*

SOMETIMES LESS IS MORE. *Using the lesser amount of powdered sugar will result in a thicker whip.*

I LIKE ICE BATHS. *For my whip that is! Rather than chilling the bowl and beaters, I often just place the mixing bowl in a large bowl that contains part water and part ice. This helps keep the bowl and coconut cream cool, even if I'm not working quickly.*

FRUIT WHIP

MAKES ABOUT 1¼ CUPS

Freeze-dried fruit adds a fruity infusion without moisture, which actually helps thicken as it flavors this whipped coconut cream. For more tricks, see my Whip Tips on page 424.

> 1 cup freeze-dried fruit (strawberry, blueberry, apple, pomegranate, etc.)
> 1 cup coconut cream
> 1 teaspoon vanilla powder or pure vanilla flavoring (can substitute vanilla extract)
> Pinch salt
> ¼ to ⅓ cup powdered confectioners' sugar, to taste

1. Chill a medium mixing bowl and a whisk or beaters in the freezer for 10 minutes.
2. Put the freeze-dried fruit in your spice grinder or food processor. Process until powdered, about 30 seconds.
3. Put the coconut cream, fruit powder, vanilla, and salt in your chilled mixing bowl. Whisk or beat with a hand mixer until the mixture is smooth, creamy, and just slightly fluffy, about 1 minute.
4. Sift in the powdered sugar and whisk or beat with your hand mixer to combine.
5. Store in an airtight container in the refrigerator for up to 3 days. It will thicken more as it chills.

COCOA WHIP

MAKES ABOUT 1¼ CUPS

This cocoa whip is so good that you might be tempted to eat it with a spoon! See my Whip Tips on page 424 for foolproof results.

> 1 cup coconut cream
> ¼ to ⅓ cup powdered confectioners' sugar, to taste
> 2½ to 3 tablespoons cocoa powder, to taste
> 1 teaspoon vanilla powder or pure vanilla flavoring (can substitute vanilla extract)
> Pinch salt

1. Chill a medium mixing bowl and a whisk or beaters in the freezer for 10 minutes.
2. Put the coconut cream in your chilled bowl and whisk or beat with a hand mixer until the mixture is smooth, creamy, and just slightly fluffy, about 1 minute.
3. Sift in the powdered sugar and cocoa. Add the vanilla and salt. Whisk or beat with a hand mixer on low speed to incorporate the ingredients.
4. Store in an airtight container in the refrigerator for up to 1 week. It will thicken more as it chills.

QUICK CHOCOLATE CHUNKS

MAKES 3 OUNCES

This chocolate works great for snacking, homemade bark, or no-bake recipes, or as a trail mix add-in. It can also be melted for a chocolate coating on bars.

1½ ounces food-grade cocoa butter, finely chopped or grated (3 tablespoons melted)
¼ cup cocoa powder
1 to 3 tablespoons agave nectar or powdered confectioner's sugar (see Variations below)
¼ teaspoon vanilla powder or pure vanilla flavoring
Pinch salt

1. Put the cocoa butter in a medium mixing bowl. Pour a few inches of hot water into a larger bowl and place the cocoa butter bowl inside it. Be careful not to get any water in the cocoa butter. Let the cocoa butter melt, whisking occasionally.
2. Sift the cocoa powder and powdered sugar (if using) into the cocoa butter and whisk to combine. Add the agave nectar (if using), vanilla, and salt and whisk until very smooth.
3. Pour the liquid chocolate into silicone molds and refrigerate for 30 minutes, or until set.
4. Pop the chocolate out of the molds to enjoy or chop and use in no-bake recipes.
5. Store in an airtight container at room temperature for up to 1 week, or in the refrigerator or freezer for optimum freshness and to enjoy later.

VARIATIONS

COCONUT OIL: Use ¼ cup melted coconut oil in place of the cocoa butter and skip step 1. This version will tend to soften and possibly melt at warmer room temperatures, so store it in the refrigerator or freezer.

BITTERSWEET: Use just 1 tablespoon agave nectar. If you prefer powdered sugar, use 1½ tablespoons, but agave nectar will give you a smoother result.

SEMI-SWEET: Use 3 tablespoons powdered sugar. If you prefer agave nectar, use 2 tablespoons, but be aware that it will produce much softer chocolate.

SUGAR-FREE: Replace the sweetener with a very small amount of pure stevia powder or your favorite powdered sugar-free sweetener, to taste.

MYLK CHOCOLATE

MAKES 5 OUNCES

This rich, creamy chocolate works great for snacking, homemade bark, or no-bake recipes, or as a trail mix add-in. It can also be melted for a chocolate coating on bars.

2 ounces food-grade cocoa butter, finely chopped or grated (¼ cup melted)
6 tablespoons powdered confectioners' sugar, or to taste
3 tablespoons cocoa powder
¼ cup dairy-free coconut milk powder
¾ teaspoon vanilla powder or pure vanilla flavoring
Pinch salt

1. Put the cocoa butter in a medium mixing bowl. Pour a few inches of hot water into a larger bowl and place the cocoa butter bowl inside it. Be careful not to get any water in the cocoa butter. Let the cocoa butter melt, whisking occasionally.
2. Sift the powdered sugar and cocoa powder into the cocoa butter and whisk to combine. Add the coconut milk powder, vanilla, and salt and whisk until very smooth.
3. Pour the liquid chocolate into silicone molds and refrigerate for 30 minutes, or until set.
4. Pop the chocolate out of the molds to enjoy or chop and use in no-bake recipes.
5. Store in an airtight container at room temperature for up to 1 week, or in the refrigerator or freezer for optimum freshness and to enjoy later.

....

CASHEW VARIATION

Omit the coconut milk powder. Put the powdered sugar, cocoa powder, and 3 table-spoons raw cashews in your spice grinder. Process until powdered. Sift this mixture into your cocoa butter and proceed with the recipe as directed.

....

WHITE CHOCOLATE

MAKES 4 OUNCES

This sweet, creamy chocolate tastes very "natural" compared to the chemical-laden brands from the store. And of course, it's dairy free, too! This chocolate works best in no-bake recipes or homemade bark, or for infusing recipes with white chocolate flavor.

2 ounces food-grade cocoa butter, finely chopped or grated (¼ cup melted)
¼ cup powdered confectioners' sugar, or to taste
1½ tablespoons dairy-free coconut milk powder
¼ teaspoon pure vanilla powder or paste *or* 1-inch piece vanilla bean

1. Put the cocoa butter in a medium mixing bowl. Pour a few inches of hot water into a larger bowl and place the cocoa butter bowl inside it. Be careful not to get any water in the cocoa butter. Let the cocoa butter melt, whisking occasionally.

2. Sift the powdered sugar into the cocoa butter and whisk to combine. Add the coconut milk powder and vanilla powder, paste, or seeds scraped from the vanilla bean piece. Whisk until very smooth.

3. Pour the liquid white chocolate into silicone molds and refrigerate for 30 minutes, or until set.

4. Pop the white chocolate out of the molds to enjoy or chop and use in no-bake recipes.

5. Store in an airtight container at room temperature for up to 1 week, or in the refrigerator or freezer for optimum freshness and to enjoy later.

....

CASHEW VARIATION

Omit the coconut milk powder. Put the powdered sugar and ¼ cup raw cashews in your spice grinder. Process until powdered. Sift this mixture into your cocoa butter and proceed with the recipe as directed. This makes a thicker white chocolate coating for dipping truffles and dairy-free ice cream.

....

PEANUT BUTTER CHIPS

MAKES 4 OUNCES

Peanut powder is a great way to infuse peanut buttery flavor without adding moisture. These chips work great in no-bake recipes, melted for a peanut butter coating on bars, or tossed into trail mixes.

  2 ounces food-grade cocoa butter, finely chopped or grated (¼ cup melted)
  6 tablespoons peanut powder
  ⅓ cup powdered confectioners' sugar, or to taste
  Generous pinch salt

1. Put the cocoa butter in a medium mixing bowl. Pour a few inches of hot water into a larger bowl and place the cocoa butter bowl inside it. Be careful not to get any water in the cocoa butter. Let the cocoa butter melt, whisking occasionally.

2. Put the peanut powder, powdered sugar, and salt in your spice grinder. Process for 30 seconds.

3. Sift the peanut mixture into the cocoa butter and whisk until smooth. For even smoother results, pour the mixture into your blender and blend until smooth, about 30 seconds.

4. Pour the peanut butter chocolate into silicone molds and refrigerate for 30 minutes, or until set.

5. Pop the peanut butter chocolate out of the molds to enjoy or chop and use in no-bake recipes.

6. Store in an airtight container at room temperature for up to 1 week, or in the refrigerator or freezer for optimum freshness and to enjoy later.

NO-BAKE CRUMBLE TOPPING

MAKES 1²/₃ CUPS

It's impossible to beat the quick preparation, fun crispy bite, and perfectly sweet flavor of this wholesome, butter-less crumble topping. It turns chopped fruit or a bowl of dairy-free yogurt into a special treat, and is also great atop dairy-free ice cream! And because it's made without any flours or eggs, you can safely enjoy it "raw."

 1 cup almond flour or almond meal
 ⅓ cup coconut sugar (can substitute brown sugar or your granulated sweetener
  of choice)
 ½ teaspoon ground cinnamon
 Pinch salt
 3 to 4 tablespoons coconut oil (can substitute organic palm oil)
 1 teaspoon pure vanilla flavoring (can substitute vanilla extract)

1. Line a medium plate with parchment paper or wax paper.
2. Put the almond flour, sugar, cinnamon, and salt in a medium bowl and whisk to combine.
3. Add the coconut oil and vanilla and whisk until coarse crumbs form. Use 3 tablespoons oil for finer crumbs, 4 tablespoons for chunkier, firmer crumbles.
4. Dump the crumble mixture onto your paper-lined plate, and spread it out a bit. Place the plate in the freezer for 10 minutes.
5. Remove the crumble from the freezer and break up any large chunks.
6. Store the mixture in an airtight container or plastic freezer bag in the freezer.

CREDITS & APPRECIATION

There are some fabulous people who contributed to this book, and I want to formally introduce you to each of them.

Sarah Hatfield is an associate editor for my website, **GoDairyFree.org**, and she is also my lead recipe tester. No one helped me more with the content of this book than Sarah. She is the mother of a milk-allergic teen, has three other non-allergic children, and is married to a wonderful baker. Her household was a big part of ensuring that these recipes were family friendly, and Sarah also contributed some of her own beloved family recipes. She even solicited her sister, Emily Vallozzi, for infant-friendly recipes and ideas. You can see more of Sarah's recipes at **GoDairyFree.org/sarah-recipes** and **NoWheyMama.com**.

Hannah Kaminsky is one of the most prolific vegan dessert recipe creators out there, with five cookbooks under her faux leather belt, at last count. Hannah helped create a few of the trickier vegan baking options in this book. She also contributed a few of her own classic sweet recipes. You can see more of her recipes and photography work at **BittersweetBlog.com**.

A few other recipes were also contributed by my friends, and talented cookbook authors, **Dreena Burton** of **PlantPoweredKitchen.com**, **Alexa Croft** of **FloAndGrace.com**, and **Cybele Pascal** of **CybelePascal.com**.

Finally, thank you to my husband, **Anthony**, very supportive friends **Tess** and **Caroline**, agent **Sharon**, and the wonderful **BenBella Books** team for making this book happen.

METRIC CONVERSIONS & EQUIVALENTS

LIQUID / DRY MEASURES	
U.S.	**METRIC**
¼ teaspoon	1.25 milliliters
½ teaspoon	2.5 milliliters
1 teaspoon	5 milliliters
1 tablespoon	15 milliliters
1 fluid ounce	30 milliliters
¼ cup	60 milliliters
⅓ cup	80 milliliters
½ cup	120 milliliters
⅔ cup	160 milliliters
¾ cup	180 milliliters
1 cup (8 fluid ounces)	240 milliliters
1 pint (2 cups)	480 milliliters
1 quart (4 cups)	960 milliliters
1 ounce (by weight)	28 grams
4 ounces (by weight)	114 grams
8 ounces / ½ pound (by weight)	227 grams
16 ounces / 1 pound (by weight)	454 grams

COOKING MEASUREMENT EQUIVALENTS	
1 tablespoon	3 teaspoons
⅛ cup	2 tablespoons
¼ cup	4 tablespoons
⅓ cup	5 tablespoons + 1 teaspoon
½ cup	8 tablespoons
1 cup	16 tablespoons
1 gallon	4 quarts
1 quart	2 pints
1 pint	2 cups

LENGTH	
U.S.	**METRIC**
⅛ inch	3 millimeters
¼ inch	6 millimeters
½ inch	12 millimeters
1 inch	2.5 centimeters
1 foot (12 inches)	30 centimeters

BAKING PANS		
U.S.	**METRIC**	**METRIC VOLUME**
8 × 5-inch (loaf)	20 × 13 centimeters	1.8 liters
9 × 5-inch (loaf)	23 × 13 centimeters	2 liters
8 × 8-inch	20 × 20 centimeters	2 liters
7 × 11-inch	18 × 27 centimeters	1.5 liters
8 × 12-inch	20 × 30 centimeters	3 liters
9 × 13-inch	23 × 33 centimeters	3.5 liters
8-inch round (cake)	20 × 4 centimeters	1.2 liters
9-inch round (cake)	23 × 4 centimeters	1.5 liters
9-inch round (pie)	23 × 3 centimeters	1 liter

REFERENCES

CHAPTER 1: WHAT IS DAIRY?

Wattiaux, Michel A. *Dairy Essentials*. Madison, WI: The Babcock Institute, 1999.

Lindmark Månsson, Helen. "Fatty Acids in Bovine Milk Fat." *Food & Nutrition Research* 52 (2008): 1. https://www.ncbi.nlm.nih.gov/pmc/articles/PMC2596709.

Newcomer, Chris, and Steven C. Murphy. "Guideline for Vitamin A & D Fortification of Fluid Milk." The Dairy Practices Council, 2001. https://phpa.health.maryland.gov/OEHFP/OFPCHS/Milk/Shared%20Documents/DPC053_Vitamin_AD_Fortification_Fluid_Milk.pdf.

Harvard T.H. Chan School of Public Health. "Vitamin A." *The Nutrition Source*, 2006. https://www.hsph.harvard.edu/nutritionsource/vitamin-a.

Ford, Clark. "Milk & Milk Products." *Food and the Consumer*. Department of Food Science and Human Nutrition, Iowa State University, Fall 2000.

Adam, Mike. "Why It Takes 2,000 Gallons of Fresh Water to Produce One Gallon of Milk." *The Natural News Network*, June 2, 2008. http://www.naturalnews.com/023341_water_milk_organic.html.

The Weston A. Price Foundation. "Which Do You Choose?" A Campaign for Real Milk, 2001. https://www.realmilk.com/safety/which-do-you-choose.

Minnesota Department of Agriculture. "MDA's Role in Preventing Antibiotic Resistance."

U.S. Department of Agriculture. "How USDA's Dairy Grading Program Works."

National Dairy Council. *Newer Knowledge of Milk and Other Fluid Dairy Products*. Rosemont, IL: National Dairy Council, 1993.

Hartley, Jo. "The Facts About Pasteurization and Homogenization of Dairy Products." *The Natural News Network*, April 9, 2008. http://www.naturalnews.com/022967_milk_pasteurization_dairy.html.

Enig, Mary G. "Milk Homogenization and Heart Disease." *Wise Traditions in Food, Farming and the Healing Arts*. Weston A. Price Foundation, Summer 2003. https://www.westonaprice.org/health-topics/know-your-fats/milk-homogenization-heart-disease.

Organic Consumers Association. "How Artificial Hormones Damage the Dairy Industry and Endanger Public Health." Food & Water Watch, June 2009. https://www.organicconsumers.org/sites/default/files/rbgh.pdf.

Francis, G. L., F. M. Upton, F. J. Ballard, et al. "Insulin-like Growth Factors 1 and 2 in Bovine Colostrum: Sequences and Biological Activities Compared with Those of a Potent Truncated Form." *Biochemical Journal* 251, no. 1 (1988): 95–103. https://www.ncbi.nlm.nih.gov/pmc/articles/PMC1148968.

Moulton, Libby. "Labeling Milk from Cows Not Treated with rBST: Legal in All 50 States as of September 29th, 2010." *Columbia Science and Technology Law Review*, October 28, 2010. http://stlr.org/2010/10/28/labeling-milk-from-cows-not-treated-with-rbst-legal-in-all-50-states-as-of-september-29th-2010.

The European Commission—Food Safety. "Report on Public Health Aspects of the Use of Bovine Somatotropin." March 15–16, 1999. https://ec.europa.eu/food/sites/food/files/safety/docs/sci-com_scv_out19_en.pdf.

Holmes, M. D., M. N. Pollak, W. C. Willett, et al. "Dietary Correlates of Plasma Insulin-like Growth Factor I and Insulin-like Growth Factor Binding Protein 3 Concentrations." *Cancer Epidemiology, Biomarkers, and Prevention* (September 2002): 852–61. https://www.ncbi.nlm.nih.gov/pubmed/12223429.

Chan, J. M., M. J. Stampfer, E. Giovannucci, et al. "Plasma Insulin-like Growth Factor-I and Prostate Cancer Risk: A Prospective Study." *Science* 279, no. 5350 (January 23, 1998): 563–66. https://www.ncbi.nlm.nih.gov/pubmed/9438850.

Yu, H., F. Jin, X. O. Shu, et al. "Insulin-like Growth Factors and Breast Cancer Risk in Chinese Women." *Cancer Epidemiology, Biomarkers, and Prevention* 11, no. 8 (August 2002): 705–12. https://www.ncbi.nlm.nih.gov/pubmed/12163322.

Dohoo, I. R., L. DesCôteaux, K. Leslie, et al. "A Meta-Analysis Review of the Effects of Recombinant Bovine Somatotropin." *The Canadian Journal of Veterinary Research* 67, no. 4 (October 2003): 252–64. https://www.ncbi.nlm.nih.gov/pmc/articles/PMC280709.

Broadwater, Neil, and Hugh Chester-Jones. "Raising Dairy Calves." Minnesota Dairy Team, 2009. https://www.extension.umn.edu/agriculture/dairy/calves-and-heifers/raising-dairy-heifer-calves-from-bith-to-six-months.pdf.

Notermans, S., J. Dufrenne, P. Teunis, et al. "A Risk Assessment Study of *Bacillus cereus* Present in Pasteurized Milk." *Food Microbiology* 14 (1997): 143–51. http://smas.chemeng.ntua.gr/miram/files/publ_359_5_10_2005.pdf.

McDonough, F. E., A. D. Hitchins, N. P. Wong, et al. "Modification of Sweet Acidophilus Milk to Improve Utilization by Lactose-Intolerant Persons." *American Journal of Clinical Nutrition* 45, no. 3 (1987): 570–74. https://www.ncbi.nlm.nih.gov/pubmed/3103415.

Qi, P. X., D. Ren, Y. Xiao, et al. "Effect of Homogenization and Pasteurization on the Structure and Stability of Whey Protein in Milk." *Journal of Dairy Science* 98, no. 5 (2015): 2884–97. doi:10.3168. https://www.ncbi.nlm.nih.gov/pubmed/25704975.

Poulsen, O. M., J. Hau, and J. Kollerup. "Effect of Homogenization and Pasteurization on the Allergenicity of Bovine Milk Analysed by a Murine Anaphylactic Shock Model." *Clinical Allergy* 17, no. 5 (1987): 449–58. https://www.ncbi.nlm.nih.gov/pubmed/3677371.

Davis, Benjamin J. K., Cissy X. Li, and Keeve E. Nachman. "A Literature Review of the Risks and Benefits of Consuming Raw and Pasteurized Cow's Milk." Department of Environmental Health Sciences Johns Hopkins Bloomberg School of Public Health, December 8, 2014. http://www.jhsph.edu/research/centers-and-institutes/johns-hopkins-center-for-a-livable-future/_pdf/research/clf_reports/RawMilkMDJohnsHopkinsReport2014_1208_.pdf.

Lerebours, E., Ndam C N'Djitoyap, A. Lavoine, et al. "Yogurt and Fermented-Then-Pasteurized Milk: Effects of Short-Term and Long-Term Ingestion on Lactose Absorption and Mucosal Lactase Activity in Lactase-Deficient Subjects." *American Journal of Clinical Nutrition* 49, no. 5 (1989): 823–27. http://www.ncbi.nlm.nih.gov/pubmed/2497632.

The a2 Milk Company. "What Is a2 Milk™?" https://thea2milkcompany.com/faq/a2-milk-2.

Jenkins, J. A., H. Breiteneder, and E. N. Mills. "Evolutionary Distance from Human Homologues Reflects Allergenicity of Animal Food Proteins." *The Journal of Allergy and Clinical Immunology* 120, no. 6 (2007): 1399–405. doi:10.1016/j.jaci.2007.08.019. https://www.ncbi.nlm.nih.gov/pubmed/17935767.

Skripak, J. M., E. C. Matsui, K. Mudd, et al. "The Natural History of IgE-Mediated Cow Milk Allergy." *Journal of Allergy and Clinical Immunology* 120, no. 5 (2007): 1172–77. doi:10.1016/j.jaci.2007.08.023. https://www.ncbi.nlm.nih.gov/pubmed/17935766.

Infante Pina, D., R. Tormo Carnice, M. Conde Zandueta. "Use of Goat's Milk in Patients with Cow's Milk Allergy." *Anales de Pediatria* 59, no. 2 (2003): 138–42. http://www.ncbi.nlm.nih.gov/pubmed/12882742.

Bellioni-Businco, B., R. Paganelli, P. Lucenti, et al. "Allergenicity of Goat's Milk in Children with Cow's Milk Allergy." *Journal of Allergy and Clinical Immunology* 103, no. 6 (1999): 1191–94. http://www.ncbi.nlm.nih.gov/pubmed/10359905.

The Word. "Mare's Milk." *New Scientist* 2608 (June 16, 2007): 58. http://www.foodsmatter.com/allergy_intolerance/goat_sheep_milks/research/mares_milk.html.

Shabo, Y., R. Barzel, M. Margoulis, et al. "Camel Milk for Food Allergies in Children." *Israel Medical Association Journal* 7, no. 12 (2005): 796–98. https://www.ima.org.il/FilesUpload/IMAJ/0/51/25828.pdf.

Ehlayel, M. S., K. A. Hazeima, F. Al-Mesaifri, et al. "Camel Milk: An Alternative for Cow's Milk Allergy in Children." *Allergy and Asthma Proceedings* 32, no. 3 (2011): 255–58. doi:10.2500/aap.2011.32.3429.

Businco, L., P. G. Giampietro, P. Lucenti, et al. "Allergenicity of Mare's Milk in Children with Cow's Milk Allergy." *Journal of Allergy and Clinical Immunology* 105, no. 5 (2000): 1031–34. http://www.ncbi.nlm.nih.gov/pubmed/10808187.

Sears, William. "Ask Dr. Sears: Advantages of Goat's Milk." *Parenting.* http://www.parenting.com/article/ask-dr-sears-advantages-of-goats-milk.

Monti, G., S. Viola, C. Baro, et al. "Tolerability of Donkey's Milk in 92 Highly Problematic Cow's Milk Allergic Children." *Journal of Biological Regulators and Homeostatic Agents* 26, no. 3 (2012): 75–82. http://www.ncbi.nlm.nih.gov/pubmed/23158519.

Polidori, P., and S. Vincenzetti. "Use of Donkey's Milk in Children with Cow's Milk Protein Allergy." *Foods* 2 (2013): 151–59. doi:10.3390/foods2020151.

CHAPTER 2: WHY WE LIVE DAIRY FREE

Prescott, S., R. Pawankar, K. J. Allen, et al. "A Global Survey of Changing Patterns of Food Allergy Burden in Children." *World Allergy Organ Journal* 6, no. 1 (2013): 21. doi:10.1186/1939-4551-6-21.

Fiocchi, Alessandro, and Vincenzo Fierro. "Food Allergy." *World Allergy Organization.* March 2017. http://www.worldallergy.org/professional/allergic_diseases_center/foodallergy.

Carroccio, A. "Milk Allergy Can Persist After Infancy." *Clinical and Experimental Allergy Study at University of Palermo* 28 (1998): 817–23.

"About Food Allergy Symptoms." Food Allergy Research & Education. https://www.foodallergy.org/symptoms.

Grimbaldeston, Metz, Yu, et al. "Effector and Potential Immunoregulatory Roles of Mast Cells in IgE-Associated Acquired Immune Responses." *Current Opinion in Immunology* 18, no. 6 (2006): 751–60. doi:10.1016/j.coi.2006.09.011. PMID 17011762.

"Lactose Intolerance." National Institute of Diabetes and Digestive and Kidney Diseases, May 2014. https://www.niddk.nih.gov/-/media/Files/Digestive-Diseases/Lactose_Intolerance_508.pdf?la=en.

Longo, G., E. Barbi, I. Berti, et al. "Specific Oral Tolerance Induction in Children with Very Severe Cow's Milk–Induced Reactions." *The Journal of Allergy and Clinical Immunology* 121, no. 2 (2008): 343–47. doi:10.1016/j.jaci.2007.10.029.

Spergel, Jonathan. "Nonimmunoglobulin E-Mediated Immune Reactions to Foods." *Allergy, Asthma & Clinical Immunology* 2 (2006): 78. doi:10.1186/1710-1492-2-2-78.

Kwon, J., J. Kim, S. Cho, et al. "Characterization of Food Allergies in Patients with Atopic Dermatitis." *Nutrition Research and Practice* 7, no. 2 (April 2013): 115–21. doi:10.4162/nrp.2013.7.2.115.

Nowak-W grzyn, Anna. "Food Protein-Induced Enterocolitis Syndrome and Allergic Proctocolitis." *Allergy and Asthma Proceedings* 36, no. 3 (2015): 172–84. doi:10.2500/aap.2015.36.3811.

Dellon, E. S., E. T. Jensen, C. F. Martin, et al. "Prevalence of Eosinophilic Esophagitis in the United States." *Clinical Gastroenterology and Hepatology* 12, no. 4 (2014): 589-96. doi:10.1016/j.cgh.2013.09.008.

Alfadda, Abdulrahman A., and Martin A. Storr. "Eosinophilic Colitis: Epidemiology, Clinical Features, and Current Management." *Therapeutic Advances in Gastroenterology* 4, no. 5 (2011): 301–309. doi:10.1177/1756283X10392443.

Moissidis, I., D. Chaidaroon, P. Vichyanond, et al. "Milk-Induced Pulmonary Disease in Infants (Heiner Syndrome)." *Pediatric Allergy and Immunology* 16, no. 6 (2005): 545–52. doi:10.1111/j.1399-3038.2005.00291.x.

Fiocchi, A., J. Brozek, H. Schünemann, et al. "World Allergy Organization (WAO) Diagnosis and Rationale for Action Against Cow's Milk Allergy (DRACMA) Guidelines." *Pediatric Allergy and Immunology* 21 (2010): 1–125. doi:10.1111/j.1399-3038.2010.01068.x.

Skripak, Justin M., Elizabeth C. Matsui, Kim Mudd, et al. "The Natural History of IgE-Mediated Cow's Milk Allergy." *Journal of Allergy and Clinical Immunology* 120, no. 5 (2007): 1172–77. doi:10.1016/j.jaci.2007.08.023.

"Milk Allergy Symptoms." Mayo Clinic. http://www.mayoclinic.org/diseases-conditions/milk-allergy/basics/symptoms/con-20032147.

Reda, Shereen M. "Gastrointestinal Manifestations of Food Allergy." *Pediatric Health* 3, no. 3 (2009): 217–29. doi:10.2217/phe.09.13.

Juntti, Hanna, and Jorma Sami Tikkanen. "Cow's Milk Allergy Is Associated with Recurrent Otitis Media During Childhood." *Acta Oto-Laryngologica* 119, no. 8 (1999): 867–73. doi:10.1080/00016489950180199.

Dehghani, S. M., B. Ahmadpour, M. Haghighat, et al. "The Role of Cow's Milk Allergy in Pediatric Chronic Constipation: A Randomized Clinical Trial." *Iranian Journal of Pediatrics* 22, no. 4 (2012): 468–74. http://www.ncbi.nlm.nih.gov/pmc/articles/PMC3533146.

"Milk Allergies." Cleveland Clinic. https://my.clevelandclinic.org/childrens-hospital/health-info/diseases-conditions/hic-Milk-Allergies.

"Anaphylaxis: MedlinePlus Medical Encyclopedia." MedlinePlus: Health Information from the National Library of Medicine. https://medlineplus.gov/ency/article/000844.htm.

Lill, Claudia, Benjamin Loader, Rudolf Seemann, et al. "Milk Allergy Is Frequent in Patients with Chronic Sinusitis and Nasal Polyposis." *American Journal of Rhinology and Allergy* 25, no. 6 (2011): 221–24. doi:10.2500/ajra.2011.25.3686. http://www.ncbi.nlm.nih.gov/pubmed/22185729.

Mansfield, L. E., T. R. Vaughan, S. F. Waller, et al. "Food Allergy and Adult Migraine: Double-Blind and Mediator Confirmation of an Allergic Etiology." *Annals of Allergy, Asthma & Immunology* 55, no. 2 (1985): 126–29. http://www.ncbi.nlm.nih.gov/pubmed/4025956.

Lockey, Richard F., and Joy McCann Culverhouse. "Anaphylaxis: Synopsis." World Allergy Organization, September 2012. http://www.worldallergy.org/professional/allergic_diseases_center/anaphylaxis/anaphylaxissynopsis.php.

"Skin Prick Tests for Food Allergies." Food Allergy Research & Education. http://www.foodallergy.org/diagnosis-and-testing/skin-tests.

Cudowska, B., and M. Kaczmarski. "Atopy Patch Test in the Diagnosis of Food Allergy in Children with Atopic Eczema Dermatitis Syndrome." *Rocz Akad Med Bialymst* 50 (2005): 261–67. http://www.ncbi.nlm.nih.gov/pubmed/16358980.

Mowszet, K., K. Matusiewicz, and B. Iwa czak. "Value of the Atopy Patch Test in the Diagnosis of Food Allergy in Children with Gastrointestinal Symptoms." *Advances in Clinical and Experimental Medicine* 23, no. 3 (2014): 403–409. http://www.ncbi.nlm.nih.gov/pubmed/24979512.

Agrawal, S. K., R. Das, M. M. Goel, et al. "Tetrazolium Reduction Test in Diagnosis of Urinary Tract Infections." *Indian Journal of Pathology and Microbiology* 29, no. 1 (1986): 61–65. http://www.ncbi.nlm.nih.gov/pmc/articles/PMC3536737.

Berni Canani, Roberto, Naseer Sangwan, Andrew T. Stefka, et al. "*Lactobacillus rhamnosus* GG-Supplemented Formula Expands Butyrate-Producing Bacterial Strains in Food Allergic Infants." *The ISME Journal* 10, no. 3 (2015): 742–50. doi:10.1038/ismej.2015.151.

"Where We Stand Today." Food Allergy Research & Education. https://www.foodallergy.org/research/overview.

Calatayud, Martorel, Muriel García, Martorell Aragonés, et al. "Safety and Efficacy Profile and Immunological Changes Associated with Oral Immunotherapy for IgE-mediated Cow's Milk Allergy in Children: Systematic Review and Meta-Analysis." *Journal of Investigational Allergology and Clinical Immunology* 24, no. 5 (2014): 298–307. http://www.jiaci.org/issues/vol24issue5/2.pdf.

"Mixed Long-Term Results Following Milk Oral Immunotherapy." The American Academy of Allergy, Asthma & Immunology. http://www.aaaai.org/global/latest-research-summaries/Current-JACI-Research/Mixed-results-milk-oral-immunotherapy.

Wang, J., and X. M. Li. "Chinese Herbal Therapy for the Treatment of Food Allergy." *Current Allergy and Asthma Reports* 12, no. 4 (2012): 332–38. http://www.ncbi.nlm.nih.gov/pubmed/22581122.

"Lactose Intolerance: What You Need to Know." Johns Hopkins Medicine. http://www.hopkinsmedicine.org/healthlibrary/conditions/digestive_disorders/lactose_intolerance_85,P00388.

Praveen, Roy. "Lactose Intolerance." Medscape, July 14, 2015. http://emedicine.medscape.com/article/187249-overview.

"Lactose Intolerance." British Nutrition Foundation, 2000.

"Lactose Intolerance." Mayo Clinic, September 2, 2016. http://www.mayoclinic.org/diseases-conditions/lactose-intolerance/basics/definition/con-20027906.

"Lactose Maldigestion Fact Sheet." National Dairy Council.

Inman-Felton, Amy E. "Overview of Lactose Maldigestion (Lactase Nonpersistence)." *Journal of the American Dietetic Association* 98 (1999): 481–89. doi:10.1016/S0002-8223(99)00120-0.

"Executive Summary: Lactose Intolerance and Health." National Center for Biotechnology Information, 2010. https://www.ncbi.nlm.nih.gov/books/NBK44620.

Scrimshaw, N. S., and E. B. Murray. "The Acceptability of Milk and Milk Products in Populations with a High Prevalence of Lactose Intolerance." *American Journal of Clinical Nutrition* 48, no. 4 (1988): 1079–159. http://www.ncbi.nlm.nih.gov/pubmed/3140651.

"Lactose Intolerance." Genetics Home Reference, May 2010. http://ghr.nlm.nih.gov/condition/lactose-intolerance.

Burger, J., M. Kirchner, B. Bramanti, et al. "Absence of the Lactase-Persistence-Associated Allele in Early Neolithic Europeans." *Proceedings of the National Academy of Sciences* 104, no. 10 (2007): 3736–41. doi:10.1073/pnas.0607187104.

O'Connell, S., and G. Walsh. "Physicochemical Characteristics of Commercial Lactases Relevant to Their Application in the Alleviation of Lactose Intolerance." *Applied Biochemistry and Biotechnology* 134, no. 2 (2006): 179–92. doi:10.1385/abab:134:2:179.

Carper, Steve. "The Really BIG List of Lactose Percentages." Steve Carper's Lactose Intolerance Clearinghouse. http://www.stevecarper.com/li/list_of_lactose_percentages.htm.

Matz, Samuel A. *Ingredients for Bakers*. McAllen, TX: Pan-Tech International, 1987.

Shepheard, Nicola. "Dairy Intolerance Real—'Not in People's Heads.'" The University of Auckland, August 14, 2017. https://www.auckland.ac.nz/en/about/news-events-and-notices/news/news-2017/08/dairy-intolerance-real.html.

"Galactosemia." Genetics Home Reference, August 2015. https://ghr.nlm.nih.gov/condition/galactosemia.

Stahler, Charles. "How Many Adults Are Vegetarian? The Vegetarian Resource Group Asked in a 2006 National Poll." *Vegetarian Journal* 4, 2006.

Barnard, N. D., J. Cohen, D. J. Jenkins, et al. "A Low-Fat Vegan Diet Improves Glycemic Control and Cardiovascular Risk Factors in a Randomized Clinical Trial in Individuals with Type 2 Diabetes." *Diabetes Care* 29, no. 8 (2006): 1777–83. doi:10.2337/dc06-0606.

D'Enfert, C., I. Reyss, C. Wandersman, et al. "Protein Secretion by Gram-Negative Bacteria. Characterization of Two Membrane Proteins Required for Pullulanase Secretion by *Escherichia coli* K-12." *The Journal of Biological Chemistry* 264, no. 29 (1989): 17462–68. http://www.ncbi.nlm.nih.gov/pmc/articles/PMC2677007.

Bunner, A. E., C. L. Wells, J. Gonzales, et al. "A Dietary Intervention for Chronic Diabetic Neuropathy Pain: A Randomized Controlled Pilot Study." *Nutrition & Diabetes*, May 26, 2015. doi:10.1038/nutd.2015.8.

"Autism and Developmental Disabilities Monitoring (ADDM) Network." Centers for Disease Control and Prevention, December 5, 2016. http://www.cdc.gov/ncbddd/autism/addm.html.

Baio, Jon. "Prevalence of Autism Spectrum Disorder Among Children." Centers for Disease Control and Prevention, March 28, 2014.

"Parent Ratings of Behavioral Effects of Biomedical Interventions." Autism Research Institute, 2005. ARI Publ. 34. https://www.autism.com/pdf/providers/ParentRatings2009.pdf.

"Fact Sheet: CDC Autism Research." Centers for Disease Control and Prevention, March 4, 2006. https://www.cdc.gov/media/transcripts/AutismResearchFactSheet.pdf.

"Biomedical and Dietary Approaches." Autism Society of America.

Larson, Nina. "Diet Changes Give Hyperactive Kids New Taste for Life in Norway." AFP and Yahoo! News, February 24, 2008, http://health.gmnews.com/news/2008-08-06/health/003.html.

Lawlor, D. A., S. Ebrahim, N. Timpson, et al. "Avoiding Milk Is Associated with a Reduced Risk of Insulin Resistance and the Metabolic Syndrome: Findings from the British Women's Heart and Health Study." *Diabetic Medicine* 22, no. 6 (2005): 808–11. doi:10.1111/j.1464-5491.2005.01537.x.

Brody, S. "The Rate of Growth of the Dairy Cow: Extrauterine Growth in Weight." *The Journal of General Physiology* 3, no. 5 (1921): 623–33. doi:10.1085/jgp.3.5.623.

Berkey, Catherine S., Helaine R. Rockett, Walter C. Willett, et al. "Milk, Dairy Fat, Dietary Calcium, and Weight Gain." *Archives of Pediatrics & Adolescent Medicine* 159, no. 6 (2005): 543. doi:10.1001/archpedi.159.6.543.

Gunther, C. W., P. A. Legowski, R. M. Lyle, et al. "Dairy Products Do Not Lead to Alterations in Body Weight or Fat Mass in Young Women in a 1-Year Intervention." *American Journal of Clinical Nutrition* 81, no. 4 (2005): 751–56.

Stein, Rob. "Study: More Milk Means More Weight Gain." *Washington Post*, June 7, 2005. http://www.washingtonpost.com/wp-dyn/content/article/2005/06/06/AR2005060601348.html.

"Dairy Data." *United States Department of Agriculture*. https://www.ers.usda.gov/data-products/dairy-data.aspx.

Geisler, Malinda. "Cheese Industry Profile." *Ag Marketing Resource Center*, May 2012. http://www.agmrc.org/commodities-products/livestock/dairy/cheese-industry-profile/

"U.S. Agriculture—Linking Consumers and Producers: What Do Americans Eat?" *USDA Agriculture Fact Book*, 1998. https://www.rma.usda.gov/ftp/publications/handbooks/FB97.PDF.

Shai, I., R. Jiang, J. E. Manson, et al. "Ethnicity, Obesity, and Risk of Type 2 Diabetes in Women: A 20-Year Follow-Up Study." *Diabetes Care* 29, no. 7 (2006): 1585–90. doi:10.2337/dc06-0057.

Colditz, Graham A. "Weight Gain as a Risk Factor for Clinical Diabetes Mellitus in Women." *Annals of Internal Medicine* 122, no. 7 (1995): 481. doi:10.7326/0003-4819-122-7-199504010-00001.

Manson, J. E., M. J. Stampfer, G. A. Colditz, et al. "Physical Activity and Incidence of Non-Insulin-Dependent Diabetes Mellitus in Women." *The Lancet* 338, no. 8770 (1991): 774–78. doi:10.1016/0140-6736(91)90664-b.

"Vitamin D and Flavonoids Examined for Impact on Breast and Ovarian Cancers." ScienceDaily, April 7, 2006. www.sciencedaily.com/releases/2006/04/060407144100.htm.

Laino, Charlene. "A Call for More Vitamin D Research." *A Cancer Journal for Clinicians* 56, no. 5 (2006): 250–51. doi:10.3322/canjclin.56.5.250.

Larsen, Hans. "Milk and the Cancer Connection." *International Health News* 76 (April 1998). http://www.notmilk.com/drlarsen.html.

"Milk Link to Ovarian Cancer Risk." BBC News, November 29, 2004. http://news.bbc.co.uk/2/hi/health/4051331.stm.

Stewart, Alison. "Hormones in Milk Are Linked to Cancer." *Consumer Health Journal*, March 2004. http://newsmine.org/content.php?ol=nature-health/health/cancer/hormones-in-milk-are-linked-to-cancer.txt.

Fairfield, Kathleen M., David J. Hunter, Graham A. Colditz, et al. "A Prospective Study of Dietary Lactose and Ovarian Cancer." *International Journal of Cancer* 110, no. 2 (2004): 271–77. doi:10.1002/ijc.20086.

"Harvard Researchers Link Prostate Cancer and Dietary Calcium." CNN, April 4, 2000. http://www.cnn.com/2000/HEALTH/cancer/04/04/prostrate.cancer.

Allen, N. E., T. J. Key, P. N. Appleby, et al. "Animal Foods, Protein, Calcium and Prostate Cancer Risk: The European Prospective Investigation into Cancer and Nutrition." *British Journal of Cancer* 98, no. 9 (2008): 1574–81. doi:10.1038/sj.bjc.6604331.

Yang, Meng, Stacey A. Kenfield, Erin L. Van Blarigan, et al. "Dairy Intake After Prostate Cancer Diagnosis in Relation to Disease-Specific and Total Mortality." *International Journal of Cancer* 137, no. 10 (2015): 2462–69. doi:10.1002/ijc.29608.

"Vegan Diet 'Cuts Prostate Cancer Risk.'" *BBC News*, June 8, 2000. http://news.bbc.co.uk/2/hi/health/782959.stm

Liebman, Bonnie. "Preventing Prostate Cancer." *Nutrition Action Health Newsletter*, July/August 2001.

Tseng, M., R. A. Breslow, B. I. Graubard, et al. "Dairy, Calcium, and Vitamin D Intakes and Prostate Cancer Risk in the National Health and Nutrition Examination Epidemiologic Follow-Up Study cohort." *American Journal of Clinical Nutrition* 81, no. 5 (2005): 1147–54.

Jacobsen, B. K., S. F. Knutsen, and G. E. Fraser. "Does High Soy Milk Intake Reduce Prostate Cancer Incidence? The Adventist Health Study." *Cancer Causes and Control* 9, no. 6 (1998): 553–57.

Chan, J. M., M. J. Stampfer, J. Ma, et al. "Dairy Products, Calcium, and Prostate Cancer Risk in the Physicians' Health Study." *American Journal of Clinical Nutrition* 74, no. 4 (October 2001): 549–54.

Kurahashi, N., M. Inoue, M. Iwasaki, et al. "Dairy Product, Saturated Fatty Acid, and Calcium Intake and Prostate Cancer in a Prospective Cohort of Japanese Men." *Cancer Epidemiology Biomarkers & Prevention* 17, no. 4 (2008): 930–37. doi:10.1158/1055-9965.epi-07-2681.

Hedlund, T. E., P. D. Maroni, P. G. Ferucci, et al. "Long-Term Dietary Habits Affect Soy Isoflavone Metabolism and Accumulation in Prostatic Fluid in Caucasian Men." *Journal of Nutrition* 135, no. 6 (2005): 1400–1406.

Adebamowo, C. A., D. Spiegelman, C. S. Berkey, et al. "Milk Consumption and Acne in Adolescent Girls." *Dermatology Online Journal* 12, no. 4 (2006): 1. http://www.ncbi.nlm.nih.gov/pubmed/17083856.

Adebamowo, C. A., D. Spiegelman, C. S. Berkey, et al. "Milk Consumption and Acne in Teenaged Boys." *Journal of the American Academy of Dermatology* 58, no. 5 (2008): 787–93. doi:10.1016/j.jaad.2007.08.049. http://www.ncbi.nlm.nih.gov/pubmed/18194824.

Danby, F. W. "Acne and Milk, the Diet Myth, and Beyond." *Journal of the American Academy of Dermatology* 52, no. 2 (2005): 360–62. doi:10.1016/j.jaad.2004.09.022.

Wangen, Stephen. "Acne: How Food Can Cause It." *Food Allergy Solutions Review*, February 2004. http://www.foodallergysolutions.com/food-allergy-news0402.html.

Adebamowo, C. A., D. Spiegelman, F. W. Danby, et al. "High School Dietary Dairy Intake and Teenage Acne." *Journal of the American Academy of Dermatology* 52, no. 2 (2005): 207–14. doi:10.1016/j.jaad.2004.08.007.

Hoyt, Garrett, Matthew S. Hickey, and Loren Cordain. "Dissociation of the Glycaemic and Insulinaemic Responses to Whole and Skimmed Milk." *British Journal of Nutrition* 93, no. 2 (2005): 175. doi:10.1079/bjn20041304.

Cordain, Loren. "Implications for the Role of Diet in Acne." *Seminars in Cutaneous Medicine and Surgery* 24, no. 2 (2005): 84–91. doi:10.1016/j.sder.2005.04.002.

Egger, J., J. Wilson, C. M. Carter, et al. "Is Migraine Food Allergy? A Double-Blind Controlled Trial of Oligo-antigenic Diet Treatment." *Pain* 21, no. 2 (1985): 205. doi:10.1016/0304-3959(85)90314-8.

Egger, J., C. M. Carter, J. F. Soothill, et al. "Oligoantigenic Diet Treatment of Children with Epilepsy and Migraine." *The Journal of Pediatrics* 114, no. 1 (1989): 51–58. doi:10.1016/s0022-3476(89)80600-6.

Grant, Ellen C. G. "Food Allergies and Migraine." *The Lancet* 313, no. 8123 (1979): 966–69. doi:10.1016/s0140-6736(79)91735-5.

"Scientists Identify Migraine Chromosome." *Deutsche Welle*, September 10, 2005.

Leira, R., and R. Rodríguez. "Diet and Migraine." *Revista de Neurologia* 24, no. 129 (1996): 534–38.

De Roest, R. H., B. R. Dobbs, B. A. Chapman, et al. "The Low FODMAP Diet Improves Gastrointestinal Symptoms in Patients with Irritable Bowel Syndrome: A Prospective Study." *International Journal of Clinical Practice* 67, no. 9 (2013): 895–903. doi:10.1111/ijcp.12128.

Molodecky, N. A., I. S. Soon, D. M. Rabi, et al. "Increasing Incidence and Prevalence of the Inflammatory Bowel Diseases with Time, Based on Systematic Review." *Gastroenterology* 142, no. 1 (2012): 46–54.e42. doi:10.1053/j.gastro.2011.11.016.

"Crohn's Disease and Ulcerative Colitis Diet and Nutrition Q & A." Crohn's & Colitis Foundation, January 17, 2014. http://www.ccfa.org/resources/diet-and-nutrition-1.html.

Botoman, V. A., G. F. Bonner, and D. A. Botoman. "Management of Inflammatory Bowel Disease." *American Family Physician* 57, no. 1 (1998): 57–68, 71–72.

Mishkin, B., M. Yalovsky, and S. Mishkin. "Increased Prevalence of Lactose Malabsorption in Crohn's Disease Patients at Low Risk for Lactose Malabsorption Based on Ethnic Origin." *American Journal of Gastroenterology* 92, no. 7 (1997): 1148–53.

Knowles, Jarol B. "Dietary Factors in Gastrointestinal Diseases." *Digestive Health Matters*, Spring 2004. http://www.digestivewellness.net/docs/IFFGD_148_dietary_factors_gastrointestinal_diseases.pdf.

Abdullah, Mohammad, Audrey Cyr, Marie-Ève Labonté, et al. "The Impact of Dairy Consumption on Circulating Cholesterol Levels Is Modulated by Common Single Nucleotide Polymorphisms in Cholesterol Synthesis- and Transport-Related Genes." *The FASEB Journal* 28, no. 1 (2014). www.fasebj.org/content/28/1_Supplement/1038.4.

Lindquist, Susan Barber. "Mayo Clinic Study Shows Increase in Parkinson's Disease Over 30 Years." Mayo Clinic, June 20, 2016. http://newsnetwork.mayoclinic.org/discussion/mayo-clinic-study-shows-increase-in-parkinsons-disease-over-30-years.

Hughes, Katherine C., Xiang Gao, Iris Y. Kim, et al. "Intake of Dairy Foods and Risk of Parkinson's Disease." *Neurology* 89, no. 1 (2017): 46–52. doi:10.1212/wnl.0000000000004057.

Bunch, T. W. "Polymyositis: A Case History Approach to the Differential Diagnosis and Treatment." *Journal of Occupational and Environmental Medicine* 34, no. 2 (1992): 105–109. doi:10.1097/00043764-199202000-00006.

Nordqvist, Christian. "Chronic Fatigue Syndrome Symptoms Reduced by Dark Chocolate Consumption." *Medical News Today*, October 1, 2007. http://www.medicalnewstoday.com/articles/84141.php.

CHAPTER 3: STRONG BONES, CALCIUM & BEYOND

Feskanich D., W. C. Willett, M. J. Stampfer, et al. "Milk, Dietary Calcium, and Bone Fractures in Women: A 12-year Prospective Study." *American Journal of Public Health* 87, no. 6 (1997).

Michaëlsson, Karl, Hans Lithell, Bengt Vessby, et al. "Serum Retinol Levels and the Risk of Fracture." *New England Journal of Medicine* 348, no. 4 (2003): 287–94. doi:10.1056/nejmoa021171.

Michaëlsson, K., A. Wolk, S. Langenskiold, et al. "Milk Intake and Risk of Mortality and Fractures in Women and Men: Cohort Studies." *BMJ* 349 (2014): g6015. doi:10.1136/bmj.g6015.

Heaney, Robert P., David A. McCarron, Bess Dawson-Hughes, et al. "Dietary Changes Favorably Affect Bone Remodeling in Older Adults." *Journal of the American Dietetic Association* 99, no. 10 (1999): 1228–33. doi:10.1016/s0002-8223(99)00302-8.

"Should You Get Your Nutrients from Food or from Supplements?" Harvard Health Publishing, May 2015, https://www.health.harvard.edu/staying-healthy/should-you-get-your-nutrients-from-food-or-from-supplements.

"Calcium: What's Best for Your Bones and Health?" Harvard T.H. Chan School of Public Health, https://www.hsph.harvard.edu/nutritionsource/calcium-full-story.

Qiu, R., W-t. Cao, H-y. Tian, et al, "Greater Intake of Fruit and Vegetables Is Associated with Greater Bone Mineral Density and Lower Osteoporosis Risk in Middle-Aged and Elderly Adults," *PLoS ONE* (Jan 2017) 12(1). doi: 10.1371/journal.pone.e0168906.

Hooshmand, S., M. Kern, D. Metti, et al., "The Effect of Two Doses of Dried Plum on Bone Density and Bone Biomarkers in Osteopenic Postmenopausal Women: A Randomized, Controlled Trial," *Osteoporos International* 27, no. 7 (July 2016): 2271-79. doi: 10.1007/s00198-016-3524-8.

Payton, M. E., K. Brummel-Smith, B. H. Arjmandi, et al., "Comparative Effects of Dried Plum and Dried Apple on Bone in Postmenopausal Women," *British Journal of Nutrition* 106, no. 6 (September 2011): 923-30. doi: 10.1017/S000711451100119X.

Devine, A., J. M. Hodgson, I. M. Dick, et al. "Tea Drinking Is Associated with Benefits on Bone Density in Older Women." *American Journal of Clinical Nutrition* 86 (October 2007): 1243–47.

Sellmeyer, D. E. "Potassium Citrate Prevents Increased Urine Calcium Excretion and Bone Resorption Induced by a High Sodium Chloride Diet." *Journal of Clinical Endocrinology & Metabolism* 87, no. 5 (2002): 2008–12. doi:10.1210/jc.87.5.2008.

Briggs, J. C., and J. F. Ficke. "Quality of Rivers of the United States, 1975 Water Year; Based on the National Stream Quality Accounting Network (NASQAN)." *U.S. Geological Survey Publications Warehouse* 436 (1977): 78–200. https://pubs.er.usgs.gov/publication/ofr78200.

Van den Berg, H. "Bioavailability of Vitamin D." *European Journal of Clinical Nutrition* 51 Suppl 1 (1997): S76–9.

"Dietary Reference Intakes: Calcium, Phosphorus, Magnesium, Vitamin D, and Fluoride." Institute of Medicine. Washington, DC: National Academies Press, 1997. doi:10.17226/5776.

"Dietary Reference Intakes for Calcium and Vitamin D." Institute of Medicine. Washington, DC: National Academies Press, 2011. doi:10.17226/13050.

"National Nutrient Database for Standard Reference (Release 28)." United States Department of Agriculture, Agricultural Research Service. https://www.ars.usda.gov/northeast-area/beltsville-md/beltsville-human-nutrition-research-center/nutrient-data-laboratory/docs/usda-national-nutrient-database-for-standard-reference.

Cranney, A., T. Horsley, S. O'Donnell, et al. "Effectiveness and Safety of Vitamin D in Relation to Bone Health." *Evidence Report/Technology Assessment* 158 (2007): 1–235.

Phillips, Kathleen. "Orange, Grapefruit Juice for Breakfast Builds Bones in Rats." *AgriLife Today*, June 5, 2006. https://today.agrilife.org/2006/06/05/orange-grapefruit-juice-for-breakfast-builds-bones-in-rats.

Deyhim, F., K. Mandadi, B. Faraji, et al. "Grapefruit Juice Modulates Bone Quality in Rats." *Journal of Medicinal Food* 11, no. 1 (2008): 99–104. doi:10.1089/jmf.2007.537.

Feskanich, D., W. C. Willett, and G. A. Colditz. "Calcium, Vitamin D, Milk Consumption, and Hip Fractures: A Prospective Study Among Postmenopausal Women." *American Journal of Clinical Nutrition* 77, no. 2 (2003): 504–11.

Pennington, Jean A., and Judith S. Spungen. *Bowes & Church's Food Values of Portions Commonly Used*. Philadelphia: Lippincott, 1998.

United States Department of Agriculture, Human Nutrition Information Service, Agriculture Handbook Number 8-11.

Weaver, Connie M., and Robert P. Heaney. *Calcium in Human Health*. New York: Humana Press, 2005.

Weaver, C. M., W. R. Proulx, and R. Heaney. "Choices for Achieving Adequate Dietary Calcium with a Vegetarian Diet." *The American Journal of Clinical Nutrition* 70, no. 3 Suppl (1999): 543S–48S. http://ajcn.nutrition.org/content/70/3/543s.full.

CHAPTER 4: INFANT & CHILDHOOD MILK ALLERGIES

Fiocchi, A., A. Assa'ad, S. Bahna, et al. "Food Allergy and the Introduction of Solid Foods to Infants: A Consensus Document. Adverse Reactions to Foods Committee, American College of Allergy, Asthma and Immunology." *Annals of Allergy, Asthma, and Immunology* 97 (2006): 10–21.

"Eight Signs Your Baby Has a Milk Allergy." Babies Online. https://www.babiesonline.com/articles/baby/eightsignsmilkallergy.asp.

Zutavern, A., I. Brockow, B. Schaaf, et al. "Timing of Solid Food Introduction in Relation to Eczema, Asthma, Allergic Rhinitis, and Food and Inhalant Sensitization at the Age of 6 Years: Results from the Prospective Birth Cohort Study LISA." *Pediatrics* 121, no. 1 (2007): e44–52. doi:10.1542/peds.2006-3553.

Fiocchi, A., J. Brozek, H. Schünemann, et al. "World Allergy Organization (WAO) Diagnosis and Rationale for Action Against Cow's Milk Allergy (DRACMA) Guidelines." *World Allergy Organization* 3, no. 4 (2010): 57–161. doi:10.1097/wox.0b013e3181defeb9.

Greer, F. R., S. H. Sicherer, and A. W. Burks. "Effects of Early Nutritional Interventions on the Development of Atopic Disease in Infants and Children: The Role of Maternal Dietary Restriction, Breastfeeding, Timing of Introduction of Complementary Foods, and Hydrolyzed Formulas." *Pediatrics* 121, no. 1 (2008): 183–91. doi:10.1542/peds.2007-3022.

Wighton, Kate. "Infant Milk Formula Does Not Reduce Risk of Eczema and Allergies, Says New Study." Imperial College London, March 9, 2016. http://www3.imperial.ac.uk/newsandeventspggrp/imperialcollege/newssummary/news_8-3-2016-17-32-45.

Kaplan, Matt. "Breast Is Best, But Watch Out for the Allergies." *New Scientist*, August 5, 2006.

CHAPTER 5: OTHER DAIRY-FREE CONCERNS

Schulte, Erica M., Nicole M. Avena, and Ashley N. Gearhardt. "Which Foods May Be Addictive? The Roles of Processing, Fat Content, and Glycemic Load." *PLoS ONE* 10, no. 2 (2015). doi:10.1371/journal.pone.0117959.

Martelli, A., A. De, M. Corvo, et al. "Beef Allergy in Children with Cow's Milk Allergy; Cow's Milk Allergy in Children with Beef Allergy." *Annals of Allergy, Asthma & Immunology* 89, no. 6, Suppl 1 (2002): 38–43. www.ncbi.nlm.nih.gov/pubmed/12487203.

Yan, L., and E. L. Spitznagel. "Soy Consumption and Prostate Cancer Risk in Men: A Revisit of a Meta-Analysis." *American Journal of Clinical Nutrition* 89, no. 4 (2009): 1155–63. doi:10.3945/ajcn.2008.27029.

"Soy Allergy." Mayo Clinic, July 11, 2014. http://www.mayoclinic.org/diseases-conditions/soy-allergy/basics/definition/con-20031370.

Barrett, Julia R. "The Science of Soy: What Do We Really Know?" *Environmental Health Perspectives* 114, no. 6 (2006): A352–58. doi:10.1289/ehp.114-a352.

Messina, Mark, and Geoffrey Redmond. "Effects of Soy Protein and Soybean Isoflavones on Thyroid Function in Healthy Adults and Hypothyroid Patients: A Review of the Relevant Literature." *Thyroid* 16, no. 3 (2006): 249–58. doi:10.1089/thy.2006.16.249.

"Extra Virgin Coconut Oil—the 'Good' Saturated Fat." *The Doctors' Prescription for Healthy Living* 7, no. 2: 35–37.

Wax, Emily. "Protein in Diet." *MedlinePlus Medical Encyclopedia*, April 25, 2015. medlineplus.gov/ency/article/002467.htm.

Mangels, Reed. "Protein in the Vegan Diet." *Simply Vegan*, 5th edition. Baltimore, MD: Vegetarian Resource Group, 2013. http://www.vrg.org/nutrition/protein.php.

Brody, S. "The Rate of Growth of the Dairy Cow: V. Extrauterine Growth in Linear Dimensions." *The Journal of General Physiology* 6, no. 3 (1924): 329–36. doi:10.1085/jgp.6.3.329.

Nutrition facts from calorie-count.com, nutritiondata.com, and product-specific labels.

CHAPTER 6: RESTAURANT DINING

"Want to Watch Calories When Dining Out?" National Restaurant Association, Table Service Restaurant Trends, 2001.

Koeller, Kim, and Robert La France. *Let's Eat Out!: Your Passport to Living Gluten and Allergy Free*. Chicago, IL: R and R Publishing, 2005.

Taylor, S. L., and S. L. Hefle. "Food Allergies and Other Food Sensitivities: A Publication of the Institute of Food Technologists' Expert Panel on Food Safety and Nutrition." *Food Technology* 55 (2001): 68–83.

CHAPTER 8: DECODING FOOD LABELS

Ylitalo, Leea, Soili Mäkinen-Kiljunen, et al. "Cow's Milk Casein, a Hidden Allergen in Natural Rubber Latex Gloves." *Journal of Allergy and Clinical Immunology* 104, no. 1 (1999): 177–80. doi:10.1016/s0091-6749(99)70131-4.

Carper, Steve. "Dairy or Nondairy? The Experts Speak." Steve Carper's Lactose Intolerance Clearinghouse. http://www.stevecarper.com/li/dairy_or_nondairy_the_experts_speak.htm.

Heber, Rabbi Dovid. "Facts on Wax: Are Vegetable and Fruit Waxes Kosher?" Star-K. www.star-k.org/articles/articles/1128/facts-on-wax-are-vegetables-and-fruit-waxes-kosher.

CHAPTER 13: HOW TO MOO-VE BEYOND BUTTER

"Fats & Oils; Smoking Points." *The New Professional Chef*, 6th edition. Hoboken, NJ: John Wiley & Sons, 1996.

Chu, Michael. "Smoke Points of Various Fats." Cooking for Engineers, June 10, 2004. http://www.cookingforengineers.com/article/50/Smoke-Points-of-Various-Fats.

RECIPE INDEX

INDEX

A

acidophilus milk, 13–14
acne, 40
AD (atopic dermatitis/atopic eczema), 20–21
addiction to dairy, 68–70
ADHD (attention deficit hyperactivity disorder), 35–36
African cuisine, 87
agar-agar, 152
agglutinin, 16
air travel, foods and, 96–97
ALCAT test, 25
alcohol
  bone strength and, 48
  dairy in alcoholic drinks, 94
allergies. *See* food allergies
almond milk beverage, 131
alpha-casein, 15
American cuisine, 87–88
amino acid-based infant formula, 63
anaphylaxis, 20, 22–23
animal proteins, allergenic, 15
antibiotics
  calcium and absorption of, 60
  in dairy products, 10–11
antibodies
  in breast milk, 63
  defined, 19
antihistamines, 27, 78
antioxidants
  calcium absorption/retention and, 47
  in ghee, 144
appliances, 124–125
arthritic pain, 45
atopic dermatitis/atopic eczema (AD), 20–21
atopy patch test, 24
attention deficit hyperactivity disorder (ADHD), 35–36
A2 milk, 15
autism, 34–35
avocados, 74

B

bakery items, shopping for, 115
baking ingredients, 114–115
balanced diet, 47
bean milk beverages, 138
beans, calcium in, 54–55
beef broth, 57
beef cross-reactivity, 70
beta-casein, 15
beverages
  alcoholic drinks, dairy in, 94
  carbonated, 9

juices, 54
  milk (*See* milk beverages)
  shopping for, 119–120
BGH (bovine growth hormone), 10. *See also* rBGH (rBST)
birthday party foods, 99
bisphosphonate medications, calcium and, 60
blood tests, for milk allergies, 24–25
bone broth, 57
bone fracture, calcium consumption and, 50–51
bone strength, 46–60
  building and maintaining, 47–49
  calcium needed for, 49–51
  calcium-rich foods for, 51–58
  calcium supplements for, 58–60
  dairy consumption and, 46–47
bottled sauces, 112, 113
bovine growth hormone (BGH), 10. *See also* rBGH (rBST)
Brazil nut milk beverage, 131
breastfeeding, 62–63. *See also* human breast milk
broth, homemade, 57
buffalo milk, 18
butter
  clarified, 143, 144
  dairy, 143
  ghee, 143, 144
  lactose levels in, 32
  nondairy, 144–145
  in restaurant meals, 82
  substitutes for, 145–150
buttermilk substitutes, 156–158
buttermylk, 157
  preparing, 157
  as yogurt substitute, 164
butter oil, 143
buttery spreads, 145
buttery sticks, 145
B vitamins, 8, 9
  B12, 8, 16, 130
  in goat's milk, 16
  in sheep's milk, 16
  in store-bought milk beverages, 130

C

caffeine, bone strength and, 48
calcium, 9
  absorption of, 59
  for bone strength, 49–51
  dietary reference intakes for, 49–50
  foods fortified with, 57
  foods rich in, 51–58

uses of, 6
and weight loss, 36
cream
dairy-free, store-bought, 160
heavy, substitutes for, 160–161
lactose levels in, 32
light, substitutes for, 159
creamer, dairy free, 154–155, 158, 161
cream of coconut, 162
Crohn's disease, 42
cultural cuisines, 83–90
African, 87
American, 87–88
Caribbean, 87
Chinese, 83–84
English pubs, 88
French, 90
German/Swiss, 90
Greek, 86–87
Indian, 88–89
Irish pubs, 88
Italian, 89
Japanese, 84
Mexican, 85
Spanish, 86
Thai, 84
Vietnamese, 84–85
when traveling, 97
"cultured" dairy products, lactose levels in, 32

D

dairy alternative market, 2
dairy case items, 118
dairy free (food label term), 102
dairy-free diet, 19–45. *See also* dairy substitutes;
    specific topics
and ADHD, 35–36
and autism, 34–35
concerns when following (*See* concerns with
    dairy-free diet)
and dairy intolerance, 32–33
for feeling good, 45
and galactosemia, 33
for general health and disease
    prevention, 38–45
and lactose intolerance, 27–32
menus for, 68–69
and milk allergies, 19–27
options with, 6
and paleo diet, 36
reasons for consuming, 3–4
saboteurs of, 69
transitioning to, 69
and vegan diet , 33–34
and weight loss, 36–38
dairy ingredient lists, 106–107
dairy intolerance, 32–33
dairy products, 6–15
addiction to, 68–70

antibiotics in, 10–11
butter, 143
defined, 6
determining lactose percentages in, 31
and homogenization, 12–13
lactose levels in, 31–32
low-fat, 37
low-lactose, 30
mammal milks, 15–18
milk, 7–9
modified milks, 13–15
organic, 9–11
and pasteurization, 11–12
raw, 11–13
synthetic hormones in, 10, 11
dairy substitutes, 128–164
butter, 143–150
buttermilk, 156–158
cheese, 151–154
chocolate, 154
creamer, 154–155
evaporated milk, 161–162
half-and-half, 158–159
heavy cream, 160–161
light cream, 159
milk beverages, 128–142
powdered milk, 156
sour cream, 162–163
sweetened condensed milk, 162
whole milk, 130
yogurt, 163–164
daycare, foods at, 99
desensitization, 26
desserts, shopping for, 117
diabetes
and vegan diet, 34
in women, dairy effects on, 37
diagnosis. *See* testing for lactose intolerance;
    testing for milk allergies
diarrhea, as sign of milk allergy, 61
dips, 115–116
disease prevention. *See* health and disease
    prevention
donkey's milk, 17
dried plums, as "super-bone" food, 49
drinks, alcoholic, 94
dry milk powders
dairy free, 156
lactose levels in, 31

E

ear infections, as sign of milk allergy, 61
eating out. *See* restaurant dining; social events
EE (eosinophilic esophagitis), 21
egg allergies, 6
eggs, 6
EGIDs (eosinophilic gastrointestinal
    disorders), 21
elemental calcium, 58

elimination test, 23, 41

ELISA (enzyme-linked immunosorbent assay), 24–25

English pub cuisine, 88

enzyme-linked immunosorbent assay (ELISA), 24–25

EoE (eosinophilic esophagitis), 21

eosinophilic esophagitis (EE, EoE), 21

eosinophilic gastrointestinal disorders (EGIDs), 21

ethnic foods. *See* cultural cuisines

European Union labeling law, 103

evaporated milk
  lactose levels in, 31
  substitutes for, 161–162

exercise
  for strong bones, 47
  to turn attention from food, 69

extra-virgin olive oil, 148–149

F

FAA (Federal Alcohol Administration), 103

FAHF-2 (food allergy herbal formula-2), 26

failure to thrive, as sign of milk allergy, 61

FALCPA (Food Allergen Labeling and Consumer Protection Act), 102–103

family gatherings, food at, 94–95

fast food, 91–92

fat(s). *See also specific types, e.g.*: oils
  in children's diets, 66
  in cow's milk, 7–8
  and homogenization of milk, 12
  and irritable bowel syndrome, 42
  in mammal milks, 18
  in milk, lactose intolerance and, 31
  plant-based sources of, 74–76
  in sheep's milk, 16
  in store-bought milk beverages, 130

fat-soluble vitamins, in cow's milk, 8–9

Federal Alcohol Administration (FAA), 103

feeling good, 45

fiber, in store-bought milk beverages, 130

fibromyalgia, 45

fish, calcium in, 56

Fisher, Jerome K., 40

504 plan, 98–99

flax milk beverage, 138

folic acid, in goat's milk, 16

food addiction, 70

Food Allergen Labeling and Consumer Protection Act (FALCPA), 102–103

food allergies. *See also specific allergies*
  animal proteins, 15
  from antibiotic residues in milk, 10
  beef, 70
  in children,m 62
  concerns in restaurant dining, 80–81
  defined, 19
  egg, 6

food intolerances vs., 27
  getting help with, 67
  as headache/migraine trigger, 40
  and homogenization, 12
  laws on allergen labeling, 102–103
  milk, 3–4, 6, 12 (See also milk allergies/ intolerances)
  and pasteurization, 12
  soy, 73

food allergy herbal formula-2 (FAHF-2), 26

food-induced pulmonary hemosiderosis (Heiner syndrome), 21

food intolerances, 19. *See also* milk allergies/ intolerances
  dairy intolerance, 32–33
  defined, 20
  food allergies vs., 27
  as headache/migraine trigger, 40
  lactose intolerance (*See* lactose intolerance)

food labels, 102–111
  confusing statements on, 103–104
  "dairy free" on, 102
  dairy ingredient lists, 106–107
  and hidden dairy ingredients, 108–111
  kosher certification, 105
  laws on food allergen labeling, 102–103
  "nondairy" on, 102
  "vegan" on, 122

food protein-induced enterocolitis syndrome (FPIES), 21

Food Safety and Inspection Service (FSIS), 103

FPIES (food protein-induced enterocolitis syndrome), 21

French cuisine, 90

fresh pasta, 119

friendly gatherings, foods at, 93–94

frozen foods, 119

fruit butters, 145

fruits
  calcium in, 54
  for infants or toddlers, 64
  as low-fat substitutes, 150

FSIS (Food Safety and Inspection Service), 103

fussiness, as sign of milk allergy, 61

G

galactose, 33, 38

galactosemia, 33, 63

gastrointestinal tests, for milk allergies, 25

genetically modified foods, 73

German cuisine, 90

ghee, 143, 144

gluten-free/casein-free (GFCF) diet, 35

goat's milk, 15, 16

grains, 117–118
  calcium in, 54
  for infants or toddlers, 64

Greek cuisine, 86–87

milk soy protein intolerance, 21
NSLP (National School Lunch
      Program), 97, 98
nut butters, 144
nut cream, as heavy cream substitute, 161
nutritional drinks, 64
nutritional yeast, 153
NuTron test, 25
nuts, 74–75
    calcium in, 52
    half-and-half substitute from, 158–159
    light cream substitute from, 159
    milk beverages from, 131–135, 137–138

O

OA (osteoarthritis), 45
oat milk beverage, 133–134
obesity, 37
oils
    as butter substitutes, 146–149
    dietary fat from, 74
    heart-healthy, 81
    high-heat, 148
    low-heat, 147
    in margarine, 145
    medium-heat, 147–148
    no-heat, 146–147
    in shortenings, 145
OIT (oral immunotherapy), 26
oligoantigenic diet, 41
olives, 75
opioid peptides, 70
oral challenges, for milk allergies, 23
oral contraceptives, 78
oral immunotherapy (OIT), 26
organic milk, 9–11
osteoarthritis (OA), 45
osteoporosis, 46–47. See also bone strength
    and mineral balance, 9
    and "super-bone" foods, 48–49
ovarian cancer, 38
oxalates, 58

P

paleo diet, 36, 144
palm fruit oil, 150
palm kernel oil, 150
palm oil, 145, 149–150
pantry items, 114
Parasol, 96
Parkinson's disease, 43
pasta, fresh, 119
pasteurization, 8, 11–12
pathogens
    and pasteurization, 11–12
    in raw milk, 13
pea milk beverage, 138
peanut butter, 144

peanut milk beverage, 134
peanuts, 74–75
pecan milk beverage, 134
phosphorus, 9, 16
phytates, 58
pine nut milk beverage, 135
pistachio milk beverage, 135
"plain language" labeling law, 102–103
plant-based food sources
    dairy-free milk beverages, 128
    of fats, 74–76
    of proteins, 76–77
play dates, foods at, 99
pork allergy, 70
potassium
    and calcium absorption/retention, 47
    in goat's milk, 16
    in sheep's milk, 16
potato milk beverage, 135–136
powdered milk, 156
prepared foods, 120
primal diet, 36
primary lactose intolerance, 28, 30
probiotics
    sources of, 164
    trace allergy aggravators in, 78
    for treatment of milk allergies, 25–26
    in yogurt and kefir, 14
processed foods, 12
produce, 112
prostate cancer, 39–40, 71
protein(s). See also casein (milk protein)
    allergenic, 15
    antibodies, 19
    in camel's milk, 17
    complete vs. incomplete, 76
    in cow's milk, 7, 73
    in donkey's milk, 17
    for infants or toddlers, 65
    in mammal milks, 18
    plant-based sources of, 76–77
    in sheep's milk, 16
    in store-bought milk beverages, 130
protein powders, 76–77
prunes, as "super-bone" food, 49
pumpkin seed milk beverage, 136

Q

quinoa milk beverage, 138

R

RA (rheumatoid arthritis), 45
radioallergosorbent test (RAST), 24
rapeseed oil, 148
raw dairy products, 11
    camel's milk, 17
    consumption of. 13
    milk, 7, 13

synthetic hormones, 10, 11
Synthroid, calcium and absorption of, 60

T

tahini, 153
tea, as "super-bone" food, 49
teethers, 65
testing for lactose intolerance, 29–30
    hydrogen breath test, 30
    lactose tolerance test, 29
    stool acidity test, 30
testing for milk allergies, 23–25
    atopy patch test, 24
    blood tests, 24–25
    elimination test and oral challenge, 23
    gastrointestinal tests, 25
    skin prick test, 23–24
Thai cuisine, 84
tiger-nut milk beverage, 137–138
tofu
    as half-and-half substitute, 158
    as heavy cream substitute, 160
    as light cream substitute, 159
    in making cheese alternatives, 153–154
    as yogurt substitute, 164
traveling, food when, 95–97
treatment
    of lactose intolerance, 30–31
    of milk allergies, 25–27
tree nut butter, 144
tree nuts, 74–75

U

ulcerative colitis, 42
USP certification, 59, 60

V

Vallozzi, Emily, 65, 66
vegan (food label term), 122
vegan diet, 33–34, 68, 69
vegan options
    dairy-free milk beverages, 128
    shopping for, 118
vegan skincare products, 77
vegan supplements, 78
Vega test, 25
vegetables
    calcium in, 52–53
    as heavy cream substitute, 160–161
    for infants or toddlers, 64
Vietnamese cuisine, 84–85
vitamin A, 8, 16
vitamin C, 8, 47
vitamin D, 8–9
    and bone fracture, 51
    and bone strength, 47–48
    for bone strength, 60
    and calcium absorption/retention, 47
    in store-bought milk beverages, 130
vitamin E, 8
    and calcium absorption/retention, 47
    in sheep's milk, 16
vitamin K, 8, 47
vitamins
and calcium absorption/retention, 47
    in cow's milk, 8
    in goat's milk, 16
    and pasteurization, 12
    in sheep's milk, 16
vomiting, as sign of milk allergy, 61

W

wallaby milk, 18
walnut milk beverage, 138
water
    calcium intake from, 57
    in children's diets, 64
    in cow's milk, 7, 9
water buffalo milk, 18
water-soluble vitamins, in cow's milk, 8
weight gain, 73–77
    plant-based dietary fat sources for, 74–76
    plant-based dietary protein sources
      for, 76–77
weight loss
    with dairy-free diet, 36–38
    with vegan diet, 34
whey
    in cow's milk, 7
    in IgE allergy, 20
    lactose levels in, 31
    in non-IgE allergies, 20
Wolf, Robb, 36
women
    calcium intake for, 49, 50
    dairy consumption and health of, 37
    ovarian cancer in, 38

Y

yak milk, 18
yogurt, 304
    dairy-free, 163
    probiotics in, 14
    substitutes for, 163–164

Z

zebra milk, 18
zinc, calcium absorption/retention and, 47

ABOUT THE AUTHOR

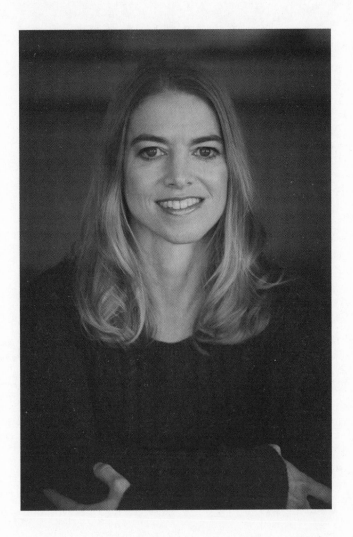

ALISA FLEMING is the founder of **GoDairyFree.org**, the leading website and online magazine for dairy-free living since 2004. She is also the author of *Go Dairy Free: The Guide and Cookbook* and editor for the international publication *Allergic Living* magazine.

Alisa is an expert in recipe creation, lifestyle topics, and informational writing for the special diet industry. She has spoken at several events and continuously works with leading natural food brands to ensure that dairy-free consumers have a never-ending supply of delicious options.

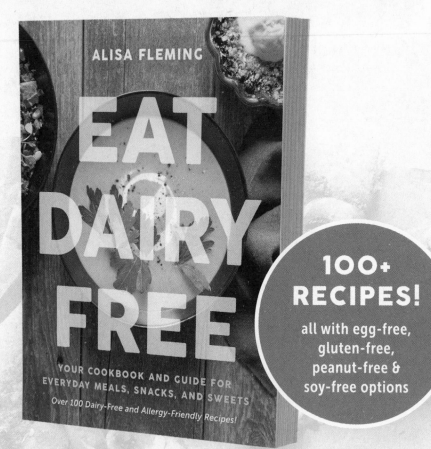

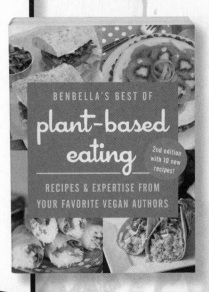